Plab
Part I

Plab
Part I

Plab
Part I

Dinesh Khanna

PEEPEE
PUBLISHERS and DISTRIBUTORS (P) LTD.

Plab Part I

Published by
Pawaninder P. Vij
Peepee Publishers and Distributors (P) Ltd.

7/31, Ansari Road, Daryaganj,
New Delhi 110002 (India)
Ph: 55195868, 9811156083
e-mail: peepee160@yahoo.co.in
e-mail: peepee160@rediffmail.com

NOTICE

As we all know the field of medicine is ever changing. The author and the publisher have taken references and information from sources which are universally accepted as reliable. All efforts have been taken to keep the informatin in the book as updated as possible. However, in view of the possibility of human error, neither the author nor the publisher claim responsibility of accuracy or even existence of the information provided in the book. All questions given in the papers are solely on the basis of memory of students appeared in previous examinations and hence variations are bound to exist in places. The book has been published in good faith to help students prepare for the exam

First Edition: **2004**

ISBN: 81-88867-27-6

Cover design by Prashant Das

Printed at
Lordson, C-5/19, Rana Pratap Bagh, Delhi-110 007

Dedicated to my son
Laksh
who has been and
will always remain close to my heart

PREFACE

This book is for all those who have made up their minds to write the PLAB (Professional and Linguistics Assessment Board exam) Part I and pursue their further studies and careers in the UK. If you dream of getting as MRCP, MRCOG (Obs and Gynae) or similar UK degrees, this book is here to make sure that your dream is realized. But the only unexhaustive favour that a parent can do his child is to teach him to help himself. So this book is here to light the fire of knowledge for you, but to keep it burning is upto you. This book will show you the direction, the road to sure success but you will be the one to walk through this road. And thats a promise that there's just no way you can fail once you do so.

The PLAB part I exam is different from Indian PG exams in that the questions asked are more clinically oriented. So it is mandatory for you to have completed one year of internship. The more clinical experience you have, the easier you'd find solving the PLAB EMQ'S.

Nevertheless, even if you aim to clear PLAB right after completing your MBBS, the gist lies in practising the maximum number of EMQ's.

This book provides you with six latest question papers of the PLAB exam with solutions and explanations that are to the point and can be relied upon. In the second section of our book, we give you six mock test papers to time and test yourself. It is only practice that can help you improve your score. So when you begin attempting a paper even if you don't get most of your answers correct, don't be disheartened. And remember,

Success doesn't mean the absence of failures,
it means the attainment of ultimate objectives.
It means winning the war, not every battle.
— Edwin C. Bliss

Another thing that must be emphasized upon here, is how to study for PLAB. Because of time constraints, we would advice you to study in a retrospective manner i.e. read the EMQ'S and consult the related theory matter. For even if you have ample time to read all the text extensively, when you solve the EMQ's after this, you do not have the orientation and when a few weeks are left for your exam, you have no time to revise everything. So what you need, is a book like this, which gives you the proper orientation, and can be revised in a short period of time.

We believe in a holistic approach. When a person works, its not just his hand that is writing or eyes that are reading; his whole body, every organ, every cell is working to get a task done. The same way, to get to your target, you ought to know your subjects in totality. The only way to do that is to practise the previous years papers and know the themes that are asked frequently pretty well.

However, nothing is permanent in life except change. Medicine is a rapidly advancing field. It is like a great Kaleidoscope before which time is ever-changing. The information provided in this book is in accordance with the standards acceptable at the time of publication. We promise to keep updating our book with the latest developments in the field of medicine.

Also, the questions here are reproduced from the memory of students who have been appearing for the PLAB exam. We regret any errors that might be making these questions slightly different from those asked in the exam.

As you turn over this page, you have just made up your mind to begin. And every beginner is a winner!

Wish you all the best!

Dinesh Khanna

ACKNOWLEDGEMENTS

Dr Puneet Kaur Kochhar

1st year resident, Deptt of Obstetrics and Gynaecology, LNJP.

This book really would not have seen the light of the day had you not been there supporting me. Thanks for taking out time from your busy PG schedule and working for the book.

My Family

I wish to thank my family members especially my parents for providing all the support I needed while working for the book. You indeed are the worlds best parents.

Mr. Pawan Vij

Thanks for providing me all the help, support and encouragement from him and from his staff I required to complete this book. Your direction helped me sail through.

CONTENTS

CONTENTS

OPD	out-patient department
OTM	Oxford Textbook of Medicine (OUP 3e, 1996)
OTS	Oxford Textbook of Surgery (OUP 2e, 2000)
P_2	pulmonary component of second heart sound
P_aCO_2	partial pressure of carbon dioxide in arterial blood
PAN	polyarteritis nodosa
PaO_2	partial pressure of carbon dioxide in arterial blood
PBC	primary biliary cirrhosis
PCP	pneumocystis carinii pneumonia
PCR	polymerase chain reaction (DNA diagnosis)
PCV	packed cell volume
PE	pulmonary embolism
PEEP	positive end-expiratory pressure
PERLA	pupils equal reactive to light and accommodation
PID	pelvic inflammatory disease
PIP	proximal interphalangeal
PL	prolactin
PND	paroxysmal nocturnal dyspnoea
POP	progesterone only pill
PPI	proton pump inhibitor,eg omeprazole lansoprazole etc
PR	per rectum (by the rectum)
PRL	prolactin
PRN	pro re nata (as required)
PRV	polycythaemia rubra vera
PSA	prostate specific antigen
PTH	parathyroid hormone
PTT	prothrombin time
PUO	pyrexia of unknown origin
PV	per vaginam (by the vagina)
qds	quater die sumendus (to be taken 4 times a day)
qid	quater in die (4 times a day) qqh: quarta quaque hora (every 4h)
RA	rheumatoid arthritis
RAD	right axis deviation on the ECG
RBBB	right bundle branch block
RBC	red blood cell
RFT	respiratory function tests
Rh	Rh; not an abbreviation, but derived from the rhesus monkey
RIF	right iliac fossa
RUQ	right upper quadrant
RVF	right ventricular failure
RVH	right ventricular hypertrophy
Rx	recipe (treat with)
S or sec	second (s)
S1, S2	first and second heart sounds
SBE	subacute bacterial endocarditis
SC	subcutaneous

SD	standard deviation
SE	side effect(s)
SL	sublingual
SLE	systemic lupus erythematosus
SOB	short of breath (SOB (O)E short of breath on exercise)
SOL	space occupying lesion
SR	slow-release (also called modified-release)
stat	statim (immediately as initial dose)
STD/STI	sexually-transmitted disease or sexually-transmitted infection
SVC	superior vena cava
SXR	skull X-ray
Sy(n)	syndrome
T_0	temperature
$T_{1/2}$	biological half-life
T3	triiodothyronine
T4	thyroxine
TB	tuberculosis
tds	ter die sumendus (to be taken 3 times a day)
TFTs	thyroid function tests (eg TSH)
TIA	transient ischaemic attack
TIBC	total iron binding capacity
tid	ter in die (3 times a day)
TOE	transoesophageal echocardiography
TPR	temperature, pulse and respiration count
TRH	thyroid-releasing hormone
TSH	thyroid-stimulating hormone
U	units
UC	ulcerative colitis
U&E	urea & electrolytes and creatinine in plasma, unless stated otherwise
UMN	upper motor neurone
URT	upper respiratory tract
URTI	upper respiratory tract infection
USG	ultrasound
UTI	urinary tract infection
VDRL	venereal diseases research laboratory
VE	ventricular extrasystole
VF	ventricular fibrillation
VMA	vanillyl mandelic acid (HMMA)
V/Q	ventilation/perfusion ratio
VSD	ventriculo septal defect
WBC	white blood cell
WCC	white cell count
wk(s)	week (s)
yr(s)	year (s)
ZN	Ziehl-Neelsen (stain for acid-fast bacilli, eg mycobacteria)

IELTS

INTERNATIONAL ENGLISH LANGUAGE TESTING SYSTEM

IELTS, the International English Language Testing System, is designed to assess the language ability of candidates who need to study or work where English is the language of communication.

IELTS is a highly dependable, practical and valid English language assessment primarily used by those seeking international education, professional recognition, bench-marking to international standards and global mobility.

It is an internationally owned and globally recognised direct English language assessment of the highest quality and integrity readily available throughout the world.

IELTS is recognised by universities and employers in many countries, including Australia, Canada, New Zealand, the UK and the USA. It is also recognized by professional bodies, immigration authorities and other government agencies.

IELTS is jointly managed by University of Cambridge ESOL Examinations (Cambridge ESOL), British Council and IDP: IELTS Australia. IELTS conforms to the highest international standards of language assessment. It covers the four language skills—listening, reading, writing and speaking.

IELTS is not recommended for candidates under the age of 16.

Test Administration

IELTS tests are administered at centres throughout the world. There are currently more than 270 centres, in over 110 countries. A full list of centres is available on the IELTS website: **www.ielts.org.**

Most centres conduct a testing session at least once a month and more often at peak times. Results are available within two weeks of the test. The candidate will receive only one copy of their test results but additional copies can be sent direct to receiving institutions.

Candidates not allowed to repeat the test within ninety days at any centre. Presently the test fees for IELTS is 5850/- Rupees.

Academic and General Training

IELTS is available in two formats—Academic and General training.

The Academic Modules assess whether a candidate is ready to study or train in the medium of English at an undergraduate or postgraduate level. Admission to undergraduate and postgraduate courses should be based on the results of these modules.

The General Training Modules emphasise basic survival skills in a broad social and educational context. General Training is suitable for candidates who are going to English speaking countries to complete their Secondary education, to undertake work experience or training programmes not at degree level, or for immigration purposes to Australia, Canada and New Zealand.

Listening

Time: Approximately 30 minutes

Candidates listen to a number of recorded texts, which increase in difficulty as the test progresses. These include a mixture of monologues and conversations and features a variety of English accents and dialects.

The recording is heard only once, but candidates are given time to read to questions and write down their answers

Academic Reading

Time: 60 minutes

There are three reading passages with tasks. Texts are taken from books, magazines, journals and newspapers, all written for a nonspecialist audience. At least one of the texts contains a detailed argument.

Academic Writing

Time: 60 minutes

For the first task, candidates write a report of around 150 words based on material found in a table or diagram, demonstrating their ability to describe and explain data.

For the second task, candidates write a short essay of around 250 words in response to an opinion or a problem. They are expected to demonstrate an ability to discuss issues, construct an argument and use the appropriate tone and register.

Speaking

Time: 11-14 minutes

The test takes the form of a face to face interview. Candidates are assessed on their use of spoken English to answer short questions, to speak at length on a familiar topic, and also to interact with the examiner.

Test format

Candidates are tested in listening, reading, writing and speaking. All candidates take the same Listening and Speaking Modules. There is choice of Reading and Writing Modules—Academic or General Training. It is the responsibility of the candidate to tell the Administrator which version, Academic or General Training, they need to take. We are required to give the Academic Training module test.

The tests are designed to cover the full range of ability from non-user to expert user, with each module consisting of tasks of ascending levels of difficulty.

The first three modules—Listening, Reading and Writing—must be completed in one day. No break is given between the three modules. The Speaking Module may be taken, at the discretion of the test centre, in the period seven days before or after the other three modules.

Preparing for the test

It is not necessary to attend a preparation course but it is, of course, a good idea to prepare thoroughly for the test.

A specimen paper booklet is available from test centres, or directly from Cambridge ESOL or IDP: IELTS Australia. This includes a full practice test with an answer key and a CD of the listening test so that candidates can get some idea of their level and familiarise themselves with the format of the test.

There is also a wide range of published preparation materials.

You can taken an IELTS preparation course at British Council Centres in India.

IELTS Test Results.

Results are issued by test centres within two weeks of the test. Test centres are not permitted to give results out over the phone nor by fax or e-mail.

A score is reported for each module of the test. The individual module scores are then averaged and rounded to produce an Overall Band Score. Overall Band Scores and Listening and Reading scores are reported in whole and half Bands; Writing and Speaking Band Scores are reported in whole Bands only.

Band 9—Expert User

Has fully operational command of the language: appropriate, accurate and fluent with complete understanding.

Band 8—Very Good User

Has fully operational command of the language with only occasional unsystematic inaccuracies and inappropriacies. Misunderstandings may occur in unfamiliar situations. Handles complex detailed argumentation well.

Band 7—Good User

Has operational command of the language, though with occasional inaccuracies, inappropriacies and misunderstandings in some situations. Generally handles complex language well and understands detailed reasoning.

Band 6—Competent User

Has generally effective command of the language despite some inaccuracies, inappropriacies and misunderstandings. Can use and understand fairly complex language, particularly in familiar situations.

Band 5—Modest User

Has partial command of the language, coping with overall meaning in most situations, though is likely to make many mistakes. Should be able to handle basic communication in own field.

Band 4—Limited User

Basic competence is limited to familiar situations. Has frequent problems in understanding and expression. Is not able to use complex language.

Band 3—Extremely Limited User

Conveys and understands only general meaning in very familiar situations. Freunet breakdowns in communication occur.

Band 2—Intermittent User

No real communication is possible except for the most basic information using isolated words or short formulae in familiar situations and to meet immediate needs. Has great difficulty in understanding spoken and written English.

Band 1—Non User

Essentially has no ability to use the language beyond possibly a few isolated words.

Band 0—Did not attempt the test

No assessable information provided.

Test Report Form

The Test Report Form includes a large number of security features, and the authenticity of any Test Report Form can be verified by the test partners. Cambridge ESOL, British Council and IDP: IELTS Australia reserve the right to cancel any IELTS Test Report Form in the event of any attempt to tamper with or misuse the information contained in it.

As a general rule it is recommended that a Test Report Form that is more than two years old should only be accepted as evidence of present level of ability if accompanied by proof that a candidate has actively maintained or tried to improve their English language of proficiency.

Test Modules

Each candidate takes four IELTS test modules, one in each of the four skills, listening, reading, writing and speaking.

Listening

The Listening Module takes around 30 minutes. There are 40 questions. There are four sections. The Listening Module is recorded on a tape and is played ONCE only.

During the test, time is given for candidates to read the questions and write down and then check their answers. Answers are written on the question paper as candidates listen. When the recording ends, ten minutes are allowed for candidates to transfer their answers to an Answer Sheet.

The first two sections are concerned with social needs. There is a converation between two speakers and then a monologue.

The final two sections are concerned with situations related more closely to educational or training contexts. There is a conversion between up to four people and then a further monologue.

A range of English accents and dialects are used in the recordings which reflects the international usage of IELTS.

Reading

The reading modules takes 60 minutes. There are 40 questions, based on three reading passages with a total of 2,000 to 2, 750 words.

All answers must be entered on an Answer Sheet during the 60 minutes test. No extra time is allowed for transferring answers.

Texts are taken from magazines, journals, books, and newspapers. Texts have been written for a non-specialist audience.

At least one text contains detailed logical argument. One text may contain non-verbal materials such as diagrams, graphs or illustrations. If texts contain technical terms then a simple glossary is provided.

Transferring answers to the Answer Sheet

Candidates are required to transfer their answers to an Answer Sheet for the Listening and Academic Reading Modules. Ten minutes extra time is allowed for transferring answers at the end of the Listening but not for the Reading. The Answer Sheet is double-sided; candidates write their Listening answer on one side and then turn over and write their Reading answers on the other side. After marking at centres, all Answer Sheets are returned to Cambridge ESOL for analysis. It is important that candidates complete their personal details at the top of the page and obey the instructions for transfer of answers. Please note the advice given for completion of the Answer Sheet.

Writing

The writing module takes 60 minutes. There are two tasks to complete. It is suggested that about 20 minutes is spent on Task 1 which requires candidates to write at least 150 words. Task 2 requires at least 250 words and should take about 40 minutes.

Answers must be given on the answer sheet and must be written in full. Notes are not acceptable as answers. Candidates should note that scripts under the required minium word limit will be penalised.

In Task 1 candidates are asked to look at a diagram or table, and to present the information in their own words. They may be asked to describe and explain data, describe the stages of a process, how something works or describe an object or event.

In Task 2 candidates are presented with a point of view of argument or problem.

Part of the test realisation is to respond appropriately in terms or register, rhetorical organisation, style and content. Appropriate responses are short essays or general reports, addressed to tutors or examiners.

Speaking

The Speaking Module takes between 11 and 14 minutes and consists of an oral interview between the candidate and an examiner. All interviews are recorded on audio cassette.

In Part 1 candidates answer general questions about themselves, their homes/families, their jobs/studies, their interests, and a range of familiar topic areas. This part lasts between four and five minutes.

In Part 2 the candidate is given a verbal prompt on a card and is asked to talk on a particular topic. The candidate has one minute to prepare before speaking at length, for between one and two minutes. The examiner then asks one or two rounding-off questions.

In Part 3 the examiner and candidate engage in a discussion of more abstract issues and concepts which are thematically linked to the topic prompt in Part 2. The discussion lasts between four and five minutes.

FAQ's ABOUT IELTS

1. What can the candidate bring into the examination room?

   Only pens, pencils and erasers. Correction fluid must not be used. You must leave anything which you do not need, or which is not allowed, either outside the examination room, or as instructed by the supervisor. Mobile phones and pagers must be switched off and placed with personal belongings in the area designated by the supervisor. Any candidate who does not switch off their phone/pager, or who retains one in their possession, will be disqualified.

2. Is the IELTS test completed in one day?

   The Listening, Reading and Writing components of the test are always completed immediately after each other and in this same order. The Speaking test can be taken up to 7 days either before or after the test date.

3. What kind of accents can be heard in the Listening and Speaking Modules?

   As IELTS is an international test, a variety of English accents are used in both of these Modules.

4. Does the listening tape provide the candidate with necessary instructions and pauses?

   Yes. At the beginning of the test, candidates receive instructions and hear a sample question. Next, candidates read Section One questions and then listen to Section One and answer the questions on the question paper as they listen. The same procedure follows for Sections Two, Three and Four. This takes approximately 30 minutes to complete. In the following final ten minutes, candidates transfer their answers onto the answer sheet.

5. Is there a similar period of ten minutes at the end of the Reading test for the transfer of answers?

   No. The Reading test is of one hour, and you must write all your answers on the answer sheet in this time.

6. Can I make some notes on the Listening and Reading question paper?

   Yes. The examiner will not see your question paper.

7. What is the Speaking test?

   The Speaking test is conducted with a one-to-one interview with a certified examiner, which is recorded on an audio-cassette.

8. What should the candidate bring for the Speaking test?

The candidate needs to bring the same identification documents they supplied on registration, as these must be checked again against the information on the application form. These documents will be checked by the administrator and the Speaking examiner prior to the candidate entering the interview room.

9. What happens if a candidate loses their Test Report Form?

At any time within two years of the date of the examination, a candidate can apply to the centre which administered the test to send 5 copies of the original Test Report Form free of charge. These Test Report Forms will not be sent to the candidates themselves, but the Universities abroad, Embassies and Consulate. For any further copies, there is an administration charge per copy. Please contact your test centre for further details.

10. When will the candidate receive their results?

Under usual test circumstances, the candidates will receive their Test Report Forms approximately two weeks after they complete their test.

11. How soon can candidates repeat the test?

Candidates are not permitted to retake the test at any centre within 90 days of their previous test date, i.e. 90 days and no fewer. Candidates are reminded that scores are unlikely to improve dramatically without English language tuition in the interim.

12. What help is available for disabled candidates?

Test centres make every effort to cater for the special needs of any disabled candidates, to enable them to best understand questions and tasks and to give their answers. Candidates with special needs should inform their test centre when applying so that appropriate arrangements can be made.

13. What happens if a candidate is delayed by circumstances beyond their control (e.g. a transportation strike)?

The test centre offers the candidate an alternative test date as soon as possible.

14. What happens if a candidate wants to postpone or cancel their application?

Candidates who request a postponement or cancellation of their test within 5 weeks of the test date will normally be charged the full fee unless they are able to provide appropriate medical evidence to support their request within 5 days of the test date.

15. What happens if a candidate is absent on the day of the test without giving prior notice?

The candidate will lose their full test fee. However, if a medical certificate is provided within 5 days of the test date then the full fee is refunded minus a local administrative deduction.

16. How strictly is IELTS marked?

Candidates should take care when writing answers on the listening and reading answer sheets as incorrect spelling and grammar are penalised. Both UK and US varieties of spelling are acceptable.

If candidates are asked to write an answer using a certain number of words and/or (a) number(s), they will be penalised if they exceed this. For example if a question specifies as answer using NO MORE THAN THREE WORDS and the correct answer is 'black leather coat', the answer 'coat of black leather' is incorrect.

In questions where candidates are expected to complete a gap, candidates should only transfer the necessary missing word(s) on to the Answer Sheet. For Example if a candidate has to complete 'in the ....' and the correct answer is 'morning ' the answer 'in the morning' would be incorrect.

Candidates should read and follow the instructions and questions very carefully. In Listening especially, care also should be taken when transferring answers on to the Answer Sheet.

17. What can candidates do if they are unhappy with their results?

Candidates may apply for an enquiry on results procedure at the centre at which they took their test within four weeks of receipt of results. There is a fee for this which is refunded should the band score change.

ADVICE AND INFORMATION

Make sure you attend on time.

Know the date, time and place of your test and arrive before the scheduled starting time. If you arrive late for any of the papers, report to the supervisor or invigilator. You may not be allowed to take the test.

Bring what you need

Take into the test room only the pens, pencils and erasers which you need for the examination. Correction fluid must not be used.

Leave anything which you do not need, or which is not allowed, either outside the test room, or as instructed by the supervisor.

You may not lend anything to, or borrow anything from, another candidate during the test.

Examination Instructions

Listen to the supervisor and do what you are asked to do.

Tell the supervisor or invigilator at once if you think you have not been given the right question paper, or if the question paper is incomplete or illegible.

Read carefully and follow the instructions printed on the question paper and on the answer sheet.

Fill in the details required on the front of your question paper and on your answer sheet before the start of the test.

Advice and assistance during the test

If you are in doubt about what you should do, raise your hand to attract attention. The invigilator will come to your assistance.

You may not ask for, and will not be given, any explanation of the questions.

If on the day of the test you feel that your work may be affected by ill health or any other reason, you must inform the invigilator at the time.

Leaving the test room

You may not leave the test room without the permission of the supervisor or invigilator.

You can not leave your seat until all papers have been collected and you have been told you can leave.

When you leave the examination room you must leave behind the question paper, your answer paper, any paper used for rough work clearly crossed through and any other materials provided for the test. Do not make any noise near the examination room.

TIPS TO IMPROVE YOUR IELTS PERFORMANCE

Listening

1. Read instructions carefully, don't just glance at them. They are not always the same as in practise or previous tests.
2. Often the speaker will give you an answer and then correct themselves-watch out for this. It's a common trick.
3. Try and anticipate what the speaker will say. This requires concentration-easy in your own language, but more difficult in English.
4. Remember if you want a high score you should aim to get all questions in parts one and two correct. Don't make any careless mistakes in the easier sections.
5. Small errors can lead to low score such as spelling, omitting (s) or incomplete times e.g. 1.30.
6. Don't panic if you think the topic is too difficult or the speaker is too fast. Relax and tune in.
7. Read, write and listen at the same time. Tricky but practise!!
8. Don't leave blanks, you might as well guess, you won't be penalised.

Reading

1. Leave a question if you can't answer. To spend a long time on one answer is disastrous. Go back later if you have time and guess if you have too.
2. Don't panic if you don't know anything about the passage. All the answers are in the passage and you don't need any specialist knowledge.
3. Remember you have no extra time to transfer your answers, many candidates think because they have extra time in listening they are able to do this in reading too. You can't.
4. Before the exam read as widely as possible e.g. Newspapers, magazines, journals. Don't limit yourself to one type of text and read articles with an academic style where possible.
5. Look at ways paragraphs are organized.
6. Try and predict content of paragraph from the opening sentence.
7. Give a paragraph you read an imaginary heading.
8. Don't concentrate on words you don't know. It is fatal and wastes valuable time.
9. Try and spend a specific period each day reading.
10. Careless mistakes cost many marks. Copy the answer correctly if it is in the passage.
11. Check spellings.
12. Only give one answer if that is all that's needed.
13. Be careful with singular/plural.

Writing

1. Highlight/circle key words.
2. Clearly divide paragraphs.
3. Don't repeat ideas in a different way.
4. Stick to the topic.
5. Be careful with timing. Don't rush Task 2, it's longer and carries more weight.
6. Paragraph simply with one idea in each paragraph.
7. Avoid informal language.
8. Learn to recognise how long 150 words is in your handwriting. You don't really have time to count.
9. Don't write too many words particularly for Task One.
10. Get used to always spending several minutes re-reading and correcting your essays.
11. Don't memorise model answers, they won't fit the question and you will make more careless mistakes.

Speaking

1. It tests your ability to communicate effectively not just your grammatical accuracy.
2. Don't learn chunks of answers. The examiner is trained to spot this and will change the question.
3. Develop your answers as much as possible.
4. Speak more than the examiner.
5. Ask for clarification if necessary.
6. Remember it is not a test of knowledge and there is no single answer, but ensure that you give your opinion. Don't worry if you feel it is not sophisticated enough.
7. The areas covered are fairly predictable and not infinite so practise at home recording ideas onto a tape recorder.

SOME IMPORTANT ADDRESSES FOR IELTS

University of Cambridge ESOL Examinations
1 Hills Road, Cambridge, CB1 2EU, United Kingdom
Tel 44 1223 553355, **Fax** 44 1223 460278, **e-mail** ielts@ucles.org.uk

British Council
Bridgewater House, 58 Whitworth Street, Manchester, M1 6BB, United Kingdom
Tel 44 161 957 7755,
Fax 44 161 957 7762,
e-mail ielts@britishcouncil.org

IDP: IELTS Australia
GPO Box 2006, Canberra, ACT 2601, Australia
Tel 61 2 6285 8222,
Fax 61 2 6285 3233,
e-mail ielts@idp.com

IELTS International
100 East Corson Street, Suite 200, Pasadena, CA 91103 , USA
Tel 1 626 564 2954,
Fax 1 626 564 2981,
e-mail ielts@ceii.org

INTRODUCTION

THE PROFESSIONAL AND LINGUISTIC ASSESSMENTS BOARD (PLAB) TEST

The PLAB test is relevant for international medical graduates. If you wish to take up a period of limited registration (which you can do only if you are in supervised employment) GMC will need evidence that you have the necessary skills and knowledge to practise medicine in the UK. The PLAB test is designed to test your ability to work safely in a first appointment as a senior house officer in a UK hospital in the National Health Service (NHS).

The test is in two parts:
Part 1 is a single paper marked by computer to a standard set by the Angoff method
Part 2 is a 14-station objective structure clinical examination (OSCE) which tests your clinical and communication skills.

You cannot enter *Part 2* until you have passed *Part 1*. You must take *Part 2* within three years of passing *Part 1*. Because there is a high demand for places, particularly for *Part 2*, you will generally have to wait between four and six months between applying for, and getting, a place. So you must make sure you apply in plenty of time.

Since November 2002 there has been a time limit for the validity of a pass in the PLAB test. This means your pass in *Part 2* will be valid for EITHER three years from 1 November 2002 OR three years from the date you passed, whichever is later. You will need to work under limited registration within three years of passing the test. If you don't, you will have to take both parts of the test again.

What you will need before you take the PLAB test

Before taking the test you must have
  i. a primary medical qualification (PMQ) for limited registration as listed in the WHO Directory of Medical Schools.
  ii. obtained the relevant scores in the IELTS test (academic module): a minimum of 7 as an overall score and in the speaking section, and 6 in each of the other sections – listening, academic reading, academic writing.
  iii. at least 12 months' postgraduate clinical experience in a teaching hospital, or another hospital approved by the medical registration authorities in the appropriate country. (You can take the test without this experience, but only for employment as a junior house officer, not an SHO).
Please bear in mind that if your pass in the IELTS test is more than two years old at the time you register, you will need to prove you have maintained your English language skills.

Training and work opportunities in the UK

There have recently been a number of articles and press comments suggesting that many international medical graduates are reporting difficulty in securing employment in the UK. There have been calls for the GMC to ration or cap the number of doctors taking the PLAB test. GMC does not believe that would be an appropriate response, even if it were practically possible to find a fair and equitable way of doing so. The GMC is primarily concerned with standard setting and compliance and not with manpower planning issues.

Please remember that you will not be granted limited registration without the offer of a job. But passing PLAB does not guarantee you a job. Before you take the PLAB test, therefore, you should make sure you are well informed about opportunities for work in the UK. There are fewer vacancies in some specialities than others, for example, and there is always a delay between passing the test and securing employment.

The GMC does not hold information about vacancies, but there are a number of other routes you can try, such as

The British Medical Journal

The Health Service Journal

Personnelnet Health

The National Advice Centre for Overseas Doctors

The first three carry job adverts, and the advice centre has general information about postgraduate training opportunities.

Fees

Booking Fees

Part 1 £145

Part 2 £430

Period of notice and cancellation fee

Part 1	*Part 2*
a. Four months or more	
£87	£258
b. Between 21 days and four months	
£101	£301
c. Less than 21 days	
£145	£430

If you want to change your test date to another one you will still be charged a cancellation fee as shown above.

There are concessions on fees for refugee doctors. But if you are a refugee doctor, and want to claim the reduced fee, you will have to pay online the full amount, and then claim back the refund that is due.

Test locations and dates

Part 1 is held at centres in the United Kingdom and in certain other countries. *Part 2* can only be taken in the UK. From time to time GMC may increase the capacity at existing venues or add further dates if necessary.

GMC has to do this so that they can cope with the fluctuating demand for places.

If you need information about accommodation in the UK, visit the British Tourist Authority website.

How to apply

Ideally, you should apply online for a test place. Before you do, make sure you have read the notes in this factsheet and Advice to Candidates.

Test Results

When you attend the examination you will be told the dates for release of the results. They are posted first on the website and then sent by post. GMC does not give results over the phone, by email, by fax or at reception.

If you want a clerical check to verify your marks you must submit a request in writing no later than three weeks after the results have been issued. There is a fee of £40.

Contacting GMC

Email: registrationhelp@gmc-uk.org
Phone: +44 (0)8453 573456
Fax: +44 (0)20 7915 3532
Write: Registration Services
General Medical Council
178 Great Portland Street
London W1W 5JE UK

The PLAB Test *Part 1:*

This information is about *Part 1* of the PLAB test. Please read it carefully and use it as a reference guide.

Part 1 of the PLAB test currently consists of an Extended Matching Question Examination. The Examination paper contains 200 questions divided into a number of themes. It lasts three hours.

From September 2004 the examination will consist of extended matching questions and single best answer questions. This number of questions will remain the same.

Before applying for the examination check the following:
i. Are there jobs available in the specialty of your choice?
ii. Do you need to take the PLAB test to obtain limited registration?
iii. Are you eligible to take the PLAB test?
iv. Have you considered living expenses while you are taking the Examination?

Passing the PLAB test is one of the ways in which you can satisfy the GMC that you have the knowledge and skills which are necessary to practise medicine in the UK.

The General Medical Council must assure itself that you have these abilities before it can grant you limited registration. Limited registration will allow you to practise in the UK in supervised employment in the National Health Service.

Before you enter the PLAB test you must have obtained:

i. A primary medical qualification acceptable for limited registration.

Please check the GMC website to see if your qualification is acceptable. Acceptable qualifications include those listed in the World Directory of Medical Schools published by the World Health Organisation. You may only apply to take the PLAB test when you have passed your final examinations.

ii. Acceptable scores in the International English Language Testing Service (IELTS) test 1 (academic modules) taken a maximum of two years before the date you take *Part 1* of the PLAB test.

You must obtain the following minimum scores in the IELTS test: Overall: 7.0, Speaking: 7.0, Listening: 6.0, Academic Reading: 6.0 and Academic Writing: 6.0. The British Council runs the IELTS test in over 100 countries. You can obtain further information on IELTS from the British Council National Advice Centre or from the IELTS website: www.ielts.org

For information about exemption from IELTS please refer to the GMC website.

iii. GMC strongly recommend that you have 12 months postgraduate clinical experience from teaching hospitals or other hospitals approved by the medical registration authorities in the appropriate country.

It is possible to enter the PLAB test without this experience but you would be at a disadvantage. Without this experience you will initially only be granted limited registration at the grade of House Officer (the grade occupied by new medical graduates).

By law, this requirement does not apply to nationals of a Member State of the European Economic Area, other than the UK, and others with enforceable European Community rights.

Before being granted limited registration you must have the offer of a job, so it is important that you find out about opportunities for work in the UK.

Passing the PLAB test will not guarantee you the offer of a job and you should be aware that there are fewer vacancies in some specialties than others. Additionally most PLAB test candidates find that there is a delay of several weeks, possibly months, between passing the test and starting a job. You should bear in mind if you are applying to take PLAB before completing your pre-registration or internship year that Pre-Registration House Officer jobs are much scarcer than Senior House Officer (SHO) jobs. You should also be aware that there is likely to be much more competition in applying for jobs in London and other major cities in the UK.

You should note that doctors who hold limited registration cannot work as General Practitioners. The General Medical Council does not have information on job opportunities. You can look for jobs in the BMJ Classified Section, or on their website: www.bmj.com

Alternatively, you can obtain information from the British Council National Advice Centre at www.britcoun.org/health/nacpme.

You can take the Examination in:

The UK	-	London
Australia	-	Sydney
Bulgaria	-	Sofia
Egypt	-	Cairo

India	-	Bangalore, Chennai, Hyderabad, Kolkata, Mumbai, New Delhi
New Zealand	-	Wellington
Nigeria	-	Lagos
Pakistan	-	Islamabad and Karachi
Russia	-	Moscow
South Africa	-	Cape Town, Johannesburg
Sri Lanka	-	Colombo
UAE	-	Dubai
West Indies	-	Kingston, Jamaica

The Examination is run approximately every two months.

Examination regulations:

The regulations, apply to all candidates taking the examination. Please ensure that you read the regulations before submitting your application.

Special arrangements for disabled candidates:

If you will need special arrangements to be made because you are disabled please request a special arrangements application form when you submit your application for the Examination. Applications for special arrangements must be made at least two months before the date of the Examination and will be considered on an individual basis. Not all applications will be successful. In particular, your ability to practise safely will be taken into account. 3. Booking a place on the examination

If you have attempted *Part 1* before, you can book a place to re-take the examination and get immediate confirmation of your booking. To take advantage of this, you will need a PIN and Password. http://www.gmc-uk.org/register/faq.htm

Name

It is important that GMC can link all their correspondence with you. You should therefore use the same name and quote your GMC reference number, if you already have one, whenever you contact the GMC.

For the purposes of the PLAB test you should use the same name, in the same order, as it appears on your passport.

If this name differs from the name on your IELTS certificate or the name on the proof of identity you intend to use at the examination Or, when you apply for limited registration, the name shown on your diploma or other evidence of qualification, you will be required to provide original documentary evidence that the names on the different documents refer to you.

GMC will accept the following evidence:
  i. Your marriage certificate
  ii. A declaration from the awarding body which granted you your IELTS certificate or your primary medical qualification, stating that both names relate to you.

If you book online, GMC will correspond by e-mail. Otherwise GMC will usually contact you by post but may use telephone, fax or e-mail if they need to contact you quickly.

IELTS result

You must insert the exact date you took the IELTS test and the scores you obtained.

You should not submit the IELTS Test report Form with your PLAB application form. GMC will require this when you apply for registration after passing both parts of the PLAB test.

Please remember that the certificate is valid for a maximum of two years from the date you took the IELTS test. If your pass in the IELTS test is more than two years old at the time you will be taking *Part 1* of the PLAB test, you will need to provide proof that you have actively maintained or tried to improve your English language skills since you passed the IELTS tests. The ways in which you can do this may include:

i.   Sending GMC proof that you have undertaken a postgraduate course of study within the last two years since you took your IELTS test. You will also need to send them your original IELTS certificate showing that you achieved the required scores.
or

ii. Sending GMC a reference completed by a UK employer or your tutor or lecturer on a postgraduate course of study within the last two years since you took your IELTS test. You will also need to send GMC your original IELTS certificate showing that you achieved the required scores.
or

iii. Sending GMC proof that you have taken the IELTS test again and attaining the required scores.

Date on which you would like to take the Examination

If you book online, you will be provided with an up to date list of all examination in which there are places available otherwise please choose your preferred centres and dates from the up-to-date list.

Payment

If you book online, you must pay by debit or credit card, otherwise the fee of £145 must be paid in advance in sterling. Personal callers to the GMC's office in London may pay fees in cash. Otherwise, fees paid in the United Kingdom must be in the form of a cheque, money order or postal order payable to 'General Medical Council'. Fees sent from other countries, or paid in other countries, must be by sterling bank draft or money order. These must be made payable to 'General Medical Council'. Please remember, where appropriate, to take bank charges into account when paying the fee.

If you have applied for asylum in the UK in accordance with existing law and your application has been granted, or you have been given exceptional leave to remain, we they waive the fee for the first two attempts at the examination. If you think you are eligible for a fee waiver, please obtain a letter from the Home Office stating that you are a refugee as defined above. This letter must be submitted with your application. If presented at a later date, they are unable to reimburse fees for examination places that have already been booked. Cancellation of a confirmed examination place will count as one of your free attempts.

Do not enclose evidence of your primary qualification or IELTS Report Form at this stage. This will be checked by the General Medical Council when you apply for limited registration.

Please check the form carefully to ensure that the information is correct, and sign and date it. Applications must be completed and signed by you only. Any discrepancies may delay your application.

If you wish to take the examination in the UK, you should submit your form together with the appropriate enclosures by post to the PLAB Test Section (Candidate Services) GMC, 178 Great Portland Street, London W1W 5JE. You may bring your form to Registration Reception between 09:00 and 16:30 from Monday to Friday.

If you wish to take the examination overseas, you should post or take your form and enclosures to the appropriate British Council office.

If you apply online, you will have immediate confirmation of your place otherwise, once your form has been processed, you will be sent a letter offering you a place in the Examination and a map showing you where the Examination centre is located.

GMC will try to give you a place in one of the Examinations of your choice. If there are no places available, GMC will write to you about other Examination dates. From time to time they add new examination dates and venues in an effort to meet demand.

If you want to cancel your place, please give the office which offered you the place as much notice as possible. You must return the letter offering you an Examination place, completed as appropriate. If you cancel early, GMC may be able to offer your place to another candidate waiting to take the Examination. You may not pass the letter offering you a place to anyone else.

If you cancel your place, you will be charged a fee. This will normally be deducted from the fee you paid to enter the Examination. The amount charged depends on the amount of notice you give.

Any changes to a confirmed booking will be treated as a cancellation which will attract the appropriate cancellation charge.

If exceptional circumstances cause GMC to postpone or cancel an Examination, or to declare the results of an Examination to be invalid, you will be entitled to a full refund of the Examination entry fee. The General Medical Council will not be liable for any other costs.

1. Taking the Examination

Part 1 of the PLAB Test is a three-hour Extended Matching Question (EMQ) examination.

2. Arrival at the Examination

You must make your own arrangements for travel and accommodation. It is important that you ensure that, having been allocated a place in the Examination, you are not prevented from attending by factors such as your ability to obtain leave from employment, or the availability of transport, or visa or other immigration formalities. For information about accommodation in the UK, please visit the British Tourist Authority website at www.visitbritain.com.

3. Duration of the Examination

The Invigilator's instructions will take about 30 minutes. The Examination will last three hours and collecting the Examination materials will take a further 30 minutes. You will be required to be at the Examination centre for a minimum of four hours.

The email confirmation sent to you if you have booked online, or if you have not the letter offering you a place will tell you the time you should arrive at the Examination. If you arrive after the first half an hour of the Examination has passed, you will not be allowed to enter the Examination hall. You will not be permitted to leave the Examination hall in the first half hour or in the last half hour of the Examination. You must remain in your seat until the Chief Invigilator permits you to leave.

Although GMC expects all Examinations to run to time, it is suggested that you allow time for unforeseen delays when booking tickets for a return journey.

Water will not be available during the Examination. Other than the material provided by the GMC, you may only have water, sweets and your passport or other form of identification on your desk during the examination.

You must take proof of your identity to the Examination together with the letter from the General Medical Council or British Council offering you a place in the Examination. These will be checked at the Examination.

The following are acceptable forms of identification. To be accepted, the identification document must bear your photograph.

   i. Your passport
  ii. Your UK Immigration and Nationality Department identification document
 iii. Your Home Office travel document
 iv. Your UK driving licence

No other identification document will be accepted. If you fail to bring one of the identification documents listed above, or if the document does not bear your photograph, you will not be permitted to take the Examination.

If the name on your identification document is different from that on the letter from the General Medical Council or British Council offering you a place in the examination, you must provide original evidence that you are the person named in that letter. GMC will accept the following evidence:

   i. Your marriage certificate.
  ii. A declaration from the awarding body which granted you your IELTS certificate or your primary medical qualification, stating that both names relate to you.
      If Examination officials are in any doubt about your identity or the authenticity of your documents the following process will take place:

The Chief Invigilator will take a polaroid photograph of you and ask you to sign it on the back to verify its authenticity. If you fail to comply with this process, you will not be permitted to take the Examination.

After the Examination you will be required to produce the correct form of identification document or evidence of change of name to the Head of the PLAB Test Section at the General Medical Council or the Examinations Manager at the British Council. He or she will carry out such investigations as he or she considers appropriate and will make a final decision about the matter. If he or she decides that the person who sat the Examination is not the person who is entitled to do so, the Examination attempt will be invalid and the matter will be reported to the Registrar of the General Medical Council so it can be considered in relation to a future application for limited registration.

5. Conduct during the Examination

You will be provided with all the materials you need during the Examination. You may not use or refer to any other materials. You should not write down details of questions to take out of the examination hall.

Doctors in the UK often have to make decisions without the opportunity to consult others. Whilst they must never do this outside the limits of their professional competence, it is important that the General Medical Council ensures that they have the knowledge and skill to take these decisions. For this reason, candidates must take the Examination without help from materials or fellow candidates. Help from materials or fellow candidates will be regarded as cheating and taken very seriously.

6. Unforeseen events during the Examination

If any unforeseen problems arise during the Examination, such as a fire alarm, you should follow the instructions of the Chief Invigilator.

7. Marking the Examination

The Examination will be marked in the UK by computer. For the first sitting of the Examination, the Professional and Linguistic Assessments Board determined the standard required to pass in accordance with a recognised method of standard setting. This standard is maintained by test equating. This means that the standard for each examination will be the same, but the pass mark may vary, reflecting the difficulty of the questions set in the Examination.

8. Notification of results

At the end of the Examination, you will be told the date on which your results will be available. This will be about four weeks after the examination. Results will be published on the website and a letter containing your results will be posted about two weeks later. The results may not be collected from the General Medical Council's offices. For Examinations GMC cannot give results by telephone, fax or e-mail because GMC cannot guarantee that they will remain confidential.

If you pass you can apply online immediately to take *Part 2* of the test by going to GMC website. To gain access to the relevant part of GMC website you will need the PIN and Password GMC previously sent to you. If you are unable to apply online you can download an application form, list of available dates and Advice to candidates for the PLAB Test *Part 2* from GMC website. You can also e-mail GMC at registrationhelp@gmc-uk.org or telephone GMC on +44 (0)8453 573456.

If you fail the Examination you may re-apply. You may not apply for PLAB *Part 2* or re-apply for *Part 1* before any previous PLAB examination results have been issued.

9. Feedback

Your results will include information about your position in relation to the pass mark and the performance of the other candidates.

GMC does not provide a detailed breakdown of whether you answered individual questions correctly or incorrectly. If you fail the Examination, it means that you have not mastered a large part of the core knowledge, skills and attitudes a senior house officer needs to practise safely.

10. Verification of results

Candidates wishing to verify any mark or marks, by means of a clerical check, should submit a request in writing to the PLAB Test Section no later than three weeks after the results have been issued. A fee of £40 must accompany your request.

GMC will aim to undertake the check and issue a response within 10 working days.

11. Complaints

A candidate who wishes to make a complaint about the examination should submit a detailed written report to the Head of the PLAB Test Section no later than three weeks after the results have been issued.

You should provide your name, address, telephone number and GMC reference number.

GMC will acknowledge your complaint, investigate it and respond within 10 working days.

12. Appeals

You may not appeal against the mark you receive for the Examination. The examiners' decision is final.

A pass in the PLAB test will demonstrate that the successful candidate has the ability to practise safely as a senior house officer (SHO) in a first appointment in a UK hospital. This is the standard laid down by the General Medical Council for the PLAB test.

The examiners and question writers are aware that you may not be familiar with British culture or the National Health Service. This has been taken into account in the design of the Examination. You should remember, however, that the UK is a multi-cultural society and you should not make assumptions about a patient on the basis of gender or ethnic origin. For example, you should not assume that women do not smoke or drink.

The doctor-patient relationship is very important in the UK. As well as preparing for the Examination by revising your knowledge and skills you must recognise that attitudes are also important. The Duties of a doctor will guide you in this area.

Part 1 of the test currently consists of an Extended Matching Question (EMQ) Examination, referred to throughout this annex as the Examination. The Examination paper will contain 200 questions divided into a number of themes and may contain photographic material. It will last three hours. From September 2004 the Examination will consist of extended matching questions and single best answer (SBA) questions. The number of questions will remain the same. The proportion of SBA questions may vary from examination to examination but no more than 30% of the paper will be composed of SBA questions.

The emphasis of the Examination is on clinical management and includes science as applied to clinical problems.

The Examination is confined to core knowledge, skills and attitudes relating to conditions commonly seen by SHOs, to the generic management of life-threatening situations, and to rarer, but important, problems.

The Examination assesses the ability to apply knowledge to the care of patients.

The subject matter is defined in terms of the skill and of the content.

Four groups of skills will be tested in approximately equal proportions:

Diagnosis: Given the important facts about a patient (such as age, sex, nature of presenting symptoms, duration of symptoms) you are asked to select the most likely diagnosis from a range of possibilities.

Investigations: This may refer to the selection or the interpretation of diagnostic tests. Given the important facts about a patient, you will be asked to select the investigation which is most likely to provide the key to the diagnosis. Alternatively, you may be given the findings of investigations and asked to relate these to a patient's condition or to choose the most appropriate next course of action.

Management/Treatment: Given the important facts about a patient's condition, you will be asked to choose the most suitable treatment including therapeutics from a range of possibilities. In the case of medical treatments you will be asked to choose the correct drug therapy and will be expected to know about side effects.

The context of clinical practice: This may include:

Explanation of disease process: The natural history of the untreated disease.

Legal ethical: You are expected to know the major legal and ethical principles set out in the General Medical Council publication Good Medical Practice.

Practice of evidence-based medicine: Questions on diagnosis, investigations and management may draw upon recent evidence published in peer-reviewed journals. In addition, there may be questions on the principles and practice of evidence-based medicine.

Understanding of epidemiology: You may be tested on the principles of epidemiology, and on the prevalence of important diseases in the UK.

Health promotion: The prevention of disease through health promotion and knowledge of risk factors.

Awareness of multicultural society: You may be tested on your appreciation of the impact on the practice of medicine of the health beliefs and cultural values of the major cultural groups represented in the UK population.

Application of scientific understanding to medicine: You may be tested on the scientific disciplines which underpin medicine. Examples include anatomy, genetics and pathology.

You will be expected to know about conditions that are common or important in the United Kingdom for all the systems outlined below.

ACCIDENT AND EMERGENCY MEDICINE

Examples: Abdominal, chest and head injuries (isolated or multiple injuries), bites and stings, bruising, burns, chest pain, collapse, cardiopulmonary resuscitation (CPR), eye problems, shock, trauma.

BLOOD

Examples: Anaemias, coagulation defects, haemoglobinopathies, purpura.

CARDIOVASCULAR SYSTEM

Examples: Aortic aneurysm, arrhythmias, chest pain, deep vein thrombosis (DVT), heart failure, hypertension, ischaemic limb, myocardial infarction, myocardial ischaemia, stroke, varicose veins.

DERMATOLOGY, ALLERGY, IMMUNOLOGY AND INFECTIOUS DISEASES

Examples: Allergy, fever and rashes, meningitis, serious infections including HIV, hepatitis B and tropical diseases, skin cancers.

ENT AND OPHTHALMOLOGY

Examples: Dysphagia, earache, epistaxis, hearing problems, hoarseness, glaucoma, 'red eye', sudden visual loss.

GASTROINTESTINAL TRACT, LIVER AND BILIARY SYSTEM, AND NUTRITION

Examples: Abdominal pain, constipation, diarrhoea, difficulty in swallowing, digestive disorders, gastrointestinal bleeding, jaundice, rectal bleeding/pain, vomiting, weight problems.

METABOLISM, ENDOCRINOLOGY AND DIABETES

Examples: Diabetes mellitus, thyroid disorders, weight problems.

NERVOUS SYSTEM

Examples: Coma, convulsions, eye problems, headache, loss of consciousness, seizures, stroke, transient ischaemic attacks, vertigo.

ORTHOPAEDICS AND RHEUMATOLOGY

Examples: Arthritis, back pain, dislocations, fractures, joint pain/swelling, sprains and strains.

PSYCHIATRY

Examples: Alcohol abuse, anxiety, assessing suicidal risk, confusion and delirium, depression, drug abuse, overdoses and self harm, post-natal problems.

RENAL SYSTEM

Examples: Haematuria, renal failure, sexual health, testicular pain, urinary calculi and infections.

RESPIRATORY SYSTEM

Examples: Asthma, breathlessness/wheeze, cough, haemoptysis, pneumonia.

DISORDERS OF CHILDHOOD

Examples: Abdominal pain, asthma, child development, childhood illnesses, earache, epilepsy, eye problems, fetal medicine, fever and rashes, joint pain/swelling, loss of consciousness, meningitis, non-accidental injury, sexual abuse, testicular pain, urinary disorders.

DISORDERS OF THE ELDERLY

Examples: Altered bowel habit, dementia, depression, digestive disorders, urinary disorders

PERI-OPERATIVE MANAGEMENT

Examples: Anti-emetics, pain relief, peri-operative monitoring, post-operative complications, pre-operative assessment.

PALLIATIVE CARE, ONCOLOGY

Examples: Blood dyscrasias, general malignancy, pain relief, terminal care.

The examination paper will contain 200 questions. You will be awarded one mark for each item answered correctly. Marks are not deducted for incorrect answers nor for failure to answer. The total score on the paper is the number of correct answers given. You should, therefore, attempt all items. Names of drugs are those contained in the most recent edition of the British National Formulary (BNF).

Some questions relate to current best practice. They should be answered in relation to published evidence and not according to your local arrangements. If necessary, you should take steps to familiarise yourself with the range of equipment routinely available in UK teaching hospitals.

You will have two marksheets on the day – a purple one for questions 1 – 100 and a pink one for questions 101 – 200. Instructions on how to complete the answer sheet are at the top of the first sheet.

EMQs

Extended matching questions are grouped into themes. Each theme has a heading which tells you what the questions are about.

Within each theme there are several numbered items, usually between three and six. These are the questions and the problems you have to solve. There are examples below.

Begin by reading carefully the instruction which precedes the numbered items. The instruction is very similar throughout the paper and typically reads 'For each patient described below, choose the SINGLE most discriminating investigation from the above list of options. Each option may be used once, more than once or not at all.'

Consider each of the numbered items and decide what you think the answer is. You should then look for that answer in the list of options (each of which is identified by a letter of the alphabet). If you cannot find the answer you have thought of, you should look for the option which, in your opinion, is the best answer to the problem posed.

For each numbered item, you must choose ONE, and only one, of the options. You may feel that there are several possible answers to an item, but you must choose the one most likely from the option list. If you enter more than one answer on the answer sheet you will gain no mark for the question even though you may have given the right answer along with one or more wrong ones.

In each theme there are more options than items, so not all the options will be used as answers. This is why the instruction says that some options may not be used at all.

Alternatively a given option may provide the answer to more than one item. For example, there might be more than one item which contains descriptions of patients, and the most likely diagnosis could be the same in both instances. In this case the option would be used more than once.

Sample Extended Matching Questions

Theme 1: Joint pain

Options:
a. Ankylosing spondylitis
b. Erythema nodosum
c. Gout
d. Hyperparathyroidism
e. Joint sepsis
f. Medial cartilage tear
g. Osteoarthritis
h. Psoriatic arthropathy
i. Pyrophosphate arthropathy
j. Reactive arthritis
k. Rheumatoid arthritis

For each patient described below, choose the SINGLE most likely diagnosis from the above list of options. Each option may be used once, more than once, or not at all.

1. A 70 year old previously healthy farmer presents with pain on weight-bearing and restricted movements of the right hip.
2. A 73 year old woman with rheumatoid arthritis on immuno-suppressive drugs presents with systemic malaise and fever. She has red, hot, swollen wrists.
3. A 66 year old woman started furosemide (frusemide) two weeks ago and now presents with a red, hot, swollen metatarso-phalangeal joint.
4. A 22 year old male soldier presents with a two week history of a swollen right knee, conjunctivitis and urethritis.
5. A 30 year old man presents with a 10 year history of back pain, worse in the morning, and one episode of iritis.

Theme 2: Investigation of confusion

Options:
a. Blood cultures
b. Chest x-ray
c. Computed tomography (CT) scan of head
d. Electrocardiogram (ECG)
e. Full blood count (FBC)

f. Mid-stream urine (MSU) culture
g. Plasma glucose concentration
h. Serum urea and electrolytes concentration
i. Stool culture
j. Thyroid function tests
k. Ultrasound abdomen

For each patient described below, choose the SINGLE most discriminating investigation from the above list of options. Each option may be used once, more than once, or not at all.

1. An 84 year old woman in a nursing home has been constipated for a week. Over the past few days she has become increasingly confused and incontinent of urine.
2. A previously well 78 year old woman has been noticed by her daughter to be increasingly slow and forgetful over several months. She has gained weight and tends to stay indoors with the heating on, even in warm weather.
3. A 64 year old man has recently been started on tablets by his general practitioner. He is brought to the Accident and Emergency Department by his wife with sudden onset of aggressive behaviour and confusion. Before starting the tablets he was losing weight and complaining of thirst.
4. A frail 85 year old woman presents with poor mobility and a recent history of falls. She has deteriorated generally over the past two weeks with fluctuating confusion. She has a mild right hemiparesis.
5. A 75 year old man with mild Alzheimer's disease became suddenly more confused yesterday. When seen in the Accident and Emergency Department, his blood pressure was 90/60 mmHg and his pulse rate was 40 beats/minute and regular.

Theme 3: Causes of pneumonia

Options:

a. Bacteroides fragilis
b. Coxiella burnetii
c. Escherichia coli
d. Haemophilus influenzae
e. Legionella pneumophila
f. Mixed growth of organisms
g. Mycobacterium tuberculosis
h. Mycoplasma pneumoniae
i. Pneumocystis carinii
j. Staphylococcus aureus
k. Streptococcus pneumoniae

For each patient described below, choose the SINGLE most appropriate causative organism from the above list of options. Each option may be used once, more than once, or not at all.

1. A 25 year old man has a three day history of shivering, general malaise and productive cough. His chest x-ray shows right lower lobe consolidation.

2. A 26 year old man presents with severe shortness of breath and a dry cough which he has had for 24 hours. He is very distressed. He has been an IV drug user. His chest x-ray shows bilateral peri-hilar hazy shadowing.

3. A 35 year old previously healthy man returned from holiday five days ago. He smokes 10 cigarettes a day. He presents with mild confusion, a dry cough and marked pyrexia. His chest examination is normal. His chest x-ray shows widespread upper zone shadowing.

4. A 20 year old previously healthy woman presents with general malaise, severe cough and breathlessness which has not improved with a seven day course of amoxicillin. Physical examination is normal. Her chest x-ray shows patchy shadowing throughout the lung fields. The blood film shows clumping of red cells and cold agglutinins are present.

5. A 55 year old farmer presents with a five day history of fever, malaise, muscle pains and headache. He has an irritating but non-productive cough.

ANSWERS

Theme 1: Joint Pain

1. g
2. e
3. c
4. j
5. a

Theme 2: Investigation of confusion

1. f
2. j
3. g
4. c
5. d

Theme 3: Causes of pneumonia

1. k
2. i
3. e
4. h
5. b

Single Best Answer Questions

Consider each of the questions and decide what you think the answer is to the lead-in question given at the end of each scenario, which typically reads 'What is the SINGLE most likely diagnosis?'. You should then look for that answer in the list of options below (each of which is identified by a letter of the alphabet). If you cannot find the answer you have thought of, you should look for the option which, in your opinion, is the best answer to the problem posed.

For each question, you must choose ONE, and only one, of the options. You may feel that there are several possible answers, but you must choose the one most likely from the option list. If you enter more than one answer on the answer sheet you will gain no mark for the question even though you may have given the right answer along with one or more wrong ones.

Sample Single Best Answer Questions

1. A 17 year boy attends the Accident and Emergency Department having been taken ill whilst playing football. He gives a history of sudden onset of left-sided chest pain followed by severe and persistent breathlessness.

What is the SINGLE investigation most likely to provide a definitive diagnosis?
a. Blood gases
b. Chest x-ray
c. Echocardiogram
d. Electrocardiogram (ECG)
e. Pulmonary function tests

2. An 85 year old man who weighs 80 kg is admitted as an emergency with fever and delirium. He gives a history of dysuria and frequency. His blood pressure (BP) is 70/50 mmHg and temperature 38.6 °C. His serum creatinine is 620 mmol/l and his serum urea is 46 mmol/l. The microbiologist recommends the prescription of gentamicin.

What is the SINGLE most appropriate dose of gentamicin?
a. 40 mg single dose
b. 40 mg once daily
c. 80 mg 8 hourly
d. 80 mg 12 hourly
e. 160 mg single dose

3. A 55 year old man presents having recently noticed a lump in his right groin. He smokes heavily, has a persistent cough and has previously had an appendicectomy.

What is the SINGLE most likely diagnosis?
a. Epigastric hernia
b. Femoral hernia
c. Incisional hernia
d. Inguinal hernia
3. Spigelian hernia

4. A 58 year old postmenopausal woman presents with a one week history of vaginal bleeding. Digital vaginal examination is normal.

What is the SINGLE most appropriate diagnostic test?
a. Cervical smear
b. Endometrial aspiration

c. Plasma oestrogen

d. Serum FSH/LH levels

e. Transvaginal ultrasound scan

5. A two year old boy is brought to the Accident and Emergency Department by his mother. He has been unable to bear weight since a fall from a chair last night. He is tender over the mid-tibia but there is no obvious limb deformity.

What is the SINGLE most likely radiographic appearance of the fracture?

a. Angulated fracture

b. Compound fracture

c. Epiphyseal fracture

d. No fracture likely

e. Spiral fracture

6. An 83 year old woman admitted with a chest infection becomes confused with poor concentration. She is restless and frightened. She is verbally abusive and has perceptual abnormalities. There is no significant previous psychiatric history.

What is the SINGLE most likely diagnosis?

a. Acute confusional state

b. Drug induced psychosis

c. Lewy body dementia

d. Multi-infarct dementia

e. Psychotic depression

7. A 32 year old woman was painting her bathroom when she experienced a sudden, severe headache, vomited and collapsed hitting her head. She has been brought to the Accident and Emergency department. She now has a Glasgow Coma Scale (GCS) score of 15, a temperature of 37.7 °C, a blood pressure of 145/85 mmHg and a pulse rate of 70 beats/minute. Her physical examination is normal apart from an abrasion over her right temple.

What is the SINGLE most appropriate initial management?

a. Admit for head injury observation

b. Carboxyhaemoglobin level

c. Computed tomography (CT) brain scan

d. Lumbar puncture

e. Skull X-ray

Answers

1. b

2. e

3. d

4. e

5. e

6. a

7. c

RECOMMENDED BOOKS TO BE READ

- Oxford Handbook of Clinical Medicine 5th Edition (OHCM)
- Oxford Handbook of Clinical Specialities 6th Edition (OHCS)

These two books are a must and must be thoroughly read. Each line is important and can give rise to a question. Though these two books cover a large area that needs to be read, some other books need to be used as well.

1. Medicine: Kumar and Clarke 14th edition or Davidson 15th edition can be used for reference purposes along with thorough readings of OHCM.
   (Oxford Textbook of Medicine can be used only for some topics such as poisoning).
2. Paediatrics: OHCS and OHCM cover a lot of topics pretty well but a textbook on the subject like Essential Paediatrics by David Hull 4th Edition or the one used during your UG days would be indeed helpful.
3. Surgery: Both OHCM and OHCS cover some areas. Bailey and Love 24th edition covers most of the other required topics.
4. Psychiatry: OHCS along with any of the Medicine books would suffice.
5. Gynaecology: OHCS along with Ten teachers in gynaecology 17th edition is sufficient. Though you can also use Lecture notes in Gynaecology for reference.
6. Obstetrics: OHCS along with Ten teachers in obstetrics 17th edition is sufficient. Though you can also use Lecture notes in obstetrics for reference.
7. ENT and Ophthalmology: Although OHCS is sufficient but textbooks read during your UG days can also help as reference books. You can also use Lecture notes in ENT and Ophthalmology for referecne purposes.
8. Orthopaedics: OHCS along with references from orthopaedics section in Bailey and Love or from Lecture notes on orthopaedics will do the job.
9. Dermatology: OHCS along with any of the Medicine textbooks for finer details is just fine. You can also refer to the Lecture notes on dermatology.

Part 2: The Objective Structured Clinical Examination (OSCE)

Aim

The aim of *Part 2* is to test your clinical and communication skills. It is designed so that an examiner can observe you putting these skills into practice.

Overall format

When you enter the Examination room, you will find a series of 16 booths, known as 'stations'. Each station requires you to undertake a particular task. Some tasks will involve talking to or examining patients, some will involve demonstrating a procedure on an anatomical model. One station will be a rest station where you will have no task to perform. One station may be a pilot station where GMC is trying out a new station. Your result in this station will not count. However, the information GMC gains from candidates' performances in pilot stations is considered valuable to them.

You will be required to perform all tasks. You will be told the number of the station at which you should begin when you enter the Examination room. Each task will last five minutes.

Your instructions will be posted outside the station. You should read these instructions carefully to ensure that you follow them exactly. An example might be:

'Mr McKenzie has been referred to you in a rheumatology clinic because he has joint pains. Please take a short history to establish supportive evidence for a differential diagnosis.'

A bell will ring. You may then enter the station. There will be an examiner in each station. However, you will not be required to have a conversation with the examiner; you should only direct your remarks to him or her if the instructions specifically ask you to do so. You should undertake the task as instructed. A bell will ring after four minutes 30 seconds to warn you that you are nearly out of time. Another bell will ring when the five minutes are up. At this point, you must stop immediately and go and wait outside the next station. If you finish before the end, you must wait inside the station but you should not speak to the examiner or to the patient during this time.

You will wait outside the next station for one minute. During this time you should read the instructions for the task in this station. After one minute a bell will ring. You should then enter the station and undertake the task as instructed.

You should continue in this way until you have completed all 16 stations. You will then have finished the OSCE.

1. Contacts
   UK Government Department of Health
   Website: www.doh.gov.uk/medicaltrainingintheuk

2. Job opportunities in the UK
   British Medical Journal Classified Section
   Website: www.bmj.com
   The British Council National Advice Centre
   Bridgewater House
   58 Whitworth Street
   Manchester
   M1 6BB
   United Kingdom
   Tel: 44 161 957 7218
   Fax: 44 161 957 7029
   Website: www.britcoun.org/health/nacpme

3. Immigration/visa requirements
   Immigration and Nationality Directorate
   Block C, Whitgift Centre
   Croydon
   Surrey
   CR9 2AR
   United Kingdom

Tel: 44 0870 606 7766
The IELTS test
The British Council National Advice Centre for Postgraduate Medical Education (NACPME)
Bridgewater House
58 Whitworth Street
Manchester
M1 6BB
United Kingdom
Tel: 44 161 957 7218
Fax: 44 161 957 7029
E-mail: ed@britcoun.org
IELTS
Website: www.ielts.org

4. Applying for and taking the Examination

The United Kingdom

The General Medical Council – PLAB Test Section
178 Great Portland Street
London
W1W 5JE
United Kingdom
Name: Candidate Services
Tel: +44 (0)8453 573456
Fax: +44 207 915 3558
E-mail: plab@gmc-uk.org

India

Chennai
British Deputy High Commission
British Council Division
737 Anna Salai
Chennai 600 002
Name: Nirupa Fernandez
Tel: 91-44-852-5002
Fax: 91-44-852-3234
E-mail: nirupa.fernandez@in.britishcouncil.org

Kolkata
British Deputy High Commission
British Council Division
5 Shakespeare Sarani

Kolkata 700 071
Name: Suchitra Mukherjee
Tel: 91-33-282 9108/9144
Fax: 91-33-282-4804
E-mail: suchitra.mukherjee@in.britishcouncil.org

Mumbai
British Deputy High Commission
British Council Division
Mittal Tower 'C' Wing
Nariman Point
Mumbai 400 021
Name: Vivek Singh
Tel: 91-22-222 3560
Fax: 91-22-285-2024
E-mail: vivek.singh@britishcouncil.org

New Delhi
British High Commission
British Council Division
17 Kasturba Gandhi Marg
New Delhi 110 001
Name: P V Chaary
Tel: 91-11 3710111/3710555
Fax: 91-11 3710 717
E-mail: pv.chaary@in.britishcouncil.org

Pakistan

Karachi
The British Council
20 Bleak House Road
Near Cant's Station
Karachi
(PO Box 10410)
Name: Karima Kara
Tel: 92 21 5670391-7
Fax: 92 21 5683694
E-mail: Karima.kara@britishcouncil.org.pk

Islamabad
PO Box 1135
House no 1

Street 61
F-6/3
Islamabad
Name: Shahnaz Farooq
Tel: 92 51 111 424 424
Fax: 92 51 111 276 683
E-mail: shahnaz.farooq@britishcouncil.org.pk

Sri Lanka

Colombo
The British Council
49 Alfred Gardens
(P O Box 753) Colombo 3
Sri Lanka
Name: Panchalika Kulatunga
Tel: 94 1 581171-2
Fax: 94 1 587079
E-mail: panchalika.kulatunga@britishcouncil.org.plc

5. The duties of a doctor registered with the General Medical Council
   Patients must be able to trust doctors with their lives and well-being. To justify that trust, we as a profession have a duty to maintain a good standard of practice and care and to show respect for human life. In particular as a doctor you must:
   - make the care of your patient your first concern;
   - treat every patient politely and considerately;
   - respect patients' dignity and privacy;
   - listen to patients and respect their views;
   - give patients information in a way they can understand;
   - respect the rights of patients to be fully involved in decisions about their care;
   - keep your professional knowledge and skills up to date;
   - recognise the limits of your professional competence;
   - be honest and trustworthy;
   - respect and protect confidential information;
   - make sure that your personal beliefs do not prejudice your patients' care;
   - act quickly to protect patients from risk if you have good reason to believe that you or a colleague may not be fit to practise;
   - avoid abusing your position as a doctor; and
   - work with colleagues in the ways that best serve patients' interests.
   In all these matters you must never discriminate unfairly against your patients or colleagues.
   And you must always be prepared to justify your actions to them.

6. Contact address

Email: registrationhelp@gmc-uk.org
Phone: +44 (0)8453 573456
Fax: +44 (0)20 7915 3532
Write: Registration Services
General Medical Council
178 Great Portland Street
London W1W 5JE
UK

7. Some useful websites

http://www.plabmaster.com
http://www.plabonline.cjb.net/
http://www.aippg.com/plab-uk/
http://www.vishwamedical.com
http://www.plabtutor.com
http://www.easyexamltd.com
http://www.plabwise.co.uk
http://www.medicbyte.com
http://www.mcqs.com
http://www.fischtest.co.uk
http://www.onexamination.com
http://www.plabisgood4u.com
http://www.pastest.co.uk
http://www.7plus7.com
http://www.medvarsity.com
http://www.londondeanery.ac.uk
http://www.flash-med.com
http://www.icmeindia.com
http://www.servicelinksintl.com/plab.htm
http://www.mo-media.com/plab
http://www.mdlinks.net/plab.htm
http://www.rxpgonline.com
http://www.overseasdoctors.com
http://www.telmedpack.com/doctors
http://www.123doc.com

Section A

Section A

January 2004
Question Paper

One

Theme 1: Causes of dysphagia

Options:

a. Parkinsonism
b. Motor neurone disease
c. Stroke
d. Achalasia
e. Chagas' disease
f. Oesophageal carcinoma
g. Reflux oesophagitis
h. Pharyngeal pouch
i. Scleroderma
j. Foreign body

For each presentation below, choose the SINGLE most appropriate cause of dysphagia from the above list of options. Each option may be used once, more than once, or not at all.

1. A man complaints of dysphagia. He is unable to protrude his tongue and has difficulty in speaking. He is unable to move his all 4 limbs.

2. A man complaints of sudden dysphagia, he cannot protrude his tongue and has difficulty in speaking.

3. A 110 Kg lady complains of many years of heart burn but now complains of painful dysphagia. Barium swallow does not show any stricture.

4. A man complaints of dysphagia, he has foetor oris and there is occasional regurgitation of undigested food particles.

5. A man complains of sudden dysphagia while eating meat and chips. There is dribbling of saliva.

Theme 2: Diagnosis of fractures

Options:

a. Fracture distal end of radius
b. Metacarpal fracture
c. Supracondylar fracture of humerus
d. Scaphoid fracture
e. Posterior dislocation of shoulder joint.
f. Anterior dislocation of shoulder joint
g. Perilunate fracture
h. Pulled elbow

For each presentation below, choose the SINGLE most appropriate diagnosis from the above list of options. Each option may be used once, more than once, or not at all.

1. A man complained of pain in hand after punching a wall yesterday.
2. A young girl fell from a tree and now complains of pain in the arm. Her radial pulse cannot be felt.
3. A man having seizures came to the A & E complaining of pain in the shoulder. There was no obvious visible deformity.
4. An old lady complained of pain in the wrist and hand after she fell on an outstretched hand. Her wrist and hand are swollen.
5. A 3 year old girl tripped while holding her mothers hand. She has not used her arm since then.

Theme 3: Diagnosis of rectal conditions

Options:

a. Anal fissure
b. Perianal haematoma
c. Crohn's disease
d. Proctalgia fugax
e. Rectal carcinoma
f. Ischaemic colitis
g. Haemorrhoids

For each presentation below, choose the SINGLE most appropriate diagnosis from the above list of options. Each option may be used once, more than once, or not at all.

1. A patient with chronic constipation, and severe pain when defecating. Pain is severe and cannot undergo rectal examination.
2. Patient with severe anal pain and a swelling in the perianal region.
3. Patient with weight loss and change in bowel habits. Sigmoidoscopy shows ulcer.
4. Patient presents with bleeding rectum. He also complains of abdominal pain and weight loss. On examination anal skin tags are noted.
5. A patient complains of sudden deep shooting pain in perianal region.

Theme 4: Contraception: Mechanism of action

Options:

a. Disruption of corpus luteum
b. Inhibits ovulation
c. Prevents implantation
d. Inhibits tubal motility
e. Spermicidal
f. Causes miscarriage
g. Inhibits ovulation and thickens cervical mucus.

For each contraceptive below, choose the SINGLE most appropriate mechanism of action of contraceptive from the above list of options. Each option may be used once, more than once, or not at all.

1. Depo–Provera.
2. OCP.
3. Post-coital pill.
4. Vaginal sponge.
5. Mirena coli.

Theme 5: Cell of origin

Options:

a. Adipocyte
b. Neuroglial cells
c. Plasma cells
d. Megakaryoblast
e. Skeletal muscle
f. Lymphocytes
g. Erythroblast
h. Monocytes
i. Schwann cells
j. Neutrophil precursors
k. Astrocytes

For each pathology below, choose the SINGLE most appropriate origin from the above list of options. Each option may be used once, more than once, or not at all.

1. Lipoma.
2. Glioblastoma multiforme.
3. Myeloma.
4. AML.
5. Rhabdomyosarcoma.

Theme 6: Cause of ascites

Options:

a. Carcinomatosis peritonei
b. Subacute bacterial peritonitis
c. Nephrotic syndrome
d. Portal vein occlusion
e. Cirrhosis
f. Tuberculosis
g. Protein losing enteropathy
h. Budd–Chiari syndrome
i. Congestive cardiac failure

For each presentation below, choose the SINGLE most appropriate cause of ascites from the above list of options. Each option may be used once, more than once, or not at all.

1. A man with some cancer developing ascites.
2. A patient presents with ascites with numerous neutrophils.
3. Immigrant from India developing exudative ascites and loss of weight .
4. A patient presents with dyspnoea, orthopnoea, wheeze and cough. On examination he has ascites, tachycardia and inspiratory crepts.
5. A patient presents with chronic stigmata of liver disease and ascites.

Theme 7: Psychiatry: Management

Options:

a. Sedation
b. Psychiatric referral
c. ECT
d. TCA
e. Lithium
f. Desensitization

For each presentation below, choose the SINGLE most appropriate management from the above list of options. Each option may be used once, more than once, or not at all.

1. A boy with learning disabilities and staff are concerned about increasing number of head bangings.
2. A man with schizophrenia hears voices telling him to have bleach.
3. A 17 year old girl whose parents are separated, is brought to the A & E after she took 5 tablets of diazepam.
4. A man is admitted to a surgical ward after an accident where he sustained a minor injury. After a few days he is unresponsive to the staff.
5. A 27 year old has 2 small children. She has no family support. She is recovering from influenza and her washing machine has broken down. She comes to A & E saying she took 8 aspirin tablets.

Theme 8: Pain relief

Options:

a. Oral paracetamol
b. IV morphine
c. SC morphine
d. Oral morphine
e. Oral diclofenac
f. Codeine and paracetamol
g. IM diclofenac
h. Carbamazepine

For each presentation below, choose the SINGLE most appropriate analgesic from the above list of options. Each option may be used once, more than once, or not at all.

1. A 8 year old boy is being investigated for failure to thrive, complains of ear pain.
2. A young lady felt dizzy and she fell down. She has swelling in her ankle and pain, but she is able to walk.
3. A child presenting with signs and symptoms of appendicitis.
4. A patient with signs and symptoms of myocardial infarction.
5. A patient with carcinoma bronchus, now complains of pain and it is intolerable to paracetamol and brufen.
6. A patient presents with post herpetic neuralgia.

Theme 9: Investigation in ophthalmic conditions

Options:

a. Carotid doppler
b. Temporal lobe MRI
c. ESR
d. Carotid angiography
e. MRI pituitary fossa
f. Temporal artery biopsy
g. X-ray skull
h. X-ray orbit

For each presentation below, choose the SINGLE most appropriate investigation from the above list of options. Each option may be used once, more than once, or not at all.

1. A patient presents with typical history of temporal arteritis.
2. Patient with intermittent episodes of amaurosis fugax.
3. A patient presents with upper quadrantanopia.
4. A patient presents with signs and symptoms of acromegaly.

Theme 10: Ear treatment

Options:

a. Amoxicillin
b. Oral aciclovir
c. Topical aciclovir
d. Paracetamol
e. Flucloxacillin
f. Immediate referral to specialist
g. Routine referral to specialist

For each presentation below, choose the SINGLE most appropriate management from the above list of options. Each option may be used once, more than once, or not at all.

1. A diabetic patient with features suggestive of furunculosis.
2. A patient had syringing done and complains of sudden acute pain now.
3. A patient with varicella and has vesicles on the pinna and the eardrum.
4. A patient with a chronic history and on examination has a scarred eardrum and has a mass seen.
5. A child presents with otitis media.

Theme 11: Pre-operative investigation

Options:

a. Cancel the operation
b. ECG recording for 24 hours
c. Cardiology opinion
d. Ambulatory BP measurement
e. CXR
f. Blood sugar

For each presentation below, choose the SINGLE most appropriate pre-operative investigation from the above list of options. Each option may be used once, more than once, or not at all.

1. A patient has been admitted for a prostatectomy and his BP is 190/110 the previous day.
2. A patient with controlled angina since 10 years. Has had 2 attacks of angina in the last one week. He is posted for a prostatectomy.
3. A patient with COPD posted for prostatectomy.

Theme 12: Obstetrics and gynaecology: Treatment

Options:

a. Calcium supplement
b. HRT
c. Vaginal lubricant
d. Vaginal oestrogen
e. Subcutaneous oestrogen
f. Biphosphonates
g. Condoms
h. Vitamin D
i. Exercise

For each presentation below, choose the SINGLE most appropriate management from the above list of options. Each option may be used once, more than once, or not at all.

1. A 55 year old female who attained menopause 2 years ago. Family history of osteoporosis present. She is worried and has come for counselling.
2. A 32 year old patient with family history of osteoporosis and she has lactose intolerance.
3. A patient who has postmenopausal dyspareunia, urine culture is negative. She is not willing to take systemic hormones.
4. A postmenopausal woman presents after hysterectomy with family history of osteoporosis. She does not want to take oral medicines.

Theme 13: Non accidental injury

Options:

a. Refer to childcare centre
b. Nutritional assessment
c. Coagulation screen
d. Register with child care
e. EUA
f. Inform police
g. CT scan

For each presentation below, choose the SINGLE most appropriate management from the above list of options. Each option may be used once, more than once, or not at all.

1. A child is brought with a fracture femur, no evidence of trauma.
2. A bruise is noted on a child's hand. Mother had stopped the child from running across the road.
3. A child of unemployed parents, examination reveals no improvement from last check up.
4. A child brought with bleeding per vaginum and her vagina is sore and shows excoriations.
5. An 18 year old mother brings her one year old child to the A & E. Child is drowsy and left pupil is dilated.

Theme 14: Rheumatology diagnosis

Options:

a. Rheumatoid arthritis
b. Psoriatic arthritis
c. Enteropathic arthritis
d. Osteoarthritis
e. Ankylosing spondylitis
f. Chondromalacia patella
g. Gout
h. Pseudogout
i. Multiple myeloma

For each presentation below, choose the SINGLE most appropriate diagnosis from the above list of options. Each option may be used once, more than once, or not at all.

1. A 45 year old female with symmetrical arthropathy presents with pain which is worse on getting up.
2. A 25 year old man complains of backache and morning stiffness. He gives no history of trauma or lifting weights.
3. A patient presents with punched out erosions on X-rays and backache.
4. An elderly on thiazide diuretics for his hypertension, new complains of pain and swelling in his foot which is hot to touch. He gives no history of trauma.
5. A 45 year old female with painful movements at the joints which are worse in the evening. She also complains of some swelling in her fingers.

Theme 15: Relation to obesity

Options:

a. Type I DM
b. Type II DM
c. Alcohol
d. Cushing's disease
e. COPD
f. Obstructive sleep apnoea
g. Asthma
h. Hypothyroidism
i. Polycystic ovary disease

For each presentation below, choose the SINGLE most appropriate diagnosis from the above list of options. Each option may be used once, more than once, or not at all.

1. Weight loss would help night sleep in this condition and improve marital harmony.
2. Weight loss would help to stop the medication.
3. Stopping this would help in weight loss and vitamin deficiency.
4. Surgery in this condition will help in weight loss.

Theme 16: Psychiatry: Diagnosis

Options:

a. Acute confusional state
b. PTSD
c. Drug induced psychosis
d. Mania
e. Schizophrenia
f. Obsessive compulsive disorder
g. Major depression
h. Panic attack
i. Postnatal psychosis

For each presentation below, choose the SINGLE most appropriate diagnosis from the above list of options. Each option may be used once, more than once, or not at all.

1. A person who has undergone surgery for some condition and is receiving medicines for pain relief. On third post operative day he has features of delirium tremens.
2. A kosovian who gets startled easily when he hears any loud noises etc. He recently saw a shootout in the colony in which a child died.
3. A person who is being stopped by the police and goes on talking jumping from one topic to another.
4. A man runs to the police station saying that his house is not safe, but on checking that's not the case.

Theme 17: Surgery

Options:

a. Femoral hernia
b. Indirect inguinal hernia
c. Direct inguinal hernia
d. Maldescended testis
e. Hydrocele of canal of Nuck
f. Saphena varix
g. Lipoma
h. Richter's hernia
i. Incisional hernia

For each presentation below, choose the SINGLE most appropriate diagnosis from the above list of options. Each option may be used once, more than once, or not at all.

1. A lump that is seen below and lateral to the pubic tubercle.
2. A mass attached to the spermatic cord.
3. Young lady with lump is groin with no cough impulse. It does not reduce on lying down. It transilluminates also.
4. A GIT hernia involving only the wall of the gut.

Theme 18: Trauma to an organ

Options:

a. Urethra
b. Bladder
c. Spleen
d. Pancreas
e. Kidney
f. Diaphragm
g. Aorta
h. Liver

For each presentation below, choose the SINGLE most likely traumatized organ from the above list of options. Each option may be used once, more than once, or not at all.

1. A person who met with a accident and is in A & E with pain in right upper quadrant and hypotension.
2. A builder falls astride on a scaffolding bar.
3. A person presents after an accident. When nasogastric tube was tried, it was not successful.
4. A person presents after an accident with fullness in the loin and pain.

Theme 19: Scientific basis in nephrology

Options:

a. Obstruction
b. Papillary necrosis
c. Hypercalcaemia
d. Infection
e. Dehydration

For each presentation below, choose the SINGLE most appropriate cause from the above list of options. Each option may be used once, more than once, or not at all.

1. A patient with signs and symptoms suggestive of sarcoidosis.
2. A patient of ankylosing spondylitis on NSAIDs for many years.
3. A marathon runner develops renal colic.
4. A person having recurrent attacks of urinary tract infection.
5. A patient with chronic UTI develops stones in the kidney.

Theme 20: Investigation in seizure

Options:

a. Check drug level
b. EEG
c. CT scan
d. MRI
e. Blood sugar
f. LFTs
g. U&E
h. Telemonitoring

For each presentation below, choose the SINGLE most appropriate investigation from the above list of options. Each option may be used once, more than once, or not at all.

1. A child has had one episode of grand mal epilepsy, now presents with another attack.
2. A girl who is being treated for absence seizures, has had recurrent seizures and she is obese.
3. A child is unwell since the last few days, is brought to A & E with seizures. Child is irritable.

Theme 21: Seizures: Diagnosis

Options:

a. Febrile convulsion
b. Petit mal seizure
c. Grand mal seizure
d. Complex seizure
e. Pseudoseizure

For each presentation below, choose the SINGLE most appropriate diagnosis from the above list of options. Each option may be used once, more than once, or not at all.

1. A person who has been treated for carcinoma now comes with pain and numbness in his left leg and then starts jerking limbs without losing his consciousness.
2. A child having otitis media presents with seizure.
3. A child at school suddenly stops mid-sentence for a few seconds and then starts off where she stopped.
4. A person with a seizure involving jerking of all 4 limbs. Incontinence is noted.

Theme 22: Investigation in haematuria

Options:

a. ASO titre
b. Creatinine clearance
c. USG
d. Cystoscopy

For each presentation below, choose the SINGLE most appropriate investigation from the above list of options. Each option may be used once, more than once, or not at all.

1. An 8 year old boy comes with complaints of fever, oliguria and oedema.
2. A person presents with haematuria, he says there is family history of the same.
3. A diabetic patient with pitting oedema.

Theme 23: Psychiatry: Diagnosis

Options:

a. Low mood
b. Chronic fatigue syndrome
c. Thought broadcasting
d. Thought insertion
e. Insight
f. Judgment
g. Paranoid delusion
h. Postnatal psychosis
i. Post traumatic stress disorder
j. Mania

For each presentation below, choose the SINGLE most appropriate diagnosis from the above list of options. Each option may be used once, more than once, or not at all.

1. A lady who lacks energy and has dishevelled hair and appearance.
2. A woman who is admitted and feels that the staff knows what she is thinking.
3. A patient keeps on talking and he jumps from one topic to another.
4. A 50 year old woman complains of pain in the legs and hands. All investigations and examination are normal.

Theme 24: Prevention of respiratory asthma

Options:

a. Avoid smoke
b. Avoid allergen
c. Avoid pets

For each presentation below, choose the SINGLE most appropriate preventive measure from the above list of options. Each option may be used once, more than once, or not at all.

1. A 6 year old boy presents with recurrent bouts of asthma, parents are smokers.
2. A boy presents with recurrent attacks on playing football.
3. A child presents with acute attacks of asthma, her brother rears rabbits during holidays.

Theme 25: Loss of consciousness

Options:

a. CO poisoning
b. Hypoglycaemia
c. Meningitis
d. Subdural haematoma
e. Subarachnoid haemorrhage
f. Intracerebral haemorrhage

For each presentation below, choose the SINGLE most appropriate diagnosis from the above list of options. Each option may be used once, more than once, or not at all.

1. An alcoholic who has had recurrent falls with fluctuating consciousness.
2. A person who has been hypertensive since last 10 years and not on any treatment, presents with sudden loss of consciousness.
3. A student at hostel in the university has come back home, he has fever and rash.
4. An 8 year old child with diabetes was found lying unconscious in his home.
5. A student at the hostel was found unconscious in his room. He had installed a fireplace that day itself.
6. A person with a severe headache like he has been hit at the back of his head.

Theme 26: Urinary system

Options:

a. Post operative retention
b. Catheterise
c. Suprapubic catheterization
d. Tuberculosis
e. Transitional cell carcinoma

For each presentation below, choose the SINGLE most appropriate management/ diagnosis from the above list of options. Each option may be used once, more than once, or not at all.

1. Post-operative hernia patient has difficult in voiding urine.
2. A person in a mining accident comes with anuria.
3. A person in an accident with blood seen at the tip of the urethra.
4. A patient with frequency and haematuria. On cystoscopy red patches are seen, no infection and no signs of inflammation.

Theme 27: Trauma: Management

Options:

a. Control bleeding with external pressure
b. Vascular access and infuse normal saline
c. Vascular access and infuse blood
d. Intubate and ventilate
e. Maintain open airway
f. Needle thoracocentesis
g. Splint fracture

For each presentation below, choose the SINGLE most appropriate management from the above list of options. Each option may be used once, more than once, or not at all.

1. A 10 year old boy fell onto broken glass and is bleeding form his wrist.
2. A girl has been hit by a car, neck is immobilised. She is receiving 100% oxygen. Breathing is noisy.
3. A child fell from a horse. Her neck is immobilised and she has been given oxygen. She has a swollen thigh, and she has cool peripheries.
4. A 15 year old girl had cut her wrists and bled profusely. She is pale and tachycardic.
5. A boy was involved in an accident in which another person was killed. He is brought to A& E with a oxygen mask. He is talking. He is pale and tachycardic.

Theme 28: Infection: Diagnosis

Options:

a. Lymphoma
b. TB
c. Brucellosis
d. Lyme disease
e. Plasmodium falciparum
f. Plasmodium vivax
g. Plasmodium ovale
h. Rabies

For each presentation below, choose the SINGLE most appropriate diagnosis from the above list of options. Each option may be used once, more than once, or not at all.

1. An 8 year old boy from Somalia has complaints of haemoptysis, cough and fever.
2. A patient with cervical lymph nodes has night sweats and low grade fever.
3. A person working in a farm comes with splenomegaly and fever.
4. A patient with intermittent fever with chills and rigors, splenomegaly and seizures.
5. A girl went out in the forest for a walk and had a tick bite. She presents with fever now.

Theme 29: Dyspepsia

Options:

a. Proton pump inhibitors
b. Endoscopy
c. Antacids
d. Endoscopic biopsy
e. Oesophageal dilatation
f. Radiotherpay
g. Chemotherapy
h. Triple therapy

For each presentation below, choose the SINGLE most appropriate diagnosis/ management from the above list of options. Each option may be used once, more than once, or not at all.

1. A patient with long history of dyspepsia since 10 years, takes cimetidine but no relief.
2. A patient who has been on triple therapy for *H. pylori* comes now with complaints of dyspepsia.
3. A pregnant woman presents with dyspepsia.
4. Endoscopy done on a patient with long history of dyspepsia, shows Barrett's oesophagus.
5. A patient presents with dyspeptic symptoms. Endoscopy has been done and *H. pylori* status found positive.

Theme 30: Prenatal screening

Options:

a. Duchenne's muscular dystrophy
b. Spina bifida
c. Down's syndrome
d. Cystic fibrosis
e. Sickle cell anaemia

For each presentation below, choose the SINGLE most appropriate diagnosis from the above list of options. Each option may be used once, more than once, or not at all.

1. Mom with previous male child affected with this disorder want to know whether this child is also affected.
2. Pregnant lady with high alpha-fetoprotein want to know whether the child is having this condition.
3. Pregnant lady with high HCG and low AFP want to know whether is affected with this condition.
4. To prevent from this condition mother takes folate prior to conception and during pregnancy.
5. Mom with previous child affected with recurrent chest infections and abdominal symptoms wants to know whether this child is affected.

Theme 31: Causes of bleeding following delivery

Options:

a. Cervical lacerations
b. Vaginal lacerations
c. Uterine atony
d. Rupture of uterus
e. Cervical polyp
f. DIC

For each presentation below, choose the SINGLE most appropriate cause of bleeding from the above list of options. Each option may be used once, more than once, or not at all.

1. A lady previous history of one Caesarean section, has profuse bleeding after vaginal delivery.
2. A lady has excess vaginal bleeding after delivery of twins.
3. A lady who has 5 children, has profuse bleeding after delivery.
4. A lady who delivered without episiotomy is noted to have excess bleeding.
5. A lady with abruptio placentae, has heavy bleeding.

Theme 32: Treatment of conjunctivitis

Options:

a. Topical fusidic acid
b. Oral indomethacin
c. Oral tetracycline
d. Sodium cromoglycate
e. Oral aciclovir
f. Topical betamethasone
g. Topical chloramphenicol

For each pathology below, choose the SINGLE most appropriate treatment from the above list of options. Each option may be used once, more than once, or not at all.

1. Allergic conjunctivitis.
2. Ophthalmia neonatorum.
3. Trachoma.
4. Reiter's disease.

Theme 33: Diagnosis of arrhythmia

Options:

a. Ventricular fibrillation
b. Ventricular tachycardia
c. Supraventricular tachycardia
d. Atrial fibrillation
e. Atrial flutter
f. Ventricular ectopics
g. Wenckebach phenomenon

For each presentation below, choose the SINGLE most appropriate diagnosis from the above list of options. Each option may be used once, more than once, or not at all.

1. A patient 3 weeks post MI complains of palpitations. He is otherwise normal.
2. A 27 year old lady complains of recurrent episodes of palpitations along with spells of dizziness. Her BP and pulse are normal.
3. A 39 year old man known hypertensive complains of palpitations which he has noticed. to decrease on applying pressure over carotids.
4. A 32 year old man who is an athlete by profession complains of palpitations. He is otherwise well and his rhythm is normal.

Theme 34: Dementia: Diagnosis

Options:

a. Alzheimer's dementia
b. Alcoholic dementia
c. Huntington's chorea
d. Creutzfeldt–Jakob's disease
e. Pick's disease
f. Lewy body dementia
g. Multi infarct dementia
h. HIV
i. Frontotemporal dementia

For each presentation below, choose the SINGLE most appropriate diagnosis from the above list of options. Each option may be used once, more than once, or not at all.

1. A 40 year old lady with right handed involuntary writhing movement with strong family history.
2. A 55 year old man with no previous history of disease brought to A&E by his wife who says that he has become progressively more forgetful, tends to lose his temper and is emotionally labile.
3. A 77 year old man with weakness in his arm and leg from which he recovered within few days with short term memory loss, has extensor plantar response. He has had similar episodes 2 years ago and became unable to identify objects and make proper judgements.
4. A 70 year old man with early loss of memory, disinhibition with visuospatial orientation preserved.

Theme 35: Diagnosis of skin conditions

Options:

a. Meningococcal septicaemia
b. Herpes zoster
c. Erythema nodosum
d. Spider naevi
e. Neurofibromatosis
f. Psoriasis
g. Bullous pemphigoid
h. Dermatitis herpetiformis

For each presentation below, choose the SINGLE most appropriate diagnosis from the above list of options. Each option may be used once, more than once, or not at all.

1. A patient with multiple nodular lesions all over the body.
2. A patient with lesions present over trunk and face suffers from a chronic illness.
3. A patient with chest pain and malaise presents with this condition over his trunk.
4. A student in hostel with fever headache and rash presents to A&E.
5. A patient with bilateral hilar lymphadenopathy and cough presents with raised skin lesions in shin.

Theme 36: Diagnosis of skin conditions

Options:

a. Lichen planus
b. Sebborhoeic dermatitis
c. Candidial dermatitis
d. Psoriasis
e. Impetigo
f. Cavernous haemangioma
g. Kaposi sarcoma
h. Bullous pemphigoid
i. Erythema chronicum migrans

For each presentation below, choose the SINGLE most appropriate diagnosis from the above list of options. Each option may be used once, more than once, or not at all.

1. An infant with red rash sparing skin folds.
2. A patient with rashes over the extensor surfaces of the forearm.
3. A patient with yellow lesion with crust present over the body which spread by skin to skin contact.
4. A boy with raised lesion over the face which disappear as age advances.

Theme 37: Diagnosis of hearing loss

Options:

a. Ménière's disease
b. Wax impaction
c. Acoustic neuroma
d. Acute otitis media
e. Presbyacusis
f. Otosclerosis
g. Otitis externa
h. Ototoxicity

For each presentation below, choose the SINGLE most appropriate diagnosis from the above list of options. Each option may be used once, more than once, or not at all.

1. A patient with intermittent tinnitus, giddiness and vertigo with unilateral sensorineural hearing loss.
2. A patient with poor hygiene with unilateral conductive hearing loss.
3. A 50 year old man with unilateral sensorineural hearing loss and facial numbness.
4. A 55 year old man with bilateral sensorineural hearing loss.
5. A man with bilateral impaired hearing. His father was also affected with impaired hearing in his middle-age.

Theme 38: Investigation of swollen Joints

Options:

a. Urate crystals on joint aspirate
b. High serum calcium
c. Joint aspirate and culture
d. Positive rheumatoid factor
e. Positive antinuclear antibody
f. Pyrophosphate crystals on joint aspirate
g. ESR
h. X-ray hip
i. Positive blood culture

For each presentation below, choose the SINGLE most appropriate investigation from the above list of options. Each option may be used once, more than once, or not at all.

1. A 35 year old woman has pain and stiffness in her hands, wrists, elbows with early morning stiffness.
2. A 60 year old lady with rheumatoid arthritis developed sudden painful red hot knee and is febrile.
3. A 70 year old lady with stiffness of her shoulders and hips finds it difficult to comb her hair.
4. A 75 year old man has had painful hip for many years but his right hip has become painful with no history of trauma.
5. A hypertensive suddenly developed painful swollen knee.

Theme 39: Diagnosis of rectal bleeding

Options:

a. Angiodysplasia
b. Inflammatory bowel disease
c. Haemorrhoids
d. Diverticulosis
e. Carcinoma rectum
f. Carcinoma caecum
g. Fissure in ano

For each presentation below, choose the SINGLE most appropriate diagnosis from the above list of options. Each option may be used once, more than once, or not at all.

1. A patient with myocardial infarction develops sudden severe bleeding per rectum. PR examination is normal.
2. A young patient with chronic diarrhoea presents with bleeding per rectum.
3. A 40 year old man with painful defecation and blood in stool.
4. A 70 year old man with chronic diarrhoea and left iliac fossa pain develops bleeding per rectum. He is also anaemic.

One *January 2004 Answers*

Theme 1: Causes of dysphagia

1. **(b)** Motor neurone disease
2. **(c)** Stroke
3. **(g)** Reflux oesophagitis
4. **(h)** Pharyngeal pouch
5. **(j)** Foreign body

Theme 2: Diagnosis of fractures

1. **(b)** Metacarpal fracture
2. **(c)** Supracondylar fracture of humerus
3. **(e)** Posterior dislocation of shoulder joint
4. **(g)** Perilunate fracture
5. **(f)** Anterior dislocation of shoulder joint

Theme 3: Diagnosis of rectal conditions

1. **(a)** Anal fissure
2. **(b)** Perianal haematoma
3. **(e)** Rectal carcinoma
4. **(c)** Crohn's disease
5. **(d)** Proctalgia fugax

Theme 4: Contraception: Mechanism of action

1. **(g)** Inhibits ovulation and thickens cervical mucus
2. **(b)** Inhibits ovulation
3. **(a)** Disruption of corpus luteum
4. **(e)** Spermicidal
5. **(c)** Prevents implantation

Theme 5: Cell of origin

1. **(a)** Adipocyte
2. **(k)** Astrocytes
3. **(c)** Plasma cells
4. **(j)** Neutrophil precursors
5. **(e)** Skeletal muscle

Theme 6: Cause of ascites

1. **(a)** Carcinomatosis peritonei
2. **(b)** Subacute bacterial peritonitis
3. **(f)** Tuberculosis
4. **(i)** Congestive cardiac failure
5. **(e)** Cirrhosis

Theme 7: Psychiatry : Management

1. **(a)** Sedation

2. **(b)** Psychiatric referral
3. **(b)** Psychiatric referral
4. **(b)** Psychiatric referral
5. **(b)** Psychiatric referral

Theme 8: Pain Relief

1. **(a)** Oral paracetamol
2. **(e)** Oral diclofenac
3. **(g)** IM diclofenac
4. **(b)** IV morphine
5. **(d)** Oral morphine
6. **(h)** Carbamazepine

Theme 9: Investigation in ophthalmic conditions

1. **(c)** ESR
2. **(d)** Carotid angiography
3. **(b)** Temporal lobe MRI
4. **(e)** MRI pituitary fossa

Theme 10: Ear treatment

1. **(e)** Flucloxacillin
2. **(f)** Immediate referral to specialist
3. **(b)** Oral aciclovir
4. **(g)** Routine referral to specialist
5. **(a)** Amoxicillin

Theme 11: Pre-operative investigation

1. **(d)** Ambulatory BP measurement
2. **(c)** Cardiology opinion
3. **(e)** CXR

Theme 12: Obstetrics and gynaecology: Treatment

1. **(b)** HRT
2. **(a)** Calcium supplement
3. **(d)** Vaginal oestrogen
4. **(e)** Subcutaneous oestrogen

Theme 13: Non accidental Injury

1. **(b)** Nutritional assessment

2. **(c)** Coagulation screen
3. **(a)** Refer to childcare centre
4. **(e)** EUA
5. **(g)** CT scan

Theme 14: Rheumatology diagnosis

1. **(a)** Rheumatoid arthritis
2. **(e)** Ankylosing spondylitis
3. **(i)** Multiple myeloma
4. **(g)** Gout
5. **(d)** Osteoarthritis

Theme 15: Relation to obesity

1. **(f)** Obstructive sleep apnoea
2. **(b)** Type II DM
3. **(c)** Alcohol
4. **(d)** Cushing's disease

Theme 16: Psychiatry : Diagnosis

1. **(c)** Drug induced psychosis
2. **(b)** PTSD
3. **(d)** Mania
4. **(e)** Schizophrenia

Theme 17: Surgery

1. **(a)** Femoral hernia
2. **(d)** Maldescended testis
3. **(e)** Hydrocele of canal of Nuck
4. **(h)** Richter's hernia

Theme 18: Trauma to an organ

1. **(h)** Liver
2. **(a)** Urethra
3. **(f)** Diaphragm
4. **(e)** Kidney

Theme 19: Scientific basis in nephrology

1. **(c)** Hypercalcaemia
2. **(b)** Papillary necrosis
3. **(e)** Dehydration
4. **(a)** Obstruction
5. **(d)** Infection

Theme 20: Investigation in seizure

1. **(c)** CT Scan
2. **(a)** Check drug level
3. **(c)** CT Scan

Theme 21: Seizures : Diagnosis

1. **(e)** Pseudoseizure
2. **(a)** Febrile convulsion
3. **(b)** Petit mal seizure
4. **(c)** Grand mal seizure

Theme 22: Investigation in haematuria

1. **(a)** ASO titre
2. **(c)** USG
3. **(b)** Creatinine clearance

Theme 23: Psychiatry : Diagnosis

1. **(a)** Low mood
2. **(c)** Thought broadcasting
3. **(j)** Mania
4. **(b)** Chronic fatigue syndrome

Theme 24: Prevention of respiratory asthma

1. **(a)** Avoid smoke
2. **(b)** Avoid allergen
3. **(c)** Avoid pets

Theme 25: Loss of consciousness

1. **(d)** Subdural haematoma
2. **(f)** Intracerebral haemorrhage
3. **(c)** Meningitis
4. **(b)** Hypoglycaemia
5. **(a)** CO poisoning

6. **(e)** Subarachnoid haemorrhage

Theme 26: Urinary system

1. **(a)** Post operative retention
2. **(b)** Catheterise
3. **(c)** Suprapubic catheterization
4. **(e)** Transitional cell carcinoma

Theme 27: Trauma Management

1. **(a)** Control bleeding with external pressure
2. **(d)** Intubate and ventilate
3. **(c)** Vascular access and infuse blood
4. **(c)** Vascular access and infuse blood
5. **(c)** Vascular access and infuse blood

Theme 28: Infection: Diagnosis

1. **(b)** TB
2. **(a)** Lymphoma
3. **(c)** Brucellosis
4. **(e)** Plasmodium falciparum
5. **(d)** Lyme disease

Theme 29: Dyspepsia

1. **(a)** Proton pump inhibitors
2. **(b)** Endoscopy
3. **(c)** Antacids
4. **(d)** Endoscopic biopsy
5. **(h)** Triple therapy

Theme 30: Prenatal screening

1. **(a)** Duchenne's muscular dystrophy
2. **(b)** Spina bifida
3. **(c)** Down's syndrome
4. **(b)** Spina bifida
5. **(d)** Cystic fibrosis

Theme 31: Causes of bleeding following delivery

1. **(d)** Rupture of uterus

2. **(c)** Uterine atony
3. **(c)** Uterine atony
4. **(b)** Vaginal lacerations
5. **(f)** DIC

Theme 32: Treatment of conjunctivitis

1. **(d)** Sodium cromoglycate
2. **(g)** Topical chloramphenicol
3. **(c)** Oral tetracycline
4. **(b)** Oral indomethacin

Theme 33: Diagnosis of arrhythmia

1. **(b)** Ventricular tachycardia
2. **(c)** Supraventricular tachycardia
3. **(c)** Supraventricular tachycardia
4. **(g)** Wenckebach phenomenon

Theme 34: Dementia: Diagnosis

1. **(c)** Huntington's chorea
2. **(a)** Alzheimer's dementia
3. **(g)** Multi infarct dementia
4. **(i)** Frontotemporal dementia

Theme 35: Diagnosis of skin conditions

1. **(e)** Neurofibromatosis
2. **(d)** Spider naevi
3. **(b)** Herpes zoster
4. **(a)** Meningococcal septicaemia
5. **(c)** Erythema nodosum

Theme 36: Diagnosis of skin condition

1. **(c)** Candidial dermatitis
2. **(d)** Psoriasis
3. **(e)** Impetigo
4. **(f)** Cavernous haemangioma

Theme 37: Diagnosis of hearing loss

1. **(a)** Ménière's disease
2. **(b)** Wax impaction
3. **(c)** Acoustic neuroma
4. **(e)** Presbyacusis
5. **(f)** Otosclerosis

Theme 38: Investigations of swollen joints

1. **(d)** Positive rheumatoid factor
2. **(c)** Joint aspirate and culture
3. **(g)** ESR
4. **(f)** Pyrophosphate crystals on joint aspirate
5. **(a)** Urate crystals on joint aspirate

Theme 39: Diagnosis of rectal bleeding

1. **(a)** Angiodysplasia
2. **(b)** Inflammatory bowel disease
3. **(g)** Fissure in ano
4. **(e)** Carcinoma rectum

One / *January 2004 Explanation*

Theme 1: Causes of dysphagia

1. This is a case of Motor neurone disease. Bulbar palsy accounts for ¼th of MND patients. There is palsy of tongue, muscles of chewing/swallowing and facial muscles due to loss of function of brainstem motor nuclei. MND generally presents in those > 40 years of age with stumbling (spastic gait, foot drop), weak grip or as aspiration pneumonia. Upper motor signs include weakness, spasticity, brisk reflexes, upgoing plantars. Lower motor signs include weakness, wasting, fasciculation of tongue, abdomen, back or thigh.

2. Strokes result from ischaemic infarction or bleeding in the brain. Chief causes are thrombosis in situ, atheroembolism, heart emboli and CNS bleed. Patients may present with contralateral hemiplegia, contralateral sensory loss, homonymous hemianopia, dysphasia, quadriplegia, locked–in–syndrome, pure motor, pure sensory or mixed signs (depending upon the part involved).

3. Gastro oesophageal reflux diseases is due to dysfunction of the lower oesophageal sphincter. It is associated with smoking, alcohol, hiatus hernia, pregnancy, obesity, big meals, systemic sclerosis. Patient generally presents with heartburn, acid brash, water brash, odynophagia and nocturnal asthma. Barium swallow does not show any strictures.

4. Pharyngeal pouch is a protusion through Killian's dehiscence. Patients suffering from this condition are usually elderly. It is twice as common in men as in women. Initially symptoms are identical with those of a foreign body in the throat. Later regurgitation of undigested food at unpredictable times is the chief complaint. Still later patient can complaint of gurgling noises in the neck especially on swallowing. Such pouches can sometimes be seen to enlarge when the patient drinks. Patients have progressive loss of weight due to semi-starvation.

5. The sudden presentation of the dysphagia while eating meat and chips is suggestive of impaction of piece of meat in the oesophagus.

Theme 2: Diagnosis of fractures

1. Fractures of the shaft or neck of one or more of the medial four metacarpals are produced by the knukles striking objects (i.e. by punching), or by blows on the dorsum of the hand. Fractures of a single shaft are splinted by the adjacent metacarpals. Such fractures suffer little displacement. Fractures through the neck also result only in recession of the knuckle and a minimal loss of extension at the metacarpophalangeal joint.

2. Supracondylar fracture is most commonly due to fall on an outstreched hand with elbow slightly flexed. The possibility of interruption of blood supply to the forearm in such cases is high. It can occur at the time of injury if the brachial artery is contused or lacerated by the anterior aspect of the proximal fragment of the humerus. In such a condition, the radial pulse will not be palpable. More commonly the radial pulse is obliterated by swelling and flexion of the elbow following reduction.

3. Posterior dislocation of the shoulder although rare, may be caused by seizures. It is usually hard to diagnose the condition in an AP view radiography ('light–bulb' appearance of humeral head). Lateral radiographs are always required. Such patients are referred to the orthopaedician.

4. A fall on the palm of the outstreched and dorsiflexed hand may dislocate the whole carpus backwards in relation to the radius and lunate. This is a perilunate dislocation of the wrist. Clinically the patient will have stiff wrist and finger with swollen and tender wrist. If the lunate has dislocated it may compress the median nerve. Isolated dislocation of the lunate can usually be treated by closed reduction. If this fails, open reduction is mandatory. Avascular necrosis of the lunate (Kienbock's diseases) may occur after this injury. Trans-scaphoid perilunate dislocation should be treated by open reduction and internal fixation.

5. This sounds like a pulled elbow but is actually anterior dislocation of the shoulder joint. The question mentions that 'she has not used her arm since then'. This suggests that the pathology lies proximal to the arm. Anterior dislocation of the shoulder presents with loss of shoulder contour i.e. flattening of deltoid, anterior bulge from the head of the humerus which is palpable in the axilla. Treatment options include Kocher's method and scapular manipulation.

Theme 3: Diagnosis of rectal conditions

1. Anal fissure or Fissure-in-ano, is a midline longitudinal split in squamous lining of the lower anus often present with a mucosal tag at the external aspect-'the sentinel pile'. Mostly it is due to hard faeces or constipation. Defecation or PR examination is very painful, as in this patient.

2. The presentation in this patient is suggestive of a perianal haematoma. They are also known as thrombosed external pile. But both are misnomers because it is actually a clotted venous saccule. It is seen as a 2–4 mm 'dark blue berry' beneath the skin. It can be evacuated via a small incision under LA.

3. Rectal carcinoma is the 4th most common malignancy in women. Local spread occurs circumferentially and within 2 years complete encirclement would have taken place. Spread via the venous system occurs late. Patients present with bleeding which is the earliest and most common symptom alongwith a sense of incomplete defecation (tenesmus). Alteration in the bowel habit, weight loss and pain abdomen at a later stage are also seen. 90% of all neoplasms can be felt digitally. Procto-sigmoidoscopy will always show the carcinoma. A histological examination will not only confirm the diagnosis but also stage it. A sphincter saving operation (anterior resection) is usually done for tumours of upper 2/3rd of the rectum. For tumours involving the lower 1/3rd of the rectum, a permanent colostomy (abdominoperineal excision) is often required.

4. Crohn's disease is an inflammatory GI condition characterized by transmural granulomatous inflammation. Mostly seen in the terminal ileum and proximal colon with skin lesions in between. Smoking increases the risk 3–4 folds. Patients present with abdominal pain, weight loss, diarrhoea, aphthous ulcers, abdominal tenderness, RIF mass and perianal abscesses or tags. Small intestinal obstruction or toxic dilatation can occur as complications. One must investigate by sigmoidoscopy, rectal biopsy and barium enema which may show cobble stoning, 'rose thorn' ulcers. Predni-solone is used for mild attacks. For severe attacks, patient needs to be admitted and given IV hydrocortisone $\pm$ metronidazole $\pm$ rectal hydrocortisone.

5. Proctalgia fugax is a disease characterized by attacks of severe idiopathic pain arising in the rectum. The pain is described as stabbing cramp-like. It often occurs when the patient is in bed at night. It seems to occur commonly in patients suffering from anxiety or undue stress and is also said to afflict young doctors! It is probably due to segmental cramp in the pubococcygeus muscle. It is unpleasant and incurable but fortunately harmless.

Theme 4: Contraception: Mechanism of action

1. Depot progesterone is given as an injectable contraceptive given intramuscularly. Two preparations are available: Depo-provera (medroxy progesterone acetate) and Noristerat (norethisterone enanthate). It acts by making cervical mucus thick and viscid, thus preventing sperm penetration and also by inhibiting ovulation. However, failure rate is higher than that for combined OCPs and there are chances of irregular bleeding and occasional amenorrhoea.

2. Chief mechanism of action of combined OCPs is inhibition of ovulation. Both oestrogen and progesterone act synergistically on the hypothalamo-pituitary axis and prevent the release of GnRH from the hypothalamus through a negative feedback mechanism. Thus, there is no peak release of FSH and LH from the anterior pituitary. So, follicular growth is either not initiated or if initiated, ovulation does not occur.

3. Levonorgestrel with or without ethinyl oestradiol is used as morning-after pill. It is to be initiated within 72 hours of unprotected intercourse. The earlier it is taken after unprotected intercourse, the fewer are the chances of pregnancy. The mechanism of action is not exactly known but it probably involves disruption of ovulation or corpus luteal function depending upon the time in the menstrual cycle when it is taken.

4. Vaginal sponge is made of synthetic polyurethane impregnated with non oxynol-9 as spermicide. It acts as a surfactant which either immobilises or kills the sperms. The sponge is inserted immediately before the coitus into the vagina to cover the cervix. It should not be removed for 6 hours after intercourse. The sponge is for single use only over a 24 hour period.

5. Mirena coil is an IUCD which carries levonorgestrel. IUCDs (Intra Uterine Contraceptive Devices) induce histological and biochemical changes in the endometrium by causing a non-specific inflammatory reaction. They also increase tubal motility, which results in quick migration of the fertilized ovum into the uterine cavity before the endometrium is receptive. Both these processes result in failure of implantation.

Theme 5: Cell of origin

1. Lipomas are fatty lumps, benign in nature. They are seen wherever fat can expand. They have smooth margins with slight flatulence.

2. Malignant astrocytomas, in adults, are found most frequently in cerebral hemispheres. They are rapidly growing and diffusely infiltrating. They commonly undergo necrosis. The most malignant forms are often designated glioblastoma multiforme.

3. Myeloma is a malignant proliferation of plasma cells with diffuse bone marrow infiltration and focal osteolytic lesions.

4. AML is a neoplastic proliferation of blast cells derived from marrow myeloid elements. Blast cells may be few in the peripheral blood, therefore the diagnosis depends on bone marrow biopsy.

5. Rhabdomyosarcoma is a soft tissue tumour which is very aggressive and responsive to chemotherapy. Rhabdomyosarcoma shows evidence of skeletal muscle fibres with cross-striations.

Theme 6: Cause of ascites

1. Malignant diseases causing ascites include secondary carcinomatosis, lymphomas, leukaemias and primary mesothelioma. Malignant ascites is usually treated with repeated paracentesis of small volumes of fluid. If the underlying malignancy is unresponsive to systemic therapy, peritoneovenous shunts may be inserted.

2. Diagnostic paracentesis (50–100 ml) should be a part of the routine evaluation of patients with ascites. Cloudy fluid with a predominance of polymorphonuclear cells and a positive Gram's stain are characteristic of bacterial peritonitis. Abdominal pain and tenderness may occur but cases often present with general malaise, fever, hypotension or hepatic encephalopathy.

3. A high protein (exudative i.e. > 25 gm/L) ascites is usually found with malignancy, tuberculosis, pancreatitis or myxoedema. The mention of 'immigrant from India' and 'loss of weight' are suggestive of tuberculous origin of ascites. The ascitic fluid in tuberculosis may be clear, turbid, haemorrhagic or chylous with WCC > 1000 in which > 70% are lymphocytes.

4. Ascites in cases of congestive cardiac failure is straw coloured with variable amount of protein content (15–53 gm/L). The WCC is < 1000 which is usually mononuclear.

5. The pathogenesis of ascites in cases of cirrhosis includes increased central sympathetic outflow, portal hypertension, hypoalbuminaemia and reduced plasma oncotic pressure. The serum albumin concentration, in cirrhosis, is usually at least 10 gm/L higher than that of ascitic fluid. The ascitic fluid is straw coloured or bile stained with protein content < 25 gm/L, WCC counts < 250 and are predominantly mesothelial cells.

Theme 7: Psychiatry: Management

1. The child in this case is a threat for himself and should be hospitalized and sedated.

2. This is a patient with schizophrenia. Schizophrenia is a common mental disorder which typically presents in adulthood with delusions, hallucinations and disordered thought. The 1st rank symptoms seen in ~70% of patients are (i) Thought insertion (as in this patient) (ii) Thought broadcast (iii) Thought withdrawal (iv) Passivity (v) Hearing voices commenting on the actions of the patients (vi) Primary delusions (vii) Somatic hallucinations. Such patients require psychiatric evaluation.

3. All patients with suicidal tendencies should be referred to a psychiatrist.

4. Although, the presentation is not typical, this looks like a case of delirium. The main feature in delirium is impaired consciousness with onset over hours to days. Patients may be disoriented, agitated, drowsy or quiet and unresponsive. Its causes include various drugs (e.g benzodiazepines, opiates), hypoglycaemia, alcohol withdrawal, trauma and surgery.

5. The presentation of the patient with ingestion of 8 aspirin tablets and a poor family history are suggestive of a suicide attempt. All patients who have attempted suicide or have suicidal tendencies should be referred to a psychiatrist.

Theme 8: Pain relief

1. Failure to thrive implies poor weight gain. Poverty is the main cause of failure to thrive in developing countries. In UK the cause may be difficulty at home, emotional deprivation, unskilled feeding, child abuse or simply an idiosyncratic growth pattern. This child may be suffering from simple otitis externa which can be due to local trauma. Considering the analgesic 'ladder', paracetamol should be first tried in the patient.

2. This seems to be a simple case of sprain in the ankle. This require rest, simple analgesia e.g. diclofenac with/without topical NSAIDs.

3. Prompt appendicectomy with metronidazole 1 gm 8 hourly and cefuroxime 1.5 gm 8 hourly 3 doses IV starting 1 hour pre-operatively is the standard management protocol in patients with appendicitis. Since patient is usually anorexic in such cases and is also kept nil orally before the surgery, a painkiller should be given by a parenteral route.

4. Prehospital management of patients with myocardial infarction includes aspirin 300 mg PO, analgesia e.g. morphine 5–10 mg IV with metoclopramide 10 mg IV. Sublingual GTN is also given unless the patient is hypotensive.

5. The analgesic ladder: 1st step–non-opioid – aspirin, paracetamol, NSAIDs; 2nd step– weak opioid– codeine, dihydrocodeine, dextropropoxyphene; 3rd step– strong opioid–morphine, diamorphine, hydromorphine with or without co-analgesics. As in this case step 1 has failed to provide relief to the patient to the extent that the pain is intolerable, step 3 needs to be considered.

6. Patients with herpes who develop herpetic neuralgia require oral analgesics or low dose amitriptyline for control of pain. Patients with post herpetic neuralgia may require carbamazepine, phenytoin or capsaicin cream.

Theme 9: Investigation in ophthalmic conditions

1. This is a patient of Giant cell arteritis. The typical patient will present with sudden painless loss of vision, malaise, jaw claudication and with tender scalp on temporal arteries. ESR > 40 is suggestive. Temporal artery biopsy report may be false positive in some cases and therefore is not a reliable investigation. Management includes oral prednisolone promptly as the other eye is at risk.

2. Amaurosis fugax implies transient loss of vision. Patients complain 'curtain descending over the eye'. It is usually seen in central retinal artery occlusion and giant cell arteritis and may lead to permanent loss of vision. Occlusion is often thrombo-embolic. Risk factors include diabetes, smoking, hyperlipidaemia, heart valve diseases, atherosclerosis. Carotid angiography is required to know the aetiology, site and extent of the occlusion.

3. Visual loss according to the site involved in the visual pathway
    i. Ipsilateral complete loss of vision– Optic nerve atrophy
    ii. Bitemporal hemianopia– central chiasma– Pituitary tumour
    iii. Binasal hemianopia– Lateral chiasma
    iv. Contralateral superior quadrantopia– Temporal lobe
    v. Contralateral inferior quadrantopia– Parietal lobe
    vi. Homonymous hemianopia–Optic tract or radiation, visual cortex or anterior occipital lobe involvement.

4. Acromegaly presents between 30–50 years. Patients have coarse oily skin, large tongue, prominent supraorbital ridge, prognathism, increase in shoe size, thick spade like hands, deep voice, arthralgia, proximal muscle weakness, parastheisae due to carpal tunnel syndrome, progressive heart failure, goitre and sleep apnoea in some. Investigations required are oral GTT, serum IGF–1 and MRI pituitary fossa. Trans-sphenoidal surgery is the treatment of choice. Dopamine agonists can be used as adjuncts.

Theme 10: Ear treatment

1. Furunculosis is an acutely painful staphylococcal abscess arising in a hair follicle. Diabetes is an important predisposing factor. Flucloxacillin is the drug of choice especially if there is cellulitis.
2. This is possibly a case of ruptured tympanic membrane due to syringing. All patients with ruptured tympanic membrane should be immediately referred to an ENT specialist.
3. Herpes zoster oticus is a viral infection involving geniculate ganglion of facial nerve. It is characterized by appearance of vesicles on the tympanic membrane, deep meatus, concha and retroauricular sulcus.
4. In serous otitis media, the middle fibrous layer of the tympanic membrane gets absorbed leaving a thin drumhead which easily gets collapsed with eustachian tube insufficiency. Such cases require tympanoplasty and must be referred to an ENT specialist.
5. Otitis media means inflammation in the middle ear. Acute otitis media presents with rapid onset of pain and fever, often after a viral URTI. Chronic otitis media is also known as serous or secretory otitis media or glue ear, which implies inflammation with middle ear fluid of several months duration. Treatment is with analgesics and appropriate antibiotics e.g. amoxicillin.

Theme 11: Pre-operative investigation

1. In some patients dramatic elevations of blood pressure occur when measurements are carried out by a doctor. Although there is no conclusive evidence but it is probable that average blood pressure measured by ambulatory monitoring are better predictors of cardiovascular status.
2. An ECG is generally required pre-operatively in all patients who are > 65 years of age or have poor exercise tolerance, or have history of myocardial ischaemia, hypertension, rheumatic fever or other heart disease. He seems to be a patient of unstable angina since the patient has had two attacks of angina in last one week. Such patients would require a complete cardiology work up and hence a cardiology opinion needs to be taken here.
3. A pre-operative CXR is required in all those patients with known cardiorespiratory disease, pathology or symptoms or if the patient is above 65 years of age.

Theme 12: Obstetrics and gynaecology: Treatment

1. Oestrogen not only helps in flushes and atrophic vaginitis, it also postpones menopausal bone loss. The patient in this case does not have osteoporosis but has a family history of osteoporosis therefore HRT is indicated. In this patient it has been clearly mentioned that the patient is 2 years post menopausal. Around 80% of the UK women at the age of 50 retain their uterus. In our patient also there is no mention of hysterectomy being done. She needs to have continuous or cyclic progestogen along with oestrogen given orally or via transdermal therapy. HRT also increases bone density in established osteoporosis and decreases fractures.

2. Prevention of osteoporosis requires exercise, calcium rich diet, HRT in post menopausal women and avoiding smoking and excess alcohol intake. Treatment of osteoporosis includes HRT in postmenopausal women, biphosphonates, vitamin D and calcium rich diet. The patient in this case has family history of osteoporosis therefore has increased risk of osteoporosis. Patient has lactose intolerance which suggests lack of milk products in diet and hence poor calcium intake. Therefore she must take calcium supplements.

3. Menopause problems are related to falling oestrogen levels. Atrophy of oestrogen dependent tissues such as genitalia and breasts take place. Vaginal dryness can lead to vaginal and urinary infections, dyspareunia, traumatic bleeding and stress incontinence. Both oral and vaginal oestrogens will help in vaginal dryness. In this case, it has been clearly mentioned that (i) she is postmenopausal (suggesting atrophic vaginitis) (ii) urine culture is negative i.e. UTI is excluded (iii) does not want systemic hormones. Therefore the only treatment left is with local vaginal oestrogen application.

4. Subcutaneous oestrogen implantation is restricted in UK to patients who have undergone hysterectomy with or without oophorectomy. It involves positioning of a pellet of oestradiol in the subcutaneous tissue, usually in the lower subcutaneous abdomen. Such implants are reviewed at 6 monthly intervals and are generally well tolerated. This mode of treatment successfully treats menopausal symptoms and also protects against bone loss.

Theme 13: Non accidental injury

1. This is probably a case of pathological fracture due to rickets. Lack of vitamin D or a disturbance of its metabolism in the growing skeleton is referred to as rickets. The causes of rickets can be broadly divided into nutritional, malabsorptive and renal. Since there are no pointers in the question to suggest malabsorption or renal cause, one should get a nutritional assessment done to help diagnose rickets.

2. Since the bruise has developed on simply holding the childs' hand, one should rule out coagulation disorders. Coagulation screen would be required in this case. Coagulation tests include prothrombin time, thrombin time and kaolin cephalin clotting time (KCCT or APTT i.e. PTT - partial thromboplastin time).

3. Failure to thrive implies poor weight gain. Poverty is the main cause in developing countries. In UK the main causes include difficulty at home, emotional deprivation or unskilled feeding. As the parents are unemployed in this case, family finances are the most likely cause for lack of growth in the child. Such children should be referred to the child care centre.

4. The presentation of the child is suggestive of either a foreign body in the vagina or a sexual assault. In both the cases the vaginal examination is required. Vaginal examination in a child is always done under GA.

5. A rise in intracranial pressure in paediatric age group can be due to meningo-encephalitis, head injury, subdural or extradural haemorrhage, hypoxia, ketoacidosis, Reye's syndrome or an intracranial tumour. The child may present with listlessness, irritability, drowsiness, headache, diplopia, tense fontanelles, decreased level of responsiveness, pupil changes (ipsilateral dilatation), rising BP and falling pulse (Cushing's reflex). CT scan of the head is required in such cases to find out the cause of increase in ICP.

Theme 14: Rheumatology diagnosis

1. Rheumatoid arthritis is a persistent, symmetrical, deforming arthropathy with peak onset in 5th decade and a M : F ratio of 3 : 1. Patients typically present with swollen painful and stiff hands and feet especially in the morning. Patients have sausage shaped fingers and MCP joint swellings which later become Boutonniere and swan neck deformities of the fingers. It is associated with carpal tunnel syndrome, keratoconjunctivitis sicca, osteoporosis and amyloidosis. Treatment is with exercise, physiotherapy, intralesional steroids and NSAIDs.

2. Patients with ankylosing spondylitis are typically young who present with morning stiffness, backache, sacroiliac pain, progressive loss of spinal movement i.e. spinal ankylosis, neck hyperextension and spino-cranial ankylosis. X-ray of the spine may shows 'bamboo' spine (i.e. squaring of the vertebrae), erosions of apophyseal joints and obliteration of sacroiliac joints. Treatment includes exercise for backache and NSAIDs for pain and stiffness.

3. Multiple myeloma is a neoplastic proliferation of plasma cell with diffuse bone marrow infiltration and focal osteolytic lesions. Peak age of incidence is 70 years, patients present with bone pain tenderness, pathological fractures, lassitude, pyogenic infection, amyloidosis, neuropathy, signs of hyperviscosity, decreased visual acuity and bleeding. Bence Jones protein may be detectable in urine. Bone radiographs show punched out lesions 'Pepper pot skull'. Treatment includes high fluid intake and melphalan as such or part of ABCM regimen (Adriamycin, Bleomycin, Cyclophosphamide, Melphalan). Biphosphonates are required if hypercalcaemia is present.

4. The patient in this case is suffering from gout. Points in favour of the diagnosis are (i) the

patient is on anti-hypertensive treatment (diuretics). It is a precipitating factor for the deposition of sodium monourate crystals in the joint and causes gout. (ii) The patient presents with pain and swelling of the joint which is hot to touch. These presentations are classically seen in the acute stage of gout.

5. Osteoarthritis is thrice as common in women as in men with mean age of onset as 50 years. Patients complain of pain on movement which is worse at the end of the day alongwith stiffness and joint instability. DIP, 1st MTP joints, cervical and lumbar spine are most commonly involved. Herberden's nodes, which are bony swellings at DIP joints may be seen. Radiographs show loss of joint space, subchondral sclerosis and cysts and marginal osteophytes. Treatment includes paracetamol for pain; if inadequate, NSAIDs may be tried. Joints replacement can be considered for end stage disease.

Theme 15: Relation to obesity

1. Weight reduction is the first step in the management of obstructive sleep apnoea syndrome which is characterized by intermittent closure or collapse of the pharyngeal airway which causes apnoeic episodes during sleep. The typical patient is a fat, middle aged man with complaints of snoring, daytime somnolence, morning headache or poor sleep quality.

2. Type II DM or NIDDM is seen in older age group patients especially who are obese. Obesity probably causes insulin resistance by the associated increased rate of release of non esterified fatty acids causing post receptor defects in insulin's action. The first step in the management of NIDDM is weight loss and exercise.

3. Weight loss and vitamin B deficiency are well known facts which occur due to alcoholism. Alcoholism can cause fatty liver, hepatitis, cirrhosis, Korsakoff's psychosis $\pm$ Wernicke's encephalopathy. Alcohol withdrawal with the help of benzodiazepines and multiple high potency vitamins given IM may reverse the effects caused due to alcoholism.

4. Cushing's disease is treated by selective removal of pituitary adenoma via a transsphenoidal or very rarely transfrontal approach. Cushing's disease is due to adrenal hyperplasia due to excess ACTH from pituitary tumour. 90% of pituitary causes are microadenomas. Cushing's disease is commoner in women with a peak age incidence at 30–50 years.

Theme: 16: Psychiatry: Diagnosis

1. The signs of alcohol withdrawal i.e. delirium tremens, include tachycardia, hypotension, tremors, seizures, visual or tactile hallucinations. The symptoms of nausea, sweating, mood changes, vomiting etc. usually appear within 6 hours of stopping alcohol. The symptoms fluctuate but peak on 3rd to 4th day of withdrawal and subside over a week. Such patients need to be admitted and given generous amounts (e.g. 10 mg 6 hourly) of diazepam in initial 3 days. Thereafter the doses are tapered off.

2. Post traumatic stress disorder is seen in patients after great psychological trauma e.g. rape, shipwreck, near death, crimes of passion etc. Patients may present with anxiety, depression, obsessive recall, compulsive guilt at one's own survival, alcohol abuse, irritability, bed wetting.

3. Flight of ideas is seen in patients with mania. Other features that may be present in patients with mania are grandiose delusions, increased need for sleep, increased sexual desire, spending sprees, euphoria, hyperactivity, increased appetite and disinhibition. Less severe states are termed hypomania. Sedation with chlorpromazine may be needed. Lithium carbonate has a prophylactic effect in prevention of recurrent mania.

4. This looks like a patient of paranoid schizophrenia. Delusions (false beliefs) are characteristic of paranoid thinking. Schizophrenia typically presents with delusions, hallucinations and disordered thought. Patients with chronic illness also show withdrawal, apathy, emotional blunting and slowness of thought. 1st rank symptoms in schizophrenia are: thought insertion, thought broadcasting, thought withdrawal, passivity, hearing voices commenting on actions, primary delusions and somatic hallucinations. Hospitalization may be required for patients who are a danger to themselves or others. Antipsychotics are used to treat acute symptoms.

Theme: 17: Surgery

1. Femoral hernias present as mass in the upper medial thigh or above the inguinal ligament where it points down the leg. They are seen more in women than in men. They are likely to be irreducible and often strangulate. The neck of the hernia can be felt below and lateral to the public tubercle.

2. 2–3% of neonates have maldescended testes. On cold days retractile testes may seem to hide in the inguinal pouch. Such testes may be 'milked down' in a warm bath or white squatting or with legs crossed. These retractile testes do not require surgery. Truly undescended testes lie in the path of descent from the abdominal cavity. Early orchidopexy (fixing testes within the scrotum) may prevent infertility and decreases the risk of neoplasia.

3. Hydrocele of canal of Nuck is a condition similar to encysted hydrocele of the cord. This condition occurs in females. The cyst lies in relation to the round ligament. Unlike a hydrocele of the cord, a hydrocele of the canal of Nuck is always at least partially present within the inguinal canal.

4. Richter's hernia is a hernia in which the sac contains only portion of the circumference of the intestine. Usually the small intestine is involved. It involves the bowel wall only and not the lumen. It may complicate femoral and rarely obturator hernias.

These 18: Trauma to an organ

1. Liver injury is perhaps indistinguishable from splenic injury but suggested by localising signs of pain, tenderness and rigidity in the right upper quadrant of the abdomen. Most of the problems of injury to liver are caused by haemorrhage, leakage of bile and devitalisation of liver tissue. The mention of hypotension in the patient is suggestive of intra-abdominal haemorrhage and is an indication for laparotomy.

2. The mode of injury in this case is suggestive of urethral injury. Rupture of the bulbar urethra is the most common urethral injury. Urethral rupture is most commonly at the junction of prostatic and membranous parts in males. The appearance of a drop of blood at the end of the urethra is suggestive of urethral rupture. The triad of signs of a ruptured bulbar urethra is retention of urine, perineal haematoma and bleeding from the external urinary meatus. Such patients requires a suprapubic catheterization as soon as possible and end-to-end reanastomosis of the ruptured urethra. CT scan is the image of choice in trauma patients presenting with haematuria. But an ascending urethrogram needs to be done to locate the site and extent of the rupture.

3. The presentation of the patient in the case is suggestive of a diaphragmatic rupture leading to herniation of stomach into the lung. The mechanism of diaphragmatic rupture is high-speed blunt trauma with a closed glottis. The rupture occurs much more commonly on the left hemidiaphragm. A contrast study will confirm the diagnosis. Thoracotomy should be performed in patients presenting acutely to repair the diaphragm, prevent respiratory embarrassment and to exclude an abdominal viscus injury.

4. In a blunt abdominal trauma, liver, spleen and kidneys are chiefly at risk of injury. In this patient, the site and presentation are suggestive of renal injury. In renal injury patient will have local loin pain and tenderness. Haematuria is the cardinal sign of a damaged kidney. An IVU should be obtained urgently to (a) assess the damage to the kidney (b) make sure that the other kidney is normal. Surgical exploration is necessary in less than 10% of the cases. Surgical exploration is indicated if either there are signs of progressive blood loss or there is an expanding mass in the loin.

These 19: Scientific basis in nephrology

1. Sarcoidosis is a multisystem granulomatous disorder. It commonly affects adults aged 20–40 years. Acute sarcoidosis presents with erythema nodosum and polyarthralgia. Pulmonary manifestations include bilateral hilar lymphadenopathy, fibrosis, pulmonary infiltrates, cough, dyspnoea and chest pain. Non-pulmonary manifestations include lymphadenopathy, hepatosplenomegaly, uveitis, Bell's palsy, neuropathy, SOL, subcutaneous nodules, cardiomyopathy, hypercalcaemia, hypercalciuria, renal stones and pituitary dysfunction. Bone X-rays show 'punched out' lesions in terminal phalanges. Indications for corticosteroid therapy include parenchymal lung disease, uveitis, hypercalcaemia and neurological or cardiac involvement. Prednisolone 40 mg/day PO for 4–6 weeks is given.

2. Papillary necrosis is a part of the spectrum of pathologies which fall under the term Analgesic Nephropathy. Initially the lesion is confined to the central part of the inner medulla and affects only the interstitial cells, thin ascending limb of Henle's loop and peritubular capillaries. Later necrosis of all medullary elements occur with partial or total papillary separation. Patients may present with proteinuria, haematuria, colic or obstruction giving rise to hydronephrosis or pyonephrosis. Infection in or around necrotic papillae may manifest as acute pyelonephritis or indolent urinary infection. Complete cessation of analgesic consumption is the only specific measure.

3. One of the risk factors for nephrolithiasis is dehydration. This case being a marathon runner, we suspect him to be having dehydration intermittently due to excessive sweating. Stones in the kidney cause loin pain and stones in the ureter cause renal colic. This pain classically radiates from the loin to the groin.

4. Recurrent urinary tract infection implies further infection with a new organism. Risk factors for recurrent urinary tract infection include obstruction and renal stones. Lower urinary tract infection commonly occurs in association with bladder outflow obstruction and may precipitate acute retention. Frequency, urgency, urge incontinence, dysuria, strangury, suprapubic pain, haematuria, and cloudy, smelly urine may be present. Urgent drainage is required if there is evidence of infection above an obstruction.

5. Another risk factor for nephrolithiasis is UTI as in this patient. Renal stones may further cause infection which may be acute or chronic or recurrent. It may present with cystitis, pyelonephritis or pyonephrosis. Antibiotics are required for such cases along with IV fluids and symptomatic treatment.

Theme 20: Investigation in seizure

1. Emergency EEG is done only if the convulsive status of the patient needs to be known. In this case, the patient present with an attack of grand mal epilepsy. Therefore emergency EEG is not required. CT scan of the head needs to be done to identify any intracranial cause of the seizure e.g. SOL, trauma, stroke or neurocysticercosis.
2. As the patient in this case is obese, probably there is an increased metabolism of the anticonvulsant. Therefore patient is having recurrent seizures. The drug dosage needs to be modified according to the serum drug levels so that therapeutic levels of the drug in the blood, can be achieved.
3. Seizure can be due to trauma, SOL, stroke, SLE, alcohol withdrawal, hypoglycaemia. hyperglycaemia, hypoxia, uraemia, hyponatraemia, hypernatraemia, hypocalcaemia, encephalitis, neurocysticercosis and HIV. Investigations required for patients presenting with seizures include U & E, LFT, blood sugar, serum calcium, phosphate, FBC, INR, toxicity screens, blood levels of medications, LP and CT scan. Out of the given options, CT scan is the answer which would help in identifying an intracranial cause of the seizure.

Theme: 21: Seizures: Diagnosis

1. Pseudoseizures or psychogenic seizures are nonepileptic behaviours that resemble seizures. The behaviour is often part of a conversion reaction precipitated by underlying psychological distress. Patients may present with side-to-side turning of the head, asymmetric and large amplitude shaking movements of the limbs, twitching of all limbs without loss of consciousness or pelvic thrusting.
2. This is a case of febrile convulsion. This condition is diagnosed if the following occur together: (a) a tonic/clonic, symmetrical seizure (b) occurring with rising temperature (c) age of child between 6 months and five years. (d) no signs of CNS infection or previous history of epilepsy (e) number of seizures < 3 and lasting < 5 min. Treatment involves giving diazepam at the time of attack. Otherwise tepid sponging or paracetamol syrup.
3. Petit mal or absences are a type of Generalized seizures. There are episodes of brief (<10 sec) pauses e.g. the patient stops talking in mid-sentence and then carries on where left off. It is generally seen in childhood. Ethosuximide with/without sodium valproate is used in the treatment.
4. Tonic clonic or classical grand mal are a type of generalized seizures. They are sudden in onset with loss of consciousness. The limbs initially stiffen (tonic phase) then jerk (clonic phase); although the patient may have either of the phase singly as well. Patients are drowsy after the attack. The tongue is usually bitten at the onset of the seizure. Sodium valproate is the first line drug therapy; carbamazepine is an alternative.

Theme 22: Investigation in haematuria

1. Acute nephritis presents with haematuria and oliguria. β haemolytic streptococcus is usually the cause. A sore throat around 2 weeks before is very suggestive of the aetiology. Patients may also have fever, hypertension. oedema or loin pain. Antistreptolysin 'O' titres are helpful in the diagnosis. Treatment includes restriction of protein if oliguric, penicillin for streptococcal infection and nitroprusside for encephalopathy.

2. Adult polycystic kidney disease is an autosomal dominant condition with genes on chromosomes 16 & 4. Patients present with renal enlargement with cysts, abdominal pain, haematuria, UTI, renal calculi, hypertension or renal failure. An abdominal USG is sufficient to diagnose.

3. The hallmark of renal lesion in diabetic nephropathy is a particular form of glomerulosclerosis which is associated with arteriolar hyalinosis and interstitial fibrosis. Albuminuria is the first clinical manifestation. Then blood pressure rises and renal failure ensues after a median interval of 10–20 years. Urinary albumin levels are measured. If albuminuria is high, an attempt to lower the blood pressure by ACE inhibitors should be made. If dipstick is positive for protein, 24 hours urinary creatinine clearance should be measured. Endogenous creatinine clearance is helpful in estimating the glomerular filtration rate. Pitting oedema in this patient is suggestive of decreased oncotic pressure due to albuminuria. Therefore creatinine clearance needs to be quantified.

Theme: 23: Psychiatry: Diagnosis

1. In clinical depression, low mood occurs with sleep difficulty, change in appetite, hopelessness, pessimism and suicidal thoughts. Patients with major depression may present with anhedonia, poor appetite, weight loss, early waking, psychomotor retardation/ agitation, decrease in sexual drive, decrease ability to concentrate, feeling of worthlessness, inappropriate guilt with recurrent thoughts of suicide. Treatment has to be multipronged with psychological cognitive therapy, antidepressants or even ECT.

2. This is a patient of schizophrenia presenting with thought broadcasting. Schizophrenia is a common mental disorder which typically presents in adulthood with delusions, hallucinations and disordered thought. The 1st rank symptoms seen in ~70% of patients are (i) Thought insertion (as in this patient) (ii) Thought broadcast (iii) Thought withdrawal (iv) Passivity (v) Hearing voices commenting on the actions of the patients (vi) Primary delusions (vii) Somatic hallucinations.

3. This is a patient presenting with flight of ideas with is usually seen in mania. Other features that may be present in patients with mania are delusions, decreased need for sleep, increased sexual desire, spending sprees, euphoria, hyperactivity, increased appetite and disinhibition.

4. Chronic fatigue syndrome is a severe disabling fatigue for more than 6 months. In such patients investigations and examinations fail to reveal any abnormality. Diagnosis of chronic fatigue syndrome is made in such a setting if 4 or more of the following criteria are met (i) impaired memory or concentration not related to alcohol or drugs (ii) unexplained muscle pain (iii) polyarthralgia (iv) unrefreshing sleep (v) post-exertional malaise for > 1 day (vi) persisting sore throat not caused by glandular

fever (vii) unexplained tender cervical or axillary lymph nodes. There is no specific treatment for this condition.

Theme: 24. Prevention of respiratory asthma

1. In the BTS guidelines for treatment of asthma in children above 5 years of age, the 1st guideline is to avoid provoking factors. Since smoke is the allergen causing asthma in this case, it should be avoided.
2. Pollens are the possible causative agents in this case which trigger recurrent attacks of asthma. Hence they should be avoided.
3. Animals' fur can also trigger attacks of asthma. The presentation of such attacks during holidays when her brother rears rabbits is suggestive of the same. Hence the child should avoid pets.

Theme: 25: Loss of consciousness

1. Following points favour the diagnosis of sub-dural haematoma : (i) more common in elderly as brain shrinkage makes bridging veins more vulnerable (ii) mostly results due to trauma which may have been mild e.g. recurrent falls (iii) presents with fluctuating level of cons-ciousness. CT Scan of the head shows a con-cave or crescent shaped hyperdense clot with or without midline shift. Treatment is with evacuation via burr holes.

2. This is a patient of stroke due to intracerebral haemorrhage. The cause for CNS bleed in this patient is hypertension which is chronic and uncontrolled. Strokes result from ischaemic infarction or bleeding in brain manifested by acute focal CNS signs and symptoms. Stroke may be due to thrombosis in situ, athero-thromboembolism, heart emboli, aneurysmal rupture or trauma. Patients may present with features depending upon the affected site.

3. Out of the given options, meningitis fits as a diagnosis in this scenario of fever with rash. In fact it suggests meningococcal meningitis. Patients with meningitis may present with stiff neck, photophobia, positive Kernig's sign, positive Brudzinski's sign and opisthotonus. Lumbar puncture should be immediately done, unless patient has focal signs, DIC, purpura or impending brain herniation. As we are sus-pecting meningococcal meningitis, Benzyl-penicillin 50 mg/kg/4 hourly should be given intravenously.

4. The mention of diabetes in the case is sug-gestive of hypoglycaemia as the cause of loss of consciousness.

   Hypoglycaemia is the commonest endocrine emergency. Plasma glucose level < 2.5 mmol/L implies hypoglycaemia.

   Symptoms are either

   • Autonomic (sweating, hunger, tremors) or
   • Neuroglycopenic (drowsiness, personality changes, fits).

   Hypoglycaemia is of two types:

   i. Fasting hypoglycaemia– The most common cause is insulin or sulfonylurea treatment in a known diabetic.

   ii. Post-prandial hypoglycaemia which is seen particularly after gastric surgery (dumping).

   Treatment is with oral sugar and a long acting starch. If the patient is in coma, IV glucose or glucagon SC is given.

5. The mention of installing a fire place in his room is suggestive of carbon monoxide poi-soning. Despite hypoxaemia the skin of the patients remains pink as carboxyhaemoglobin (COHb) displaces O_2 from haemoglobin binding sites. Patients present with headache, vomiting and tachycardia. If COHb levels are > 50%, patients may have seizures, coma and cardiac arrest. Patients should be removed from the source, given 100% O_2. Mannitol IV infusion is required in patients with cerebral oedema.

6. Spontaneous bleeding into the subarachnoid space is mostly due to rupture of saccular aneurysms. Patients are typically aged between 35–65 years. Subarachnoid haemorrhage is associated with smoking, hypertension, alcohol misuse, bleeding disorder and mycotic aneurysms post SBE or post IE. Patients present with devastating headache often occipital, vomiting, collapse and coma. Neck stiffness (Kernig's sign positive) takes around 6 hours to develop. CT scan of the head shows subarachnoid or ventricular blood. The CSF is xanthochromic (yellow) after a few hours. Treatment requires control of hypertension, analgesics for headache and surgery to clip the aneurysm to prevent rebleeds.

Theme: 26: Urinary system

1. Retention of urine can be seen after any operation especially after those on the anal canal and perineal region. Retention of urine is so common after operations on the pelvic viscera (sometimes due to damage to pelvic autonomic plexus) that it is usual to forestall it by catheterising the patients before or at the conclusions of the operation. Patients with retention should be reassured and provided privacy. Making the patients sit on the edge of the bed, sound of running water and a warm bath, all can be helpful.

2. This is a case of traumatic crush injury in which acute renal failure is commonly seen. Both rhabdomyolysis and haemolysis can cause ARF. Moreover myoglobin and haemoglobin released from muscle cells cause ARF via toxic effects on tubule epithelial cells. In such major injuries, hypovolaemia and acidosis may further contribute to the pathogenesis of ARF. Such patients need to be catheterized to assess hourly urine output. Once catheterized the cause should be treated and fluid loss rectified.

3. Urethral rupture is most commonly at the junction of prostatic and membranous parts in males. The appearance of a drop of blood at the end of the urethra is suggestive of urethral rupture. The triad of signs of a ruptured bulbar urethra is retention of urine, perineal haematoma and bleeding from the external urinary meatus. Such patients requires a suprapubic catheterization as soon as possible and end-to-end reanastomosis of the ruptured urethra CT scan is the image of choice in trauma patients presenting with haematuria. But an ascending urethrogram needs to be done to locate the site and extent of the rupture.

4. Transitional cell carcinomas may arise in the bladder, ureter or renal pelvis. They usually present after 40 years of age. Male: Female ratio is 4:1. Smoking, cyclophosphamide, phenacetin, azodyes, β naphthalene, schistosomiasis are known risk factors. Patients present with painless haematuria, frequency, urgency, dysuria or obstruction. Cystoscopy with biopsy is diagnostic.

Theme 27: Trauma management

1. The site of injury is suggestive of a cut in the radial or possibly ulnar vessels. External pressure over the site and elevation of the part should control bleeding. Formal surgical repair can be undertaken later. One should not use tourniquet as it may augment ischaemic damage.

2. All patients of trauma should be initially assessed and managed by the 'ABC' protocol.
   i. Airway: Protect cervical spine if injury possible. Check any signs of obstruction, ascertain or establish patency.
   ii. Breathing: determine respiratory rate, check bilateral chest movement, percuss and auscultate. Treat as arrest, intubate and ventilate if no respiratory effort. High concentration O_2 is given if breathing is compromised.
   iii. Circulation: pulse and BP should be checked. Evidence of haemorrhage should be looked for. Patient should be treated as for arrest, if no cardiac output.
   The mention of noisy breathing in this patient suggests airway obstruction. Patency should be established but since the neck is immobilized and it cannot be extended, patient should be intubated and ventilated to prevent aspiration.

3. The patient in this case is in a condition of shock due to blood loss. The mention of swollen thigh is suggestive of fracture of femur. Simple femoral fractures can cause bleeding into the thigh often in excess of a litre in adults. This child would immediately require a vascular access and blood transfusion.

4. The presentation of the child in this case is suggestive of injury to her radial or possibly ulnar artery. The signs, pallor and tachycardia are suggestive of shock due to blood loss. This patient would also require an immediate vascular access and blood transfusion.

5. The boy has an oxygen mask and is talking, suggests that his airway and breathing have already been taken care of. GMC is probably trying to impress upon the severity of the accident, by mentioning the death of a person involved in the same accident. The signs, pallor and tachycardia are suggestive of shock which might be due to blood loss. This boy would require an immediate vascular access and blood transfusion.

Theme: 28: Infection diagnosis

1. The presentation of the boy with complains of haemoptysis, cough and fever are suggestive of tuberculosis. The boy is from Somalia, which is endemic for tuberculosis, further supports the diagnosis. Tuberculosis is a chronic granulomatous disease of humans caused by a group of closely related obligate pathogens, the mycobacterium tuberculosis complex. In clinical specimens, the tubercle bacilli occur in small clumps and in early cultures they appear as rope-like microcolonies termed 'serpentine cords'. In all suspected cases, the relevant clinical samples e.g. sputum, pleural fluid, pleura, urine, pus, ascites, peritoneum or CSF, should be obtained for culture, to establish the diagnosis. Auramine or Ziehl–Nielsen (ZN) staining reveal acid fast bacilli. Radiography shows consolidation, cavitation, fibrosis and calcification. Immunological tests include tuberculin skin test, Mantoux test, Heaf and Tine tests. Initial phase of the treatment includes 8 weeks of administration of rifampicin, isoniazid, pyrazinamide, ethambutol or streptomycin. Continuation phase requires 2 drugs administered for 4 months viz. rifampicin and isoniazid.

2. Lymphomas are malignant proliferation of lymphocytes. They are histologically divided into Hodgkins and Non Hodgkins lymphomas. In both the types, patients present with fever, malaise, lymphadenopathy, weight loss and night sweats. Rarely alcohol induced pain may also be noted. Reed–Sternberg cells are characteristically seen in Hodgkin lymphoma. Lymph node biopsy is diagnostic. Radiotherapy and/or chemotherapy are the mainstay of the treatment.

3. Brucellosis is a Zoonosis common in Middle–east and typically affects the farmers or vets. It may present as fever, sweats, malaise, anorexia, vomiting, weight loss, hepatospleno-megaly, diarrhoea, backache, rash, orchitis or myalgia. Diagnosis is by blood culture and serology. Treatment is by Doxycycline and streptomycin.

4. The presentation of this patient with fever with chills and rigors and splenomegaly are suggestive of malaria. The mention of seizures in this case points towards cerebral malaria which is a complication seen in plasmodium falciparum infection. Diagnosis requires serial thin and thick blood films which are taken at the time of fever. Thick films help in rapid detection of malarial parasites, while thin films helps in identification of the plasmodium subtype. Treatment is with Quinine, Tetracycline or Doxycycline or Clindamycin.

5. Lyme disease is a tick borne infection caused by Borrelia burgdorferi. The patient will invariably give a history of travel to the forest. It presents as erythema chronicum migrans, arthralgia, malaise, myocarditis, heart block, meningitis, ataxia, amnesia and neuropathy. Diagnosis is by clinical signs, symptoms and serology. Treatment is by Doxycycline. To avoid getting the disease, the limbs should be properly covered and insect repellants used.

Theme: 29: Dyspepsia

1. Acid suppression is required in all patients of dyspepsia. Drugs used for acid suppression include H2-receptor antagonists such as cimetidine and ranitidine. Cimetidine is given as 800 mg PO for 8 weeks and ranitidine as 300 mg PO for 8 weeks. If these drugs fail to suppress the acid formation, proton-pump inhibitors e.g. lansoprazole 30 mg/day PO is given for 4 weeks (for duodenal ulcers) or 8 weeks (for gastric ulcers).

2. Endoscopy is advised in patients of dyspepsia if there are 'alarm' symptoms e.g. > 45 years of age, weight loss, vomiting, haematemesis, anaemia and dysphagia. Moreover endoscopy should be done if despite conservative treatment with antacids, symptoms recur and *H. pylori* status is found to be negative.

3. Gastro oesophageal reflux and dyspeptic symptoms are reported by a large number of women throughout pregnancy. Antacids containing calcium, magnesium or aluminium may be useful and are considered safe. Studies on H_2 blockers and proton pump inhibitors are either inadequate or have shown some adverse effects over animal embryos.

4. Barrett's oesophagus is seen due to chronic reflux oesophagitis in which squamous mucosa shows metaplastic change. The risk of adenocarcinoma increases 40 folds. Therefore regular endoscopy and biopsy are required for early diagnosis of the malignancy. Its treatment requires intensive antireflux measures including long term proton pump inhibitors.

5. Helicobacter pylori is present in ~ 90% of cases of duodenal ulcers and ~ 80% of cases of gastric ulcers. Gastric MALT (Mucosa associated lymphoid tissue) is also associated with *H. pylori*. It is also associated with carcinoma stomach and Ménétrier's disease. Its treatment for complete eradication include Triple therapy i.e. Lansoprazole + Clarithromycin + Amoxicillin (or Metronidazole) all for a period of 1 week.

Theme: 30: Prenatal screening

1. Duchenne's muscular dystrophy, presents in boys between 1–6 years of age. They have waddling, clumsy gait. Selective washing causes calf pseudohypertrophy. Later wheelchairs are needed. Aim is to keep the boy walking with the help of knee–ankle–foot orthoses. Creatine kinase is raised and muscle biopsy shows abnormal fibres surrounded by the fat and fibrous tissue. Spinal fixation with Luque operation or bracing helps scoliosis. But there is no specific treatment and genetic counselling is important.

2. Spina bifida which implies an incomplete vertebral arch is a myelodysplasia (neural tube defect). Babies born with spina bifida often have a small skin covered lesion (a meningocoele). A maternal serum α fetoprotein level of > 90 U/ml at 18 weeks detects almost 80% of open spina bifidas. In mothers who already have an affected baby, folic acid 5 mg/day should be given before conception (as the neural tube is formed by 4 weeks, i.e. before pregnancy may even be recognized). If there is no past history of neural tube defects, 0.4 mg of folic acid is recommended before conception to 13 weeks after. Many surgeries may be needed to rectify spina bifida.

3. Down's syndrome is a genetic disorder caused due to non disjunction leading to trisomy of chromosome 21. Maternal serum AFP, unconjugated oestriol and total human chorionic gonadotropin are assessed (the 'Triple test') in relation to maternal age, weight and gestation to estimate the risk of Down's syndrome. In an affected pregnancy, level of AFP and unconjugated oestriol tend to be low while that of HCG is high. A child with Down's syndrome will have a flat facial profile, abundant neck skin, dysplastic ears, muscle hypotonia, dysplastic pelvis (evident on X-rays), round head, protuding tongue, Brushfield's spots,

short broad hands with single palmar crease, widely spaced 1st and 2nd toes a high arched palate. Patients with Down's syndrome are associated with duodenal atresia, VSD, patent ductus, ASD, low IQ and a small stature.

4. As explained in the second question.
5. Cystic fibrosis is an autosomal recessive condition caused by mutation in cystic fibrosis transmembrane conductance regulator (CFTR) gene on chromosome 7. It leads to defective chloride secretion and increased sodium absorption across the epithelium. The changes in the composition of airway surface liquid predisposes the lung to chronic pulmonary infections and bronchiectasis. At present prenatal diagnosis is offered only to parents who are known carriers, usually because they have an affected child already. Screening can be done using fetal DNA from amniotic fluid cells or from chorionic villous sampling. Clinical features include failure to thrive, meconium ileus in neonates, cough, wheeze, recurrent chest infections, bronchiectasis, haemoptysis, respiratory failure, pancreatic insufficiency (diabetes mellitus, steatorrhoea), distal intestinal obstruction, gallstones, cirrhosis, sinusitis, nasal polyps, male infertility, etc.

Sweat test is positive in cystic fibrosis; Na > 60 mmol/L and sweat Cl >70 mmol/L on two occasions. Management is symptomatic.

Theme: 31: Causes of bleeding following delivery

1. Around 70% of uterine ruptures in UK are due to dehiscence of previous caesarean section scars. Other risk factors include obstructed labour in multiparous, oxytocin infusion, pervious cervical surgery, high forceps delivery, internal version and breech extraction. Postpartum indicators of uterine rupture are continuous PPH with a well-contracted uterus, if bleeding continuous postpartum after cervical repair and presence of shock. Treatment is with high flow O_2, blood transfusion and surgical repair (for small rupture) or hysterectomy.

2. Primary postpartum haemorrhage is blood loss of greater than 500 ml in the first 24 hours after delivery. Uterine atony is the cause in 90% of the cases. Factors predisposing to poor uterine contractions include past history of atony with PPH, retained placenta, ether or halothane anaesthesia, large placental site (e.g. twins, large baby), low placenta, over distended uterus, abruption, uterine malformations, fibroids, prolonged labour and older mothers. Treatment includes oxytocin IV, high flow O_2 and haemaccel or blood transfusion.

3. As explained above

4. Episiotomy is performed not only to prevent third degree perineal tears but also to hasten birth of a distressed baby, for instrumental or breech delivery and to protect a premature head. Perineal tears are classified by the degree of the damage caused. Tears are more likely to occur with big babies, precipitant labour, babies with poorly flexed heads, shoulder dystocia, when forceps are used or if the suprapubic arch is narrow. First degree tears do not involve muscle. Second degree tears involve perineal muscles. Third degree tears can extend into the rectum. The lady in

question must have had vaginal laceration and perineal tear during the delivery.

5. Disseminated intravascular coagulation in pregnancy is always secondary to stimulation of coagulation by procoagulant substance release in the maternal circulation. Known triggers include retention of a dead fetus, pre-eclampsia, placental abruption, endotoxic shock, amniotic fluid embolism, placenta acc-reta, H. mole, acute fatty liver of pregnancy. Thromboplastins are released into the circulation, fibrin and platelets are consumed. Management involves giving O_2 at 15 L/min, blood transfusion, fresh frozen plasma transfusion and/or platelet transfusion.

Theme: 32: Treatment of conjunctivitis

1. The conjunctiva is red and inflamed in conjunctivitis. It is usually bilateral. Eyes may itch, burn and lacrimate. Photophobia and purulent discharge may be present. Conjunctivitis may be viral, bacterial or allergic. For allergic conjunctivitis antihistamine drops or sodium cromoglycate drops help.

2. Ophthalmia neonatorum implies purulent discharge from the eye of a neonate < 21 days old. It is mostly due to Neisseria gonorrhoea but chlamydiae, herpes virus, staphylococci, streptococci, pneumococci and *E. coli* can also cause ophthalmia neonatorum. Chloram-phenicol 0.5% eye drops are given within 1 hour of birth in cases of gonococcal infections.

3. Trachoma is caused due to chlamydia tracho-matis. It mainly spreads by flies especially in hot, dry and dusty climates. Patients may present with lacrimation, intense erythema, follicles underneath both lids, pannus, corneal ulceration and entropion. Tetracycline 1% eye ointment and 500 mg/24 hours PO for 10 days is the treatment of choice.

4. Reiter's syndrome encompasses a triad of urethritis, conjunctivitis and seronegative arthritis. Patients may have iritis, keratoderma blenorrhagica, mouth ulcers, circinate balanitis, plantar fascitis. Neutrophils and macrophages containing neutrophils (Peking cells) can be seen in the synovial fluid. Treatment is with rest, splinting the affected joints and NSAIDs.

Theme 33: Diagnosis of arrhythmia

1. This is a case of late malignant ventricular arrhythmia. They occur 1–3 weeks post MI. Hypokalaemia, hypoxia and acidosis predispose to such complications. Avoid hypokalaemia which is the most easily avoidable cause. Large MIs should have a holter monitoring before discharge.

2. Supraventricular tachycardia is a narrow complex tachycardia with an ECG rate of > 100 beats per minute and QRS complex of duration > 120 milliseconds. P waves are either absent or inverted after the QRS complex. Vagal manoeuvres (carotid sinus massage, Valsalva manoeuvre) transiently increase AV block and may unmask an underlying atrial rhythm. If this fails adenosine 3 mg bolus is given. If that also fails, verapamil 5 mg IV over 2 min is given. DC cardioversion if nothing helps. Maintenance therapy consists of β blockers or verapamil.

3. As explained above.

4. Wenckebach block implies mobitz type 1 second-degree AV block. It is characterized by progressive PR interval prolongation prior to block of an atrial impulse. This type of block can also be observed in normal individuals with heightened vagal tone. Although it can progress to complete heart block, this is uncommon, except in the setting of acute inferior wall myocardial infarction.

Theme 34: Dementia: Diagnosis

1. Huntington's chorea is an autosomal dominant condition with full penetrance. It is usually seen in middle aged individuals. Signs are progressive in patients: Chorea→ irritability →dementia with or without seizures→death. It is due to too few corpus striatum GABA-nergic and cholinergic neurons. The life span of these patients is much shorter. No treatment can prevent progression. Counselling of the patient and the family should be done.

2. Alzheimer's dementia is the most common form of dementia in UK. Suspect AD in any enduring, acquired deficit of memory and cognition. Onset may be from 40 years though it may be seen earlier in patients suffering from Down's syndrome. On histological examination plaques with neurofibrillary tangles and cortical β-amyloid protein are found. On MRI an increased cortical atrophy in the medial temporal lobe can be seen. In stage I of AD there is falling memory and spatial disorientation. In stage II the personality disintegrates and in stage III the patient is apathetic, wasted and bedridden.

3. This is a case of multi infarct or vascular dementia in which hypertension is a risk factor. Such patients are characterized by psychomotor slowing, reduced attention, loss of executive function and personality changes.

4. Frontotemporal dementia is characterized by atrophy of frontal and temporal lobes. There are no features of Alzheimer's pathology. Patients present with early change in personality with disinhibition, hyperorality, stereotyped behaviour and emotional apathy. Spatial orientation is preserved.

Theme 35: Diagnosis of skin conditions

1. Neurofibromatoses are autosomal dominant conditions. Type 1 neurofibromatosis i.e. von Recklinghausen's disease is characterized by cafe-au-lait spots (flat coffee coloured skin patches), freckles in axillae, groin and neck base. Dermal neurofibromatosis implies small violaceous nodules appearing at puberty. Nodular neurofibromas arise from nerve trunks. Lisch nodules which are hamartomas on the iris are also seen in Type 1 neurofibromatosis.

   Type 2 neurofibromatosis are associated with bilateral vestibular schwannomas (acoustic neuromas). Cafe-au-lait spots are fewer. Juvenile posterior subcapsular lenticular opacity develops before other manifestations.

2. The typical physical findings in liver disease include icterus, hepatomegaly, hepatic tenderness, splenomegaly, spider naevi, palmar erythema and excoriations. Spider naevi can be seen both in acute and chronic liver diseases. They are especially prominent in patients with cirrhosis. Spider naevi are superficial, tortuous arterioles filling from the centre outwards. They occur only on arms, face and upper trunk. They may be difficult to defect in dark-skinned individuals.

3. Reactivation of the primary infection causes shingles. Patients present with pain in a dermatomal distribution which precedes malaise and fever. Some days later macules, papules and vesicles develops in the same dermatome. Thoracic and ophthalmic dermatomes are the most vulnerable. Rising antibody titres and culture or electron microscopy of the vesicle fluid confirms the diagnosis. Indications for aciclovir therapy include ophthalmic involvement, motor involvement, age > 50 years and immunocompromised status.

4. Out of the given options, meningitis fits as a diagnosis in this scenario of fever with rash. In fact it suggests meningococcal meningitis. Patients with meningitis may present with stiff neck, photophobia, positive Kernig's sign, positive Brudzinski's sign and opisthotonus. Lumbar puncture should be immediately done, unless patient has focal signs, DIC, purpura or impending brain herniation. As we are suspecting meningococcal meningitis, Benzylpencillin 50 mg/kg/4 hourly should be given intravenously.

5. Erythema nodosum implies painful, red, raised lesions on shins (may or may not be present on thighs or arms). They are seen in sarcoidosis, streptococcal infections, TB, leprosy, sulfonamide use, Pill use, dapsone therapy, Crohn's disease, UC, BCG vaccination and leptospirosis.

Theme 36: Diagnosis of skin conditions

1. Nappy rash can be due to various reasons. A red, desquamating rash, sparing the skin folds is due to moisture retention and not due to ammonia. It requires frequent changes of nappy, careful drying, emollient cream application and most importantly local hygiene. Candida is isolatable from almost half of all cases of nappy rash.

2. Psoriasis is a chronic inflammatory skin disorder. Patients have symmetrical well defined red plaques with silvery scales on extensor aspects of elbows, knees, scalp and sacrum. Nails show pitting, oncholysis, thickening and subungal hyperkeratosis. Guttate (small plaque) psoriasis is seen in the young especially if associated with concurrent streptococcal infection. Kobner phenomenon, Auspitz sign, pepper pot nail pitting and 'grease-spots' can also be seen. Treatment is by removing possible triggers, topical tar, dithanol, calcipotriol and tacalcitol application.

3. Impetigo is a common superficial bacterial infection of the skin caused by group A β-haemolytic streptococci or staphylococcus aureus. The primary lesion is a superficial pustule that ruptures and forms a characteristic yellow-brown honey-coloured crust. Bullous impetigo implies lesions caused by staphylococcus which may be tense, clear bullae. Ecthyma is a variant of impetigo that generally occurs in the lower extremities and cause punched out ulcerative lesions. Treatment involves gentle debridement of adherent crusts, in conjunction with oral antibiotics.

4. Haemangiomas are primarily composed of capillaries and are characterized by endothelial cell proliferation. These may be either superficial (strawberry) or deep (cavernous). The natural course of haemangiomas includes proliferative and involutional phases that result in complete and spontaneous regression in most cases. The lesions proliferate in the first 6 months of life. Involution starts after 1 year of age with complete resolution in 90% cases by 9 years of age. Most haemangiomas do not require any treatment. Steroids can be given in extensive disfiguring lesions. Most promising treatment is with the use of laser.

Theme 37: Diagnosis of hearing loss

1. Ménière's disease is a condition in which there is dilatation of the endolymphatic space of the membranous labyrinth causing vertigo with prostation, nausea, vomiting, tinnitus with/without progressive sensorineural hearing loss. Treatment of acute vertigo requires cyclizine. Surgical decompression of the endolymphatic sac may relieve vertigo, prevent progress of disease and conserve hearing.

2. The presentation of unilateral conductive deafness associated with poor hygiene is almost diagnostic of wax impaction. Its treatment would include softening the wax with oil drops daily for a week and then syringing the ear or suction with the help of a microscope.

3. Acoustic neuromas are slow growing, benign lesions that behave as an SOL. Also known as Vestibular Schwanomma, they cause ipsilateral tinnitus ± sensorineural deafness by compressing the cochlear nerve. Giddiness is also common Trigeminal nerve compression may cause tingling and numbness on one side of the face, as in this case. MRI is the best investigation but CT can also show enlargement or erosion of the internal auditory meatus. Surgical treatment is difficult.

4. Presbyacusis i.e. senile deafness is loss of acuity for high-frequency sounds. The condition starts before 30 years of age and progresses with age. Deafness is gradual in onset and is usually not noticed until the speech is affected. Hearing is most affected in the presence of background noise. Hearing aids are advised to such patients.

5. Otosclerosis is an autosomal dominant hereditary disorder with incomplete penetration. Half of the patients have a family history of the disease. In this condition the vascular spongy bone replaces the normal lamellar bone of otic capsule origin especially around the oral window which fixes the stapes foot plate.

Symptoms are usually seen in adulthood and are exacerbated due to pregnancy, menstruation and menopause. Hearing is often better with background noise. Surgical treatment involves stapedectomy or stapedotomy.

Theme 38: Investigation of swollen joints

1. This is a patient of rheumatoid arthritis. Rheumatoid factor is negative at the beginning but becomes positive in 80% of cases. Rheumatoid arthritis is a persistent, symmetrical, deforming arthropathy with peak onset in 5th decade and a M : F ratio of 3 : 1. Patients typically present with swollen painful and stiff hands and feet especially in the morning. Patients have sausage shaped fingers and MCP joint swellings which later become Boutonniere and swan neck deformities of the fingers. It is associated with carpal tunnel syndrome, keratoconjunctivitis sicca, osteoporosis and amyloidosis. Treatment is with exercise, physiotherapy, intralesional steroids and NSAIDs.

2. Septic arthritis should be considered if the patient appears ill and the presentation is of sudden onset. Features may be masked in immunocompromised patients or in patients with underlying joint disease. Aspirate the joint and look for pus (culture and gram stain). Sepsis may completely destroy a joint within 24 hours of onset. WBCs in the aspirate are suggestive of sepsis but not diagnostic. If septic arthritis is suspected, flucloxacillin and benzypenicillin should be administered until sensitivities are known.

3. ESR is a nonspecific indicator of the presence of disease. ESR rises with age and anaemia. An increased ESR is seen in myeloma, giant cell arteritis, rheumatoid arthritis, renal disease, sarcoidosis, abdominal aneurysm, metastatic prostatic carcinoma, leukaemia, lymphoma and infections.
Note: ESR is lowered in polycythaemia, sickle cell anaemia and cryoglobulinaemia.

4. This patient is suffering from pseudogout. Joint should be aspirated and looked for pyrophosphate crystals. Joint crystals are weakly positive birefringent in plane polarized light. Pseudogout is less severe and longer acting than gout. It affects different joints but mainly affects knees. Old age, dehydration, intercurrent illness, hyperparathyroidism, myxoedema, haemochromatosis, acromegaly, hypophosphataemia and hypomagnesaemia are associated risk factors. Treatment is symptomatic with NSAIDs.

5. The patient in this case is suffering from gout. Joint should be aspirated and looked for urate crystals. Points in favour of the diagnosis are (i) the patient is a hypertensive and must be on some antihypertensive. Diuretics may be the antihypertensive used, which is a precipitating factor for the deposition of sodium monourate crystals in the joint, (ii) the patient presents with pain and swelling of the knee joint which may be seen in the acute stage of gout.

Theme 39: Diagnosis of rectal bleeding.

1. Angiodysplasia is a vascular malformation which is associated with ageing. Angiodysplasias occur particularly in the ascending colon and caecum of elderly patients over 60 years of age. The malformations consist of dilated tortuous submucosal veins. Inspection of the mucosa is unremarkable. Bleeding is usually chronic and intermittent. There is an association with aortic stenosis (which can present as angina, dyspnoea, heaving apex beat). Colonoscopy may show the characteristic lesion in the caecum or ascending colon. Superior and inferior mesenteric angiography shows the site and extent of the lesion. To localize and confirm the source of haemorrhage, ^{99m}Tc labelled red cells are used.

2. Ulcerative colitis is an inflammatory disorder of the colonic mucosa and it never spreads proximal to the ileocaecal valve. It is more common in non smokers than smokers!. Patients typically present with gradual onset of diarrhoea mixed with blood and mucus. It is also associated with aphthous ulcers, erythema nodosum, pyoderma gangrenosum, conjunctivitis, sacroilitis and cholangiocarcinoma. Toxic dilatation of the colon can occur. Sigmoidoscopy shows inflammed, friable mucosa. Barium enema shows loss of haustra and granular mucosa. Treatment is with prednisolone and sulfasalazine.

3. Anal fissure or Fissure-in-ano, is a midline longitudinal split in squamous lining of the lower anus often present with a mucosal tag at the external aspect–'the sentinel pile'. Mostly it is due to hard faeces or constipation. Defecation or PR examination is very painful, as in this patient.

4. Rectal carcinoma is the 4th most common malignancy in women. Local spread occurs circumferentially and within 2 years complete encirclement would have taken place. Spread via the venous system occurs late. Patients present with bleeding which is the earliest and most common symptom alongwith a sense of incomplete defecation (tenesmus). Alteration in the bowel habit, weight loss and pain abdomen at a later stage are also seen. 90% of all neoplasms can be felt digitally. Proctosigmoidoscopy will always show the carcinoma. A histological examination will not only confirm the diagnosis but also stage it. A sphincter saving operation (anterior resection) is usually done for tumours of upper 2/3rd of the rectum. For tumours involving the lower 1/3rd of the rectum, a permanent colostomy (abdominoperineal excision) is often required.

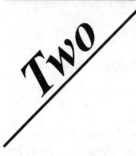

PLAB

November 2003 Question Paper

Theme 1: Management of sprains and injuries

Options:

a. Cast
b. Paracetamol
c. Suture repair
d. No weight bearing, use crutches
e. NSAIDs
f. Manipulation
g. Observe
h. Morphine

For each presentation below, choose the SINGLE most appropriate management from the above list of options. Each option may be used once, more than once, or not at all.

1. Dislocated patella and patient is on inhaled analgesic (Nitrous oxide).
2. A patient has past history of rupture of Tendo Achilles, which was managed medically. Now he has presented with rupture again. Medical treatment is not helping now.
3. Following a fall, a pregnant lady complains of pain below ankle. On examination there is mild swelling and bruising but no fracture is noted on X-rays.
4. After a rugby match, a player complains of pain following knee injury. There is no fracture noted on X-rays.
5. A 4 year old presents with trauma and knee in pain despite paracetamol.

Theme 2: Management of cardiac conditions

Options:

a. Surgical ablation of tracts
b. Verapamil
c. Digoxin
d. Enalapril
e. Amiodarone
f. DC cardioversion
g. Adenosine
h. Atropine
i. Lignocaine

For each presentation below, choose the SINGLE most appropriate management from the above list of options. Each option may be used once, more than once, or not at all.

1. A patient with heart failure presents to you with fibrillation.
2. A patient having SVT with BP 90/60. Sinus massage and adenosine have failed.
3. A patient with MI presents with recurrent ventricular tachycardia.
4. A patient presents with WPW syndrome, with no response to drugs.
5. A patient presents with VT which was controlled with lidocaine. He now needs maintenance.

Theme 3: Chest trauma: Diagnosis

Options:

a. Aortic rupture
b. Tension pneumothorax
c. Spontaneous pneumothorax
d. Splenic rupture
e. Liver trauma
f. Diaphragmatic rupture

For each presentation below, choose the SINGLE most appropriate diagnosis from the above list of options. Each option may be used once, more than once, or not at all.

1. A patient presents with chest trauma with absent breath sounds, tracheal shift and absent radial pulse.
2. A young and tall thin worker presents with breathlessness and hyper resonance on one side of his chest. He gives no history of trauma.
3. A patient presents with injury to sternum with steering wheel. X-rays show widened mediastinal shadow.

Theme 4: Acute abdomen: Diagnosis

Options:

a. X-ray KUB
b. Chest X-ray
c. X-ray abdomen
d. Pregnancy test
e. Sigmoidoscopy
f. Laparoscopy
g. Urine RE
h. Colonoscopy
i. Conservative approach

For each presentation below, choose the SINGLE most appropriate investigation from the above list of options. Each option may be used once, more than once, or not at all.

1. A patient presents with sudden onset vomiting and pain abdomen. He also adds that he has not passed wind for past many hours now. He is afebrile.
2. A patient presents with signs of perforation following diverticulitis.
3. Appendicular mass in afebrile child.
4. Carcinoma colon investigation.
5. A 23 year old female presents with left sided abdominal pain for the last 4 hours. Her last period was 7 weeks back.
6. A female presents with pain in the loin which seems to be running down the groin.

Theme 5: Investigation in abdominal conditions

Options:

a. USG Abdomen
b. Catheterization
c. Ascending urethrogram
d. Splenectomy
e. Laparoscopy
f. Observation
g. Abdominal tapping
h. Laparotomy
i. Blood transfusion
j. Get an expert opinion
k. IVU
l. MRI

For each presentation below, choose the SINGLE most appropriate investigation from the above list of options. Each option may be used once, more than once, or not at all.

1. A rugby player was hit in the back and comes with loin pain and haematuria.
2. A young man with one episode of frank haematuria. He was stable but presented with anuria now.
3. A person with anuria brought to A & E after injury with bruising on the perineum. The PR examination was normal.
4. A patient with history of RTA has fracture of left lower ribs, left sided abdominal pain and progressive guarding of left hypochondrium. Vitals are stable.
5. A middle aged man is brought to A & E with pain in left upper abdomen after a blow there. On examination his pulse rate is 110/min and BP is 90/60.

Theme 6: Prognosis and natural course of respiratory disease

Options:

a. 80% change of having wheeze in adult life
b. 50% chance of becoming normal by 6 years
c. If untreated leads to abscess
d. Very bad prognosis
e. 70% chance of getting clubbing in adulthood
f. Complaints end by the age of two
g. Complaints end by proper feeding
h. Prognosis not known
i. Extrinsic allergic alveolitis
j. Double auto antibody
k. 10% chance of COPD
l. 60% chances of developing COPD in future

For each presentation below, choose the SINGLE most appropriate prognosis/ diagnosis from the above list of options. Each option may be used once, more than once, or not at all.

1. A mother brought here 6-month old girl with difficulty in breathing and vomiting related to feeds.
2. A 5 year old boy having exercise and cold induced wheeze, mother has eczema.
3. A 2 year old boy gets respiratory wheeze whenever having cold.
4. A child was playing normally, suddenly developed breathlessness and monophonic wheeze.
5. A 6 month old boy with nocturnal wheeze, which is not controlled by steroids.
6. A child presents with sudden onset stridor, generalized itch and swellings of lips.
7. Investigation of Sjögren's syndrome.
8. Allergic symptoms in bird fancier lung.
9. A child presents with purulent sputum and cough. On examination he is febrile.

Theme 7: Anatomy of the heart

Options:

a. Left atrium
b. Right atrium
c. Left ventricle
d. Right ventricle
e. Mitral valve
f. Tricuspid valve
g. Coronary arteries
h. Interatrial septum
i. Interventricular septum
j. Sinoatrial node
k. Bundle of His
l. AV node
m. Bronchopulmonary dysplasia

For each presentation below, choose the SINGLE most appropriate anatomical area affected from the above list of options. Each option may be used once, more than once, or not at all.

1. Location of endocarditis in an IV drug abuser.
2. Location of patent foramen ovale.
3. Blood spurts into left atrium and increases left atrial pressure.
4. Site of cardiac aneurysm.
5. Increased pulmonary airway resistance and vascular resistance.
6. Structure responsible for the heart rhythm in complete heart block.

Theme 8: Diagnosis of peripheral vascular disease

Options:

a. Mural thrombus
b. Acute thrombus
c. Buerger's disease
d. Diabetes
e. DVT

For each presentation below, choose the SINGLE most appropriate diagnosis from the above list of options. Each option may be used once, more than once, or not at all.

1. A young smoker presents with peripheral vascular disease.
2. A patient with AF, pulselessness and pallor of the extremities.
3. A patient with history of MI presents with claudication and angina.
4. An elderly male with gangrene following chiropody.
5. A pregnant lady with sudden breathlessness and calf pain.

Theme 9: Haematology: Diagnosis

Options:

a. Macrocytic anaemia
b. Sickle cell anaemia
c. Iron deficiency anaemia
d. Aplastic anaemia
e. Spherocytosis

For each presentation below, choose the SINGLE most appropriate diagnosis from the above list of options. Each option may be used once, more than once, or not at all.

1. A lady presented with sore tongue.
2. An old man with bruising on chest, infection and low haemoglobin level.
3. A lady presenting with menorrhagia.
4. A young boy has pallor and jaundice. Spleen is found to be enlarged on palpation.
5. A patient who is a known case of carcinoma stomach presents with anaemia.

Theme 10: Types of emboli

Options:

a. Thrombus emboli
b. Fat emboli
c. Amniotic fluid emboli
d. Malignant emboli
e. Atheromatous emboli
f. Septic emboli
g. Paradoxical emboli
h. Fibrin emboli
i. Bone fragment emboli
j. Air emboli

For each presentation below, choose the SINGLE most appropriate type of embolus from the above list of options. Each option may be used once, more than once, or not at all.

1. A patient with DVT, was complicated by cerebral and extremity emboli. On echocardiography he was noted to have a patent foramen ovale.

2. A 28 year old with known congenital heart disease, develops small tender subcutaneous nodules in the pulp of the digits. On examination the nodules were red and tender. The patient was noted to have splenomegaly and a new heart murmur.

3. A 30 year old in her 3rd trimester of pregnancy presents with chest pain and dyspnoea increasing in severity over the last 24 hrs. She has no lower limb pain or swelling.

Theme 11: Investigation in bites

Options:

a. HIV antibodies
b. Skin swab culture
c. Lyme's serology
d. Blood film for malarial parasite, thick smear
e. Skin prick
f. Immunization

For each presentation below, choose the SINGLE most appropriate investigation from the above list of options. Each option may be used once, more than once, or not at all.

1. A girl goes for a walk in a forest. She returns with a red lesion after being bitten by an insect.

2. A middle aged police officer who is bit by an IV drug user.

3. A man returned from Zambia with fevers and rigors.

Theme 12: Enzyme defect

Options:

a. Creatinine phosphokinase
b. Troponin - T
c. Phenylalanine hydroxylase
d. Aspartate aminotransferase
e. Alanine aminotransferase
f. MM isoenzyme of creatinine kinase
g. MB isoenzyme of creatinine kinase
h. BB isoenzyme of creatinine kinase
i. Cystathionine synthetase
j. Lactic dehydrogenase

For each presentation below, choose the SINGLE most appropriate enzyme involved from the above list of options. Each option may be used once, more than once, or not at all.

1. The enzyme that occurs in high concentration in the sarcoplasm of skeletal muscle.

2. The enzyme that regulates the calcium mediated contractile process of striated muscle and is most specific for minor degrees of myocardial necrosis.

3. A Middle Eastern male child with fair complexion adopted soon after his premature birth, is noted to have delayed milestones at 8 months of age. He is also noted to have eczema. At 2 years of age the child has severe mental retardation with no pyramidal or extrapyramidal signs. Mental retardation is this child is more likely to be a defect in an enzyme.

4. A 20 year old male with mild mental retardation has had 2 successive strokes within a year. On examination he had a marfanoid habitus, with long limbs and pectus excavatum.

5. Liver congestion is most commonly associated with the elevation of this enzyme.

Theme 13: Bone investigations

Options:

a. DSA scan
b. Serum electrophoresis
c. MRI spine
d. CT scan
e. Serum calcium
f. X-ray of spine

For each presentation below, choose the SINGLE most appropriate investigation from the above list of options. Each option may be used once, more than once, or not at all.

1. A patient presents with back pain and high ESR.

2. A patient presenting with back pain, X-ray features simulating sacroilitis.

3. A man presenting with foot drop. On X-ray, there is narrowing of the disc space between 4th and 5th lumbar vertebrae. The foot drop does not resolve in 2 weeks.

Theme 14: Diabetes mellitus

Options:

a. Excess insulin
b. Relative deficiency of insulin
c. Absolute deficiency of insulin
d. Deficiency of catecholamines
e. Excess of catecholamines
f. Deficiency of glucocorticoids
g. Excess of glucocorticoids
h. Hypoglycaemia
i. Hyperglycaemia

For each presentation below, choose the SINGLE most appropriate cause from the above list of options. Each option may be used once, more than once, or not at all.

1. A female presenting with all signs and symptoms of Cushing's disease.
2. An old man presenting with signs and symptoms of hypoglycaemia.
3. A young man, obese presents with hyperglycaemia but no ketosis.

Theme 15: Cause of hypertension

Options:

a. Renal artery stenosis
b. Conn's syndrome
c. Phaeochromocytoma
d. Pregnancy
e. Cushing's syndrome
f. Steroid induced

For each presentation below, choose the SINGLE most appropriate cause from the above list of options. Each option may be used once, more than once, or not at all.

1. A young patient had hypertension with bruit in abdomen.
2. A patient presents with hypertension, pallor and palpitations.
3. A 45 year old obese women with moon facies, hirsutism and hypertension.
4. A patient with hypertension, hypokalaemia and altered serum phosphate level.

Theme 16: Diagnosis of thyroid disease

Options:

a. Drug induced
b. Hypothyroidism
c. Treated hyperthyroidism
d. Anaplastic carcinoma
e. Papillary carcinoma
f. Thyrotoxicosis
g. Follicular carcinoma

For each presentation below, choose the SINGLE most appropriate diagnosis from the above list of options. Each option may be used once, more than once, or not at all.

1. A patient presents with tremors, diarrhoea and heat intolerance.
2. A patient presents with weight gain, constipation and cold intolerance.
3. Thyroid disease following amiodarone for arrhythmias.
4. An elderly lady presents with a hard fixed thyroid swelling.

Theme 17: Prenatal screening: Diagnosis

Options:

a. Down's syndrome
b. Cystic fibrosis
c. Duchenne's muscular dystrophy
d. Spina bifida
e. Spinal muscular atrophy
f. Patau's syndrome
g. Klinefelter's syndrome
h. Weber's syndrome
i. Multiple sclerosis
j. Neural tube defects

For each presentation below, choose the SINGLE most appropriate diagnosis from the above list of options. Each option may be used once, more than once, or not at all.

1. Raised HCG and low Alpha fetoprotein.
2. Raised Alpha fetoprotein and very high HCG.
3. A pregnant mother with a history of some disease in previous child, now wants to know whether this child will have it or not.
4. A pregnant mother is given folic acid supplements to prevent this condition.
5. This disease is related with increased risk of Alzheimer's disease.
6. Previous child has recurrent infection, and parents want to know whether next child will have it.

Theme 18: CT findings in hearing loss: Diagnosis

Options:

a. Acoustic neuroma
b. Metastatic breast carcinoma
c. Paget's disease of bone
d. Otosclerosis
e. Noise induced deafness
f. Otitis media with effusion
g. Cholesteatoma
h. Higher frequency hearing loss

For each presentation below, choose the SINGLE most appropriate diagnosis from the above list of options. Each option may be used once, more than once, or not at all.

1. A 19 year old boy with mass in the antrum and resolution of some bone is noted.
2. A 9 year old boy whose CT scan of petrous bone shows air on mastoid cells. Malleus, incus and stapes are normal. Fluid collection is present.
3. A 40 year old lady whose CT scan of petrous bone shows normal malleus and incus, but cochlea shows rarefaction and densities.
4. A 60 year old man with normal CT scan (with contrast) of the petrous bone.

Theme 19: Causes of epistaxis

Options:

a. Septal perforation
b. Hypertension
c. Orf
d. Coagulopathy
e. Nasopharyngeal carcinoma

For each presentation below, choose the SINGLE most appropriate cause of epistaxis from the above list of options. Each option may be used once, more than once, or not at all.

1. A sheep farmer presents with epistaxis.
2. A boxer presents with gurgling sound and epistaxis.
3. A chrome factory worker presents with epistaxis.
4. An old man presents with epistaxis.
5. A young girl with history of bleeding following dental extraction.

Theme 20: ENT: Diagnosis

Options:

a. Carcinoma maxillary antrum
b. Sarcoidosis
c. Nasal polyposis

For each presentation below, choose the SINGLE most appropriate diagnosis from the above list of options. Each option may be used once, more than once, or not at all.

1. A man presents with swelling over cheek and epistaxis, nasal stuffiness and facial paraesthesia.
2. A Sheepkeeper gets a polyp in the nose.

Theme 21: Diagnosis of GI conditions

Options:

a. Achalasia
b. GORD
c. Oesophagitis
d. Peptic ulcer
e. Duodenal ulcer
f. *H.pylori*
g. Strongyloides stercoralis

For each presentation below, choose the SINGLE most appropriate diagnosis from the above list of options. Each option may be used once, more than once, or not at all.

1. A patient presents with pain in the epigastrium. Endoscopy confirms spiral shaped organisms.
2. Change of epithelium from squamous to columnar is noted in a patient suffering from chronic epigastric discomfort.
3. A female with pain in epigastrium at night, relieved by eating, presents with upper GI bleeding.

Theme 22: Upper GI bleeding

Options:

a. Triple therapy
b. Antimitochondrial antibodies
c. Oesophagitis
d. Barium meal
e. X-ray abdomen
f. USG abdomen
g. Gastric erosions

For each presentation below, choose the SINGLE most appropriate management/ diagnosis investigation from the above list of options. Each option may be used once, more than once, or not at all.

1. A patient of upper GI bleeding with primary biliary cirrhosis.
2. A patient of upper GI bleeding with *H. pylori* positive status requires treatment.
3. A patient of upper GI bleeding with spiral forms in microscopy requires further investigation.
4. A patient of upper GI bleeding presents with retching and vomiting.
5. A patient presents with dyspepsia with NSAIDs and tarry stools.

Theme 23: Pre-operative investigation

Options:

a. Do nothing
b. ECG
c. Echocardiography
d. Full blood count
e. Sickle cell screening
f. Chest X-ray
g. Serological tests for hepatitis
h. Coagulation screen

For each presentation below, choose the SINGLE most appropriate pre-operative investigation from the above list of options. Each option may be used once, more than once, or not at all.

1. A man with irregular pulse presenting with hernia.
2. A man on list for hernia who takes recreational drug intravenously.
3. A fit British man is admitted for bilateral inguinal hernia.
4. An Afro-carribean man with bilateral inguinal hernia.
5. A lady with a history of dental extraction with bleeding for 2 hours, now febrile and coming for some surgery.

Theme 24: Palliative care/analgesia

Options:

a. Paracetamol
b. IV morphine
c. IV benzodiazepines
d. Subcutaneous morphine through syringe driver
e. IM morphine
f. Steroids
g. Radiotherapy
h. TENS
i. Oral benzodiazepines
j. Oral morphine

For each presentation below, choose the SINGLE most appropriate palliative care/analgesia from the above list of options. Each option may be used once, more than once, or not at all.

1. A man with carcinoma of bronchus, presents with anorexia and breathlessness after surgery.
2. A man with prostatic carcinoma is in critical stage. He wants pain relief as opioids have failed.
3. A man with pancreatic cancer in last stages, suffering from pain and not responding to IV morphine.
4. A patient with carcinoma breast complaining of oedema and pain in her arm.
5. A patient with carcinoma stomach with pain. Patient is already on oral morphine which does not provide relief.
6. A man with carcinoma of bronchus with metastases, critical stage, and high doses of opiate did not help.

Theme 25: Management of chronic renal failure

Options:

a. Erythropoietin
b. Captopril
c. Haemodialysis
d. Beta-blockers
e. Calcium channel blockers

For each presentation below, choose the SINGLE most appropriate management from the above list of options. Each option may be used once, more than once, or not at all.

1. A patient with renal failure and pulmonary oedema.
2. A patient with renal failure and serum potassium level of 7.0 mmol/L.
3. A patient with end stage renal failure with anaemia.
4. A patient with renal failure due to polycystic kidney and hypertension.

Theme 26: Urological investigations

Options:

a. Serum calcium
b. Serum phosphate level
c. Parathormone level
d. Urinary cystine
e. Urinary oxalate
f. IVU
g. X-ray KUB
h. 24 hrs urine
i. Nephrostomy
j. USG
k. Urine culture
l. Isotope scan

For each presentation below, choose the SINGLE most appropriate investigation from the above list of options. Each option may be used once, more than once, or not at all.

1. A man with recurrent renal stones and high serum calcium level.
2. A man with a history of carcinoma of prostate. X-rays do not reveal anything, but IVU shows bilateral hydronephrosis.
3. A lady who has right loin pain, is febrile. She has right hydronephrosis on IVU. Next investigation may help in the management.
4. A post-operative carcinoma cervix patient, presents with anuria. Bilateral obstruction of the ureters and bilateral hydronephrosis are noted.

Theme 27: Red eye: Investigations

Options:

a. X-ray of the orbits
b. Conjunctival swab cytology
c. Fluorescein stain
d. Refer to ophthalmologist
e. Aciclovir
f. Fundoscopy
g. Measure IOP

For each presentation below, choose the SINGLE most appropriate investigation from the above list of options. Each option may be used once, more than once, or not at all

1. A worker in a metal factory complains of something in his eye.
2. A hedge gardener presenting with sudden photophobia and blepharospasm.
3. A man presents with symptoms of acute conjunctivitis and ophthalmic shingles cannot open his eyes.
4. A patient presents with purulent conjunctivitis.
5. A patient presents with headache, photophobia and diminished vision.

Theme 28: Poisoning: diagnosis

Options:

a. Paracetamol
b. Salicylates
c. Metoclopramide
d. Opiates
e. Tricyclic antidepressants
f. Digoxin
g. Diazepam

For each presentation below, choose the SINGLE most appropriate drug from the above list of options. Each option may be used once, more than once, or not at all.

1. A patient presents with pinpoint pupils and depression of respiration.
2. A woman taking tricyclics and diazepam at night is now complaining of agitation and dizziness.
3. A patient presents with visual symptoms and bradycardia.
4. A patient presents with dystonia and oculogyric crisis.
5. Ingestion of this drug causes liver failure in 3 - 4 days.

Theme 29: Drug reactions and toxicity

Options:

a. Cerebellar dysfunction
b. β-blockers
c. Vitamin B_2
d. Vitamin B_{12}
e. Tremors
f. Nephrotoxicity
g. Metoclopramide
h. Cimitidine
i. Paracetamol

For each presentation below, choose the SINGLE most appropriate toxicity/drug from the above list of options. Each option may be used once, more than once, or not at all.

1. Deficiency of this causes neurological symptoms.
2. Toxicity of lithium.
3. Extrapyramidal side effects.
4. Toxicity of carbamazepine.
5. Man with shingles in thoracic area on the 2nd day.
6. Hypotension alone.

Theme 30: Treatment of STDs

Options:

a. Single dose long acting Penicillin
b. Erythromycin
c. Doxycycline
d. Ciprofloxacin
e. Metronidazole
f. Topical clotrimazole
g. Oral nystatin
h. Steroids

For each presentation below, choose the SINGLE most appropriate treatment from the above list of options. Each option may be used once, more than once, or not at all.

1. A lady presenting with gonococcal infection.
2. A lady presenting with chlamydial infection.
3. A pregnant lady presenting with chlamydial cervicitis.
4. A lady presenting with vaginal candidiasis.
5. A lady presenting with bacterial vaginosis.

Theme 31: Gynaecology: Next step of management

Options:

a. Cervical smear
b. Cervical biopsy
c. Laparoscopy
d. Per speculum examination
e. Endometrial sampling
f. USG pelvis
g. Urine culture
h. Colposcopy

For each presentation below, choose the SINGLE most appropriate management from the above list of options. Each option may be used once, more than once, or not at all.

1. A lady was diagnosed CIN-1 cancer cervix 6 months back. She is now coming for follow up.
2. A lady with CIN-2 diagnosed 6 months back, now comes for follow up.
3. A post menopausal women presenting with bleeding and dyspareunia.
4. A pre menopausal women presenting with ectropion and bleeding.

Theme 32: Gynaecological diagnosis

Options:

a. Ectopic pregnancy
b. Stress incontinence
c. Endometrial carcinoma
d. Urge incontinence
e. True incontinence
f. UTI

For each presentation below, choose the SINGLE most appropriate diagnosis from the above list of options. Each option may be used once, more than once, or not at all.

1. An elderly lady passes small amounts of urine on sneezing.
2. A lady cannot control even upto reaching the toilet.
3. A lady complaining of dysuria and fever since a week.

Theme 33: Treatment in skin lesions

Options:

a. Hydrocortisone 2%
b. Topical hydrocortisone 1%
c. Topical antibiotics
d. Systemic steroids
e. Topical aciclovir
f. IV aciclovir
g. Oral aciclovir
h. Flucloxacillin
i. Emollients
j. Carbamazepine

For each presentation below, choose the SINGLE most appropriate treatment from the above list of options. Each option may be used once, more than once, or not at all.

1. A boy presents with eczema, weeping vesicles and redness.
2. A boy presents with eczema, intense itching and scratch marks.
3. A man presents with eczema which was not helped by 1% topical hydrocortisone.
4. A child presents with herpetic whitlow coming with some blisters over the trunk.
5. An 80 year old lady presents with herpetic rash appearing 5 days back on the back of her trunk.
6. A patient of HIV presents with herpes.
7. A patient of herpetic neuralgia.
8. A lady who is pregnant presents with shingles.

Theme 34: Convulsions in a child: Management

Options:

a. EEG
b. Drug levels
c. IV lorazepam
d. Lumbar puncture
e. Teach parents how to use rectal diazepam.

For each presentation below, choose the SINGLE most appropriate management from the above list of options. Each option may be used once, more than once, or not at all.

1. Young child presenting with high fever and fit.
2. A child presents with recurrent febrile convulsions.
3. A child presents with fever, rashes and convulsions.
4. An obese child taking valproate but seizures are not controlled.
5. Child with history of generalized convulsion 3 hours back.

Theme 35: Epidemiology in psychiatric disorders

Options:

a. Depression
b. Schizophrenia
c. Obsessive compulsive disorder
d. Anorexia nervosa
e. Anorexia bulimia
f. Anxiety
g. Starvation
h. Alcohol
i. Drug addiction

For each presentation below, choose the SINGLE most appropriate diagnosis from the above list of options. Each option may be used once, more than once, or not at all.

1. Most commonly seen in developed countries where the females are more conscious than men about weight gain.
2. The psychiatric disorder most commonly seen in young women (20 -25 years) than in older.
3. A student preparing for the exam for the last 4 weeks and having weight loss of 10 kg.
4. A businessman presents to you having trouble sleeping and poor appetite due to some changes in his business.
5. This disease is more common in females and increases as the age advances.
6. Worldwide prevalence of 0.8%, incidence in UK is 100 per million.

Theme 36: Neurological diagnosis

Options:

a. Meningioma
b. Glioma
c. Multiple sclerosis
d. Stroke
e. Hydrocephalus
f. Parkinsonism
g. MND
h. Alzheimer's dementia
i. Meningitis

For each presentation below, choose the SINGLE most appropriate diagnosis from the above list of options. Each option may be used once, more than once, or not at all.

1. A 40 year old patient having headache and vomiting is waiting for neurosurgery and radiotherapy.
2. A patient presents with dysarthria, headache and dysphagia.
3. A patient presents with hoarseness, dysphagia and lower limb paresis.
4. A patient who is wheel chaired with neurological problems, presents with blurring vision.
5. A patient who is bed ridden, presents with increasing forgetfulness.

Theme 37: Causes of confusion

Options:

a. Subdural haemorrhage
b. Hypothyroidism
c. Alzheimer's dementia
d. UTI
e. Hypoglycaemia
f. Meningitis
g. Respiratory failure
h. Vitamin B_{12} deficiency

For each presentation below, choose the SINGLE most appropriate cause of confusion from the above list of options. Each option may be used once, more than once, or not at all.

1. A patient presents with confusion with intake of drugs prescribed for his parents.
2. An alcoholic who has fallen a number of times in the past 1 month now comes with confusion.
3. A patient presents with confusion with increased forgetfulness.
4. A patient presents with confusion with incontinence.
5. A patient presents with confusion, constipation, hoarseness and hypotonia.

Theme 38: Psychiatry

Options:

a. Less coffee
b. Starvation
c. Diazepam
d. Admit
e. Methadone
f. Naltrexone
g. Acamprosate

For each presentation below, choose the SINGLE most appropriate management/diagnosis from the above list of options. Each option may be used once, more than once, or not at all.

1. A patient presents with delirium tremens and requires treatment.
2. A patient who is shaking after alcohol abstinence.
3. A student presents with more tremors before exams.
4. An old man with nutritional deficiencies.
5. An alcoholic who wants to stay away from alcohol.
6. A heroin addict wants to quit.

Theme 39: Chest pain: Diagnosis

Options:

a. Angina
b. Peptic ulcer
c. Aortic dissection
d. Herpes zoster
e. Oesophagitis
f. Pericarditis.

For each presentation below, choose the SINGLE most appropriate diagnosis from the above list of options. Each option may be used once, more than once, or not at all.

1. A middle aged man post MI presented with pain in his chest, which varies in severity with position.
2. An old man presented with pain in epigastrium, related to exertion.

Theme 40: Miscellaneous

Options:

a. Serum calcium
b. Dexa bone scan
c. Serum urate
d. Bone X-rays
e. CT chest
f. Sputum culture

For each presentation below, choose the SINGLE most appropriate investigation from the above list of options. Each option may be used once, more than once, or not at all.

1. A lady with breast cancer presents with confusion.
2. A factory worker presents with loss of weight and thickened pleura.
3. An African with supraclavicular lymph node enlargement and weight loss.

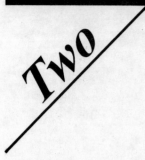
Theme 1: Management of sprains and injuries

1. **(f)** Manipulation
2. **(c)** Suture repair
3. **(b)** Paracetamol
4. **(a)** Cast
5. **(e)** NSAIDs

Theme 2: Management of cardiac conditions

1. **(f)** DC cardioversion
2. **(b)** Verapamil
3. **(i)** Lignocaine
4. **(a)** Surgical ablation of tracts
5. **(e)** Amiodarone

Theme 3: Chest trauma : Diagnosis

1. **(b)** Tension pneumothorax
2. **(c)** Spontaneous pneumothorax
3. **(a)** Aortic rupture

Theme 4: Acute abdomen: Diagnosis

1. **(c)** X-ray abdomen
2. **(b)** Chest X-ray
3. **(i)** Conservative approach
4. **(h)** Colonoscopy

5. **(d)** Pregnancy test
6. **(a)** X-ray KUB

Theme 5: Investigation in abdominal conditions

1. **(k)** IVU
2. **(k)** IVU
3. **(c)** Ascending urethrogram
4. **(a)** USG abdomen
5. **(h)** Laparotomy

Theme 6: Prognosis and natural course of respiratory disease

1. **(g)** Complaints end by proper feeding
2. **(b)** 50% chance of becoming normal by 6 years
3. **(k)** 10% chance of COPD
4. **(h)** Prognosis not known
5. **(d)** Very bad prognosis
6. **(h)** Prognosis not known
7. **(j)** Double auto antibody
8. **(i)** Extrinsic allergic alveolitis
9. **(c)** If untreated leads to abscess

Theme 7: Anatomy of the heart

1. **(f)** Tricuspid valve
2. **(h)** Interatrial septum

3. **(e)** Mitral valve
4. **(c)** Left ventricle
5. **(m)** Bronchopulmonary dysplasia
6. **(k)** Bundle of His

Theme 8: Diagnosis of peripheral vascular disease

1. **(c)** Buerger's disease
2. **(a)** Mural thrombus
3. **(b)** Acute thrombus
4. **(d)** Diabetes
5. **(e)** DVT

Theme 9: Haematology: Diagnosis

1. **(a)** Macrocytic anaemia
2. **(d)** Aplastic anaemia
3. **(c)** Iron deficiency anaemia
4. **(b)** Sickle cell anaemia
5. **(c)** Iron deficiency anaemia

Theme 10: Types of emboli

1. **(g)** Paradoxical emboli
2. **(f)** Septic embolic
3. **(c)** Amniotic fluid emboli

Theme 11: Investigation in bites

1. **(c)** Lyme serology
2. **(b)** Skin swab culture
3. **(d)** Blood film for malarial parasite, thick smear

Theme 12: Enzyme defect

1. **(f)** MM isoenzyme of creatinine kinase
2. **(b)** Troponin - T
3. **(c)** Phenylalanine hydroxylase
4. **(i)** Cystathionine synthetase
5. **(e)** Alanine aminotransferase

Theme 13: Bone investigations

1. **(b)** Serum electrophoresis
2. **(f)** X-ray of spine
3. **(c)** MRI spine

Theme 14: Diabetes mellitus

1. **(g)** Excess of glucocorticoids
2. **(a)** Excess insulin
3. **(b)** Relative deficiency of insulin

Theme 15: Cause of hypertension

1. **(a)** Renal artery stenosis
2. **(c)** Phaeochromocytoma
3. **(e)** Cushing's syndrome
4. **(b)** Conn's syndrome

Theme 16: Diagnosis of thyroid disease

1. **(f)** Thyrotoxicosis
2. **(b)** Hypothyroidism
3. **(a)** Drug induced
4. **(d)** Anaplastic carcinoma

Theme 17: Prenatal screening: Diagnosis

1. **(a)** Down's syndrome
2. **(d)** Spina bifida
3. **(c)** Duchenne's muscular dystrophy
4. **(j)** Neural tube defects
5. **(a)** Down's syndrome
6. **(b)** Cystic fibrosis

Theme 18: CT findings in hearing loss: Diagnosis

1. **(g)** Cholesteatoma
2. **(f)** Otitis media with effusion
3. **(d)** Otosclerosis
4. **(h)** Higher frequency hearing loss

Theme 19: Causes of epistaxis

1. **(c)** Orf
2. **(a)** Septal perforation
3. **(e)** Nasopharyngeal carcinoma
4. **(b)** Hypertension
5. **(d)** Coagulopathy

Theme 20: ENT: Diagnosis

1. **(a)** Carcinoma maxillary antrum
2. **(c)** Nasal polyposis

Theme 21: Diagnosis of GI conditions

1. **(f)** *H.pylori*
3. **(b)** GORD
3. **(e)** Duodenal ulcer

Theme 22: Upper GI bleeding

1. **(b)** Antimitochondrial antibodies
2. **(a)** Triple therapy
3. **(d)** Barium meal
4. **(c)** Oesophagitis
5. **(g)** Gastric erosions

Theme 23: Pre-operative investigation

1. **(b)** ECG
2. **(g)** Serological tests for hepatitis
3. **(a)** Do nothing
4. **(e)** Sickle cell screening
5. **(c)** Echocardiography

Theme 24: Palliative care/analgesia

1. **(c)** IV benzodiazepines
2. **(g)** Radiotherpay
3. **(g)** Radiotherapy
4. **(j)** Oral morphine
5. **(d)** Subcutaneous morphine through syringe driver
6. **(g)** Radiotherapy

Theme 25: Management of chronic renal failure

1. **(c)** Haemodialysis
2. **(c)** Haemodialysis
3. **(a)** Erythropoietin
4. **(b)** Captopril

Theme 26: Urological investigations

1. **(c)** Parathormone level

2. **(i)** Nephrostomy
3. **(k)** Urine culture
4. **(f)** IVU

Theme 27: Red eye: Investigations

1. **(a)** X-ray of the orbits
2. **(c)** Fluorescein stain
3. **(d)** Refer to ophthalmologist
4. **(b)** Conjunctival swab cytology
5. **(g)** Measure IOP

Theme 28: Poisoning: Diagnosis

1. **(d)** Opiates
2. **(g)** Diazepam
3. **(f)** Digoxin
4. **(c)** Metoclopramide
5. **(a)** Paracetamol

Theme 29: Drug reactions and toxicity

1. **(d)** Vitamin B_{12}
2. **(e)** Tremors
3. **(g)** Metoclopramide
4. **(a)** Hepatotoxicity
5. **(i)** Paracetamol
6. **(b)** β-blockers

Theme 30: Treatment of STDs

1. **(a)** Single dose long acting Penicillin
2. **(c)** Doxycycline
3. **(b)** Erythromycin
4. **(f)** Topical clotrimazole
5. **(e)** Metronidazole

Theme 31: Gynaecology : Next step of management

1. **(b)** Cervical biopsy
2. **(h)** Colposcopy
3. **(e)** Endometrial sampling
4. **(d)** Per speculum examination

Theme 32: Gynaecological diagnosis

1. **(b)** Stress incontinence
2. **(d)** Urge incontinence
3. **(f)** UTI

Theme 33: Treatment in skin lesions

1. **(b)** Topical hydrocortisone 1%
2. **(c)** Topical antibiotics
3. **(a)** Hydrocortisone 2%
4. **(g)** Oral aciclovir
5. **(g)** Oral aciclovir
6. **(f)** IV aciclovir
7. **(j)** Carbamazepine
8. **(f)** IV aciclovir

Theme 34: Convulsions in child: Management

1. **(c)** IV lorazepam
2. **(e)** Teach parents how to use rectal diazepam.
3. **(d)** Lumbar puncture
4. **(b)** Drug levels
5. **(a)** EEG

Theme 35: Epidemiology in psychiatric disorders

1. **(d)** Anorexia nervosa
2. **(i)** Drug addiction
3. **(f)** Anxiety
4. **(a)** Depression
5. **(a)** Depression
6. **(b)** Schizophrenia

Theme 36: Neurological diagnosis

1. **(b)** Glioma
2. **(d)** Stroke
3. **(g)** MND
4. **(c)** Multiple sclerosis
5. **(h)** Alzheimer's dementia

Theme 37: Causes of confusion

1. **(e)** Hypoglycaemia
2. **(a)** Subdural haemorrhage
3. **(c)** Alzheimer's dementia
4. **(d)** UTI
5. **(b)** Hypothyroidism

Theme 38: Psychiatry

1. **(c)** Diazepam
2. **(c)** Diazepam
3. **(a)** Less coffee
4. **(b)** Starvation
5. **(g)** Acamprosate
6. **(e)** Methadone

Theme 39: Chest pain: Diagnosis

1. **(f)** Pericarditis
2. **(a)** Angina

Theme 40: Miscellaneous

1. **(a)** Serum calcium
2. **(e)** CT chest
3. **(f)** Sputum culture

Two *November 2003 Explanation*

Theme 1: Management of sprains and injuries

1. Acute dislocation of patella occurs due to sudden contraction of the quadriceps while knee is flexed. Patient is unable to straighten the knee. Treatment consists of manipulation and reduction followed by immobilization in a cast for 3 weeks. For recurrent/habitual dislocation, treatment is operative which consists of release of tight structures on the lateral side and repair of lax structures on the medial side.

2. If the functional method of treatment (i.e. rest, ice-packs, compression and elevation) fails, or if the Achilles tendon is completely torn, the patient will require an operative sutural repair.

3. Paracetamol has been widely used in pregnancy for pain relief and antipyretic action. Its use has not been associated with congenital defects when taken in normal therapeutic doses. Aspirin, in analgesic doses increases the risk of maternal or neonatal bleeding by virtue of its antiplatelet action. It may also delay the onset of labour and increases its duration. NSAIDs can not only cause premature closure of ductus arteriosus but can also lead to renal dysfunction, intracerebral haemorrhage and necrotising enterocolitis in the newborn if given from around 24 weeks' gestation. Aspirin and NSAIDs are best avoided in pregnancy.

4. The patient may be having a meniscal tear (more frequently, the medial meniscus is torn), or an injury to any of the ligaments of the knee (mostly the anterior cruciate ligament). Treatment for both, acute meniscal tear and ligament tear, is by immobilising the knee in a Robert–Jones compression bandage for 2–3 weeks (meniscal tear) or 3–6 weeks (ligament injury). After a few weeks, the swelling subsides and adequate strength can be regained by physiotherapy.

5. The analgesic 'ladder' consists broadly of three steps. Step 1 includes non-opioid analgesics like aspirin, paracetamol and NSAIDs. Step 2 includes weak opioids like codeine, dihydrocodeine and dextropropoxyphene. Step 3 includes strong opioids like morphine, diamorphine and hydromorphine. NSAIDs which fall in the step 1 category along with paracetamol, need to be tried in this patient since paracetamol has been ineffective.

Theme 2: Management of cardiac conditions

1. Atrial fibrillation is a chronic, irregular atrial rhythm at 300–600 bpm. Common causes of atrial fibrillation are heart failure, hypertension, cardiac ischaemia, MI, mitral valve disease, hyperthyroidism, alcohol.
   It is characterized by an irregularly irregular pulse. Treatment consists of DC cardioversion done either electively following first attack of AF with an identifiable cause, or as an emergency if the patient is compromised. (Ventricular rate may be controlled by Digoxin or low dose β-blocker.

2. Supraventricular tachycardia is a narrow complex tachycardia with an ECG rate of > 100 beats per minute and QRS complex of duration > 120 milliseconds. P waves are either absent or inverted after the QRS complex. Vagal manoeuvres (carotid sinus massage, Valsalva manoeuvre) transiently increase AV block and may unmask an underlying atrial rhythm. If this fails adenosine 3 mg bolus is given. If that also fails, verapamil 5 mg IV over 2 minutes is given. DC cardioversion if nothing helps. Maintenance therapy consists of β blockers or verapamil.

3. VT is the most common regular broad complex tachycardia after MI. Hypokalaemia, hypoxia and acidosis predispose to arrhythmias. Drug of choice for VT following MI is lignocaine (or lidocaine). If this fails, DC shock may be given, followed by procainamide, if needed.

4. WPW (Wolff–Parkinson–White syndrome) is caused by congenital accessory conduction pathway between atria and ventricles. Resting ECG shows short PR interval and widened QRS complex due to slurred upstroke, or 'delta wave'. Treatment consists of surgical/radio-frequency ablation of accessory pathways.
   (Drug treatment is indicated only in symptomatic patients and is aimed at slowing the conduction rate and prolonging refractory period of the bypass tract e.g. by using flecainide, disopyramide or amiodarone.)

5. Ventricular tachycardia (VT) is a broad complex tachycardia. Acute management comprises IV lignocaine followed by IV procainamide. If no response, DC shock is given if compromised. Oral therapy consists of amiodarone loading dose followed by maintenance therapy (200 mg/24 hours).
   Side effects of amiodarone include corneal deposits, photosensitivity, hepatitis, pneumonitis, lung fibrosis, rise in free T_4, fall in free T_3, nightmares, rise in INR (warfarin potentiation).

Theme 3: Chest trauma: Diagnosis

1. This is a patient with tension pneumothorax. The mediastinum is pushed over into the contralateral hemithorax. Patients present with dyspnoea, tachycardia, hypotension, raised JVP, tracheal deviation away from the side of pneumothorax, increased percussion note, decreased air entry on the affected side. Unless the air is rapidly removed, cardio-respiratory arrest will occur.

2. Pneumothorax is collection of air in the pleural space. It often occurs spontaneous by especially in young thin men due to rupture of subpleural bulla. The patient will typically complains of sudden onset dyspnoea and pleuritic chest pain. Patient will have reduced chest expansion, hyperresonance to percussion and decreased breath sounds on the affected area. Mild pneumothorax does not require any treatment, but moderate to severe pneumothorax require aspiration.

3. A PA view chest radiograph showing widening of mediastinum (especially following chest trauma) is very suggestive of aortic rupture. Clinical signs include interscapular pain, a murmur, hoarseness and radiofemoral delay of arterial pulse.

Treatment consists of urgent exploration via a left thoracotomy through the fourth intercostal space.

Theme 4: Acute abdomen: Diagnosis

1. The diagnostic investigation for intestinal obstruction is plain abdominal X-ray which shows:
   - distended bowel loops proximal to the site of obstruction (hence, site of obstruction can also be localized).
   - Erect abdominal X-ray shows increased number of horizontal air-fluid levels.

2. Perforation following diverticulitis leads to ileus, peritonitis ± shock. Leakage of gas occurs from the bowel into the peritoneal cavity. This is seen as a gas shadow under the diaphragm in chest X-ray taken in standing position. This sign is diagnostic of intestinal perforation.

3. Appendicular mass which is a complication of acute appendicitis implies inflamed appendix surrounded by omentum. An appendicular mass in an afebrile child is managed conservatively by Ochsner–Sherren regimen i.e. patient is kept NPO, a nasogastric tube is passed and IV fluids and antibiotics started. Temperature and pulse rate is recorded 4 hourly. Clinical improvement is usually evident in 24–48 hours.

Appendix is usually removed after an interval of 6–8 weeks.

4. Adenocarcinoma of the colon is a columnar cell carcinoma originating in the colonic epithelium. Carcinoma of colon generally occurs in patients over 50 years of age. In any case of colonic bleeding in patients above 40 years of age, complete investigation of colon is required. Most tumours occur on the left side of the colon and the main symptoms are those of increasing intestinal obstruction along with pain, distension and a palpable lump. Patients may present for the first time with liver metastasis, ascites from carcinomatosis peritonei and metastases to lung, skin, bone and brain. Double contrast barium enema

shows a cancer of the colon as a constant irregular filling defect. Colonoscopy has the advantage of not only picking up the primary carcinoma but also detects synchronous polyps or even multiple carcinomas.

5. Most likely diagnosis for this patient is ectopic pregnancy since she is also having amenorrhoea since 7 weeks. However, to establish the diagnosis, pregnancy must be diagnosed as the cause of amenorrhoea (by urine pregnancy test). This is followed by an ultrasonography of pelvis to confirm the diagnosis.

An unruptured ectopic may be managed conservatively. However, a ruptured ectopic pregnancy requires urgent laparotomy.

6. Pain radiating from loin to groin, is suggestive of a ureteric colic. Investigation of choice, here, would be an X-ray KUB, to visualize any ureteric calculi.

Theme 5: Investigation in abdominal conditions

1. In a blunt abdominal trauma, liver, spleen and kidneys are chiefly at risk of injury. In this patient, the site and presentation are suggestive of renal injury. In renal injury patient will have local loin pain and tenderness. Haematuria is the cardinal sign of a damaged kidney. An IVU should be obtained urgently to (a) assess the damage to the kidney (b) make sure that the other kidney is normal. Surgical exploration is necessary in less than 10% of the cases. Surgical exploration is indicated if either there are signs of progressive blood loss or there is an expanding mass in the loin.

2. As explained above.

3. The mode of injury in this case is suggestive of urethral injury. Rupture of the bulbar urethra is the most common urethral injury. Urethral rupture is most commonly at the junction of prostatic and membranous parts in males. The appearance of a drop of blood at the end of the urethra is suggestive of urethral rupture. The triad of signs of a ruptured bulbar urethra is retention of urine, perineal haematoma and bleeding from the external urinary meatus. Such patients requires a suprapubic catheterization as soon as possible and end-to-end reanastomosis of the ruptured urethra. CT scan is the investigation of choice in trauma patients presenting with haematuria. But an ascending urethrogram needs to be done to locate the site and extent of the rupture.

4. The patient has had a splenic rupture. Points which favor this diagnosis are:
   - Splenic injury is always suspected if there is a fracture of overlying left lower ribs.
   - Presents with upper abdominal guarding and later, local bruising and abdominal distension.

The diagnosis should be confirmed by a USG (or CT Scan) to determine the site of bleeding.

5. Laparotomy is indicated in cases of (i) rupture of organ (ii) peritonitis. Organ ruptured may be spleen, aorta or an ectopic pregnancy. Such patients usually present with features of shock i.e. tachycardia, faints, hypotension [3] 20 mmHg on standing. Abdominal swelling and history of trauma are usually present. The presentation in this case is suggestive of splenic rupture causing tachycardia and hypotension.

Theme 6: Prognosis and natural course of respiratory disease

1. The child was being successively fed (breast fed) till 6 months of age. The child is weaned off from breast milk to top-feeds around 6 months of age, and may have problems in feeding around this time. The mother should be instructed to feed the child properly, which would end the problems of vomiting and difficulty in breathing related to feeds.

2. The child is suffering from early onset (atopic) asthma. In children, asthma is commonly triggered by cold air or exercise. Also, a family history of allergic disorders (e.g. allergic rhinitis or eczema) point towards this diagnosis. The child has around 50% chances of becoming normal by 6 years.

3. Wheezes (rhonchi) are caused by air passing through narrowed airways. They may be monophonic (signifying partial obstruction of one airway e.g. tumour) or polyphonic (signifying widespread narrowing of airways e.g. asthma, COPD). Most children with asthma in childhood become normal by the time they attain adulthood. 10% of such children can have respiratory symptoms even during later years.

4. This is a case of aspirated foreign body. Sudden onset of breathlessness and monophonic wheeze are suggestive of foreign body aspiration. As we do not know the duration and severity of the wheeze, prognosis cannot be commented upon. Respiratory obstruction by choking on a foreign body is a frequent cause of death. This can be prevented by performing the Heimlich manoeuvre. Back blows and chest thrusts, are instead, performed in children with foreign body aspiration.

5. Asthma implies reversible obstruction of airways. Patient may present with wheeze, dyspnoea or cough. It may be life threatening if peak flow < 33%, presence of cyanosis,

silent chest, fatigue or exhaustion, agitation or decreased level of consciousness. Steroids are used in the management protocol only when β agonists and sodium cromoglycate have not benefitted. This is a case of asthma precipitating during the nights and is not controlled by steroids. This implies a poor prognosis. Such patients must be taken to ITU, carefully monitored and intubated if required.

6. Symptoms of anaphylaxis include itching, erythema, urticaria, oedema, wheeze, laryngeal obstruction, cyanosis, tachycardia, hypotension. It is an IgE mediated hypersensitivity reaction. Management includes:

   i. Secure the airway and give 100% O_2.
   ii. Remove the cause
   iii. Raise feet to restore circulation
   iv. Give Adrenaline IM (0.5 ml of 1:1000 solution). Repeat every 5 mins, guided by pulse, BP and respiratory function, until better.
   v. Hydrocortisone 200 mg IV and chlorpheniramine 10 mg IV.
   vi. IV fluids may be required
      Anaphylactic attacks can vary in severity from person to person. Therefore the prognosis cannot be accurately predicted.

7. Sjögren's syndrome is the association of connective tissue disorder (Rheumatoid arthritis in 50%) with keratoconjunctivitis sicca or xerostomia. Conjunctival dryness can be quantified by Schirmer's test in which < 10 mm of wet filter paper in 5 min is positive. Rheumatoid factor is nearly always positive. Auto-antibodies i.e. anti-Ro (SSA) and anti-La (SSB) antibodies are variably present. Other features include neuropathy, renal involvement, hepatosplenomegaly etc. Treatment consists of hypromellose (artificial tears) ± occlusion of punctum which drains tears.

8. Bird fancier's lung is a type of extrinsic allergic alveolitis, where inhalation of allergens provokes a hypersensitivity reaction in sensitized individuals. Other examples:

   • Pigeon fancier's lung (allergen is proteins in bird droppings).
   • Farmer's and mushroom worker's lung (micropolyspora faeni, thermoactinomyces vulgaris).
   • Malt worker's lung (Aspergillus clavatus)
   • Bagassosis (Thermoactinomyces sacchari).
      Symptoms include fever, myalgia, dry cough, dyspnoea and crackles (no wheeze).

   Lung function tests reveal a reversible restrictive defect. Treatment of an acute attack:

   i. Remove the allergen and give O_2 (35–60%).
   ii. Hydrocortisone 200 mg IV
   iii. Oral prednisolone.

9. A child with purulent sputum and cough, may be having pneumonia, which if inadequately treated, leads to development of a lung abscess. Patient may present with swinging fevers, cough, purulent, foul smelling sputum, pleuritic chest pain and clubbing. Chest X-ray shows walled cavity, often with a fluid level. Bronchoscopy is done to obtain diagnostic specimens. Treatment consists of antibiotics for 4–6 weeks. Postural drainage may be required.

Theme 7: Anatomy of the heart

1. Infective endocarditis in IV drug abusers occurs mostly due to staphylococcus aureus. It gains access through the contaminated needles into the peripheral venous system. As the venous blood reaches the right side of the heart, these organisms get lodged on the tricuspid valve and grow to form vegetations here. Patient presents with fever, weight loss, anaemia, splenomegaly, clubbing, Osler's nodes, Janeway lesions, Roth's spots and splinter haemorrhages.

   Blood cultures (3 sets) taken at different times at fever peaks, are positive in 85–90%.

   Transthoracic echocardiography may show vegetations (if >2 mm in size).

   Treatment chiefly consists of antibiotics.

2. Foramen ovale is present in the interatrial septum during intrauterine period of life. It undergoes spontaneous closure after birth. However, it may remain patent in some cases leading to a persistent communication between the right and left atrium.

3. Acute mitral regurgitation tends to cause rapid increase in left atrial pressure as blood spurts back into the left atrium during ventricular contraction. Left atrial compliance is normal. Patients may present with dyspnoea, fatigue, palpitations, infective endocarditis, displaced hyperdynamic apex, RV heave, pansystolic murmur at the apex radiating to axilla, loud P_2.

   Echocardiogram is done to assess LV function. Doppler echo is done to assess size and site of regurgitation. Cardiac catheterization is done to confirm the diagnosis and rule out other valvular disease.

   Digoxin is given for AF. Diuretics improve symptoms. Surgery is done if symptoms deteriorate.

4. Left ventricle is the commonest site for cardiac aneurysm. LV aneurysm occurs as a late complication of MI (after 4–6 weeks) and presents with LVF, angina, recurrent VT or systemic embolism.

   ECG shows persistent ST segment elevation. Treatment is with anticoagulants. Consider excision.

5. Bronchopulmonary dysplasia implies chronic lung diseases of prematurity. BPD is usually due to barotrauma and oxygen toxicity but surfactant-related BPD is multifactorial. Pathophysiologic hallmark of respiratory distress syndrome is increased vascular permeability to proteins. Airway resistance may be increased due to bronchial wall oedema and cytokine-mediated bronchospasm. Pulmonary vascular resistance and pulmonary arterial pressures may also be elevated.

6. In complete heart block (third degree), the AV conduction fails completely and atria and ventricles beat independently (AV dissociation). Ventricular activity is maintained by an escape rhythm arising in the bundle of His (narrow QRS complexes) or distal conducting tissue (broad QRS complexes).

   Distal escape rhythms are slower. Complete heart block produces a slow (25–50/min) regular pulse that does not vary with exercise. Cannon waves may be visible in the neck.

Theme 8: Diagnosis of peripheral vascular disease

1. Buerger's disease (thromboangiitis obliterans) is inflammation of arteries, veins and nerves with thrombosis in middle sized arteries. It is usually seen in young males (< 40 years age), who are cigarette smokers. It may lead to gangrene.

2. Mural thrombus formed on the endocardium of the cardiac chambers (e.g. after an MI) may embolize into the systemic circulation. Such an embolus may lodge in any of the peripheral arteries leading to pulselessness and pallor of the extremities. Atrial fibrillation is an irregular atrial rhythm at 300–600 bpm. It may occur as a complication of MI or otherwise. The main risk is of embolic stroke (i.e. AF increases chances of embolization of a mural thrombus).

3. Unstable angina implies angina occurring at rest or with minimal exertion. It is associated with a greatly increased risk of MI. Although unstable angina itself is also seen as a complication of MI. The underlying pathology is usually plaque fissuring or rupture leading to platelet adhesion and hence thrombus formation. Such patients should be managed medically until symptoms subside. Angiography is done later to assess for angioplasty or surgery (CABG).

4. Patients with diabetic neuropathy present with numbness, tingling and burning worse at night. There is decreased sensation in 'stocking' distribution, absent ankle jerks and deformities. Neuropathy is patchy. Neuropathy or vascular disease in a diabetic patient puts him at high risk of foot ulceration. Foot ulcers are usually painless, punched out, in an area of thick callous with superadded infection, pus, oedema, erythema, crepitus and bad odour. Daily foot inspection, comfortable shoes, no barefoot walking, no corn-plasters and regular chiropody help. Surgery is indicated in abscess or deep infection, severe ischaemia and gangrene, spreading anaerobic infection and suppurative arthritis.

5. Points favouring the diagnosis of DVT:
   - Pregnancy is a risk factor for deep vein thrombosis (other risk factors include old age, oestrogens, surgery, malignancy, obesity, immobility, thrombophilia).
   - It presents with calf pain, mild fever, pitting oedema, increased warmth and distended veins.
   - Thrombus may dislodge from the deep veins and reach the right side of the heart. The embolus then goes into the pulmonary circulation and lodges here to cause acute pulmonary embolism, presenting with sudden breathlessness.

   Tests : Cogo's regime: compression ultrasound (repeated at 1 week) to catch early but propagating DVTs.

   D–dimer blood test.

   Compression stockings and heparin form the mainstay of treatment.

Theme 9: Haematology: Diagnosis

1. Macrocytic or megaloblastic anaemia can be seen in vitamin B_{12} and Folic acid deficiencies. The mention of sore tongue suggests vitamin B_{12} deficiency. Pernicious anaemia, parasthaesiae in fingers and toes, megaloblastic anaemia and glossitis, all are features of vitamin B_{12} deficiency.

2. Aplastic anaemia is characterized by pancytopenia with hypoplastic bone marrow. Pancytopenia includes:
   - Decreased number of RBCs evident as anaemia and low haemoglobin and hence causing fatigue.
   - Decreased number of WBCs which increases risk of infection.
   - Decreased number of platelets which increases bleeding tendencies (bruising on chest).
     Definitive treatment in young patients is Bone Marrow transplantation. Also, ciclosporin and antithymocyte globulin may be effective.

3. Menorrhagia is excessive bleeding occurring during the menstrual cycles. It leads to a chronic loss of iron thus gradually decreasing iron stores of the body and causing iron-deficiency anaemia.

4. Sickle cell anaemia results due to substitution of glutamate with valine at position 6 of beta chain of haemoglobin, leading to formation of HbS. HbS polymerizes when deoxygenated, causing RBCs to sickle. Sickle cells are fragile and haemolyse, thus leading to anaemia and jaundice. Splenomegaly may be seen in children (after 10 years, spleen shrinks due to infarction). Other features include, painful swelling of hands and feet (hand and foot syndrome), later leg ulcers, osteomyelitis, renal failure may occur. Patients may also be simply anaemic without any other features. Serum electrophoresis detects HbS.

Treatment includes Hydroxyurea if frequent crises (causes increased production of fetal haemoglobin) or simply blood transfusions to keep HbS level < 30%.

5. Carcinoma stomach is associated with blood group A, *H. pylori* infection, smoking, atrophic gastritis and Adenomatous polyps. The adenocarcinoma may be polypoid, ulcerating or leather bottle type (linitis plastica). Carcinoma stomach may cause gastrointestinal bleeding. Such chronic blood loss will result in iron deficiency anaemia.

Theme 10: Types of emboli

1. Usually, embolism from venous circulation (e.g. DVT) leads to pulmonary embolism via the right side of the heart. Likewise, emboli reaching the systemic circulation (e.g. cerebral/ peripheral arteries) arise from mural thrombus involving left side of heart. However in patients having a patent foramen ovale, a thromboembolus which originated from a deep venous thrombus, may reach the right side of the heart and traverse to the left side through the patent foramen ovale. This is then transported to the systemic circulation leading to cerebral and extremity emboli. This is known as paradoxical embolism.

2. The finger tip nodules described here are Osler's nodes developing secondary to infective endocarditis. Osler's nodes are small tender subcutaneous nodules in pulp of fingers and toes. These develop due to immune complex deposition, leading to painful pulp infarcts. Osler's nodes and Janeway lesions (painless plantar or palmar macules) are pathognomonic of IE. Other features are due to vasculitis, microscopic haematuria, Roth spots, splinter haemorrhages.

   Features of IE due to infection include fever, rigors, anaemia, malaise, splenomegaly. Cardiac lesions present as a new murmur or change in the pre-existing murmur. Septic emboli may cause abscesses in brain, heart, kidney, spleen, GIT, etc.

3. Amniotic fluid emboli lodge in pulmonary circulation, leading to pulmonary embolism. This can present with sudden onset dyspnoea, pleuritic chest pain, haemoptysis and syncope. Absence of lower limb pain or swelling rules out DVT (which is the commonest cause of pulmonary embolism).

Theme 11: Investigation in bites

1. Lyme disease is a tick-borne infection caused by Borrelia burgdorferi. It presents with erythema chronicum migrans which is a small papule developing into a large erythematous ring with central fading. It lasts 48 hours–3 months. Other features include malaise, lymphadenopathy, arthralgia, myocarditis, meningitis, ataxia, etc. Diagnosis is by clinical signs and symptoms and serology.

   Treatment for skin rash is by doxycycline 100 mg/12 hours for 10–21 days.

   For later complications, high dose IV Benzyl penicillin/cefotaxime/ceftriaxone can be given.

2. Human bites are said to be the most dangerous and can result in serious infection. Common human organism includes Eikenella corridens. Staphylococci are also common. Skin swab culture taken from the wound is thus necessary (also to determine sensitivity to antibiotics).

3. Malaria is one of the most common causes of fever and illness in the tropics. Travellers going to malaria-endemic areas can acquire the infection. Hence, chemoprophylaxis with chloroquine is advised. Chemoprophylaxis should begin a week before arrival in the malarious area and continued for at least 4 weeks or preferably 6 weeks after leaving the malarious area.

   Serial thick and thin blood films are taken at the time of fever. Thick films help in rapid detection of malarial parasites, while thin film helps in identification of the plasmodium subtype.

Theme 12: Enzyme defect

1. Creatine kinase is the preferred muscle enzyme to measure in the evaluation of myopathies. Damage to muscle causes CK to leak from the muscle fibre to serum. The MM isoenzyme predominates in skeletal muscle while CK–MB is the marker for cardiac enzyme. MM isoenzyme may be increased in trauma, muscle cramps, generalized seizures, strenuous activity, etc.

2. Troponin T (and I) are very sensitive and cardio-specific enzymes. Since troponin is not normally detectable in the blood of healthy individuals but may increase after acute MI, it is the preferred biochemical marker for MI. It is released within hours and may remain elevated for 10–14 days. Troponin also regulates calcium-mediated contractile process of striated muscle.

3. Low levels of phenylalanine hydroxylase are found in the inborn error of metabolism called phenylketonuria. Thus, phenylalanine cant be converted to tyrosine. Also, the cells are not able to effectively utilize other amino acids because of high concentration of phenylalanine. The brain cells are deprived of amino acids, which are essential nutrients for their maturation and myelination during the period of rapid neurological development. Child is usually normal in the first month of life. Neurological signs e.g. irritability, tremors, hyperkinesis, hypertonia manifest after some weeks. Development is markedly retarded, resulting in gross intellectual impairment. Other features include blond hair, blue iris and fair skin. Skin is more vulnerable to minor inflammatory lesions, rashes and eczema.

   Investigations include:

   i. Guthrie's test which is based on growth of Bacillus subtilis.

   ii. 10% ferric chloride added to patients urine gives emerald green colour.

   iii. Increased phenylalanine levels and presence of abnormal urinary metabolites of phenylalanine.

   Treatment consists of restriction of phenylalanine in diet of infants, which is to be continued till 8–10 years of age.

4. Cystathionine synthetase deficiency in the liver is the most common form of homocystinaemia. Cystathionine is not synthesized from homocysteine and serine.

   Clinical features include

   • subluxation of the lens due to deficiency of cystine.

   • recurrent thrombo-embolic episodes due to increased stickiness of platelets and activation of Hageman factor caused by accumulation of homocystine.

   • convulsions, mental retardation (due to high methionine level in brain) and osteoporosis (as cystine is required for collagen synthesis).

   Treatment consists of restriction of methionine in diet starting early in life and high doses of pyridoxine.

5. Amino transferases are increased more in hepatocellular damage, whereas alkaline phosphatase and γ–glutamyl transferase (GGT) are increased more in cholestatic conditions. Amongst the aminotransferases, alanine amino transferase (SGPT) is more specific for liver diseases, except alcoholic liver disease where aspartate aminotransferase (SGOT) increases more.

Theme 13: Bone investigations

1. The patient is most likely suffering from multiple myeloma, as:
   - It affects adults above 40 years of age. Men are affected more often than women.
   - Most common presenting complaint is severe pain in lumbar and thoracic spine. Pathological fractures, especially of the vertebrae, are common.
   - ESR is raised.
   Diagnosis may be established by serum electrophoresis, which shows an abnormal spike in the region of gamma globulin (myeloma spike).
   Other features seen in multiple myeloma are:
   - Multiple punched out lesions seen on X-rays (in skull and flat bones).
   - Increased serum calcium.
   - Urine –Bence Jones proteins (found in 30%).

2. Sacroilitis is the common presentation of ankylosing spondylitis. Thus, X-ray spine is done to look for other features pointing towards this diagnosis.
   X-ray lumbar spine shows:
   - Squaring of the vertebrae
   - Loss of lumbar lordosis
   - Bridging osteophytes
   - Bamboo spine appearance
   Also, ESR is raised
   HLA B27–positive
   Treatment is mostly conservative, consisting of NSAIDs and physiotherapy.

3. Foot-drop is commonly due to injury to common peroneal nerve or its spinal nerve roots. Since X-ray shows narrowing between L4 and L5, an MRI is done. MRI is the investigation of choice to evaluate the type and extent of compression of the cord in spinal injuries, Pott's spine etc. It also shows the condition of underlying neural tissues and thus helps in predicting the prognosis.

Theme 14: Diabetes mellitus

1. Cushing's syndrome occurs due to chronic glucocorticoid excess. The most common cause of the syndrome is cushing's disease (ACTH-dependent). This consists of adrenal hyperplasia due to excess ACTH from a pituitary tumour. It is commoner in women. Peak age is 30–50 years. Clinical features: increased weight, menstrual irregularity, amenorrhoea, moon facies, hirsutism, impotence, muscle weakness, purple abdominal striae, osteoporosis, buffalo hump, central obesity, hypertension and hyperglycaemia.
   Best screening test is overnight dexamethasone suppression test.
   24 hours urinary free cortisol is an alternative investigation (normal < 280 nmol/24 hours).
   Treatment depends on the cause.
   For adrenal or pituitary adenomas, surgery may be done, which is followed by radiotherapy and medical treatment.

2. Hypoglycaemia is the commonest endocrine emergency. Plasma glucose level < 2.5 mmol/L implies hypoglycaemia.
   Symptoms are either
   - Autonomic (sweating, hunger, tremors) or
   - Neuroglycopenic (drowsiness, personality changes, fits).
   Hypoglycaemia is of two types:
   i. Fasting hypoglycaemia– The most common cause is insulin or sulfonylurea treatment in a known diabetic.
   ii. Post-prandial hypoglycaemia which is seen particularly after gastric surgery (dumping). Treatment is with oral sugar and a long acting starch. If the patient is in coma, IV glucose or glucagon SC is given.

3. The patient is suffering from diabetes mellitus. Type I (IDDM, Insulin Dependant Diabetes Mellitus) is usually juvenile onset. It is characterized by insulin deficiency. Such patients are prone to ketoacidosis.

Type II DM (NIDDM, Non-Insulin Dependent Diabetes Mellitus) develops usually in the obese and elderly. It occurs due to impaired insulin secretion and/or insulin resistance.

Investigations include fasting venous plasma glucose (> 7 mmol/L. In cases of doubt, the 2 hour value in oral glucose tolerance test (after giving 75 g of glucose) of > 11.1 mmol/L confirms the diagnosis. NIDDM patients can be managed with diet control and oral hypo-glycaemic agents (sulfonylureas, biguanides, thiazolidinediones etc) and rarely require insulin, whereas IDDM patients are managed with insulin given subcutaneously.

Theme 15: Cause of hypertension

1. Hypertension and bruit audible in the abdomen is suggestive of renal artery stenosis.

The most common cause of hypertension is primary/essential hypertension. The most common secondary cause is renal, of which ¾th are due to renal parenchymal diseases, and ¼th are due to renovascular causes (mostly renal artery stenosis due to atheromas).

Renal artery stenosis can be diagnosed by renal arteriography.

2. Phaeochromocytoma is a rare catecholamine producing tumour, 90% of which are in the adrenal medulla.

Clinical features include episodic hypertension, restlessness, anxiety, chest tightness, pallor, weakness, palpitations, claudication, flushing, postural hypotension, vomiting, cold feet, tremors, abdominal pain, weight loss, skin mottling, pins and needles etc.

Symptoms are exacerbated by stress, stretching, surgery, sex, parturition or by cheese, alcohol and tricyclics.

Investigations include 24 hour urine for VMA, HMMA or total (or free) metadrenalines for screening.

Further investigations may include MIBG scan, abdominal CT/MRI scan for localization. Treatment is by surgical removal of the tumour.

(Remember: For BP control pre-operatively, an α-blocker e.g. phenoxybenzamine is given before β-blockers e.g. propranolol).

3. Cushing's syndrome occurs due to chronic glucocorticoid excess. The most common cause of the syndrome is cushing's disease (ACTH dependent). This consists of adrenal hyperplasia due to excess ACTH from a pituitary tumour. It is commoner in women. Peak age is 30–50 years. Clinical features: increased weight, menstrual irregularity, amenorrhoea, moon facies, hirsutism, impo-

tence, muscle weakness, purple abdominal striae, osteoporosis, buffalo hump, central obesity, hypertension and hyperglycaemia.

Best screening test is overnight dexamethasone suppression test.

24 hours urinary free cortisol is an alternative investigation (normal < 280 nmol/24 hours).

Treatment depends on the cause.

For adrenal or pituitary adenomas, surgery may be done, which is followed by radiotherapy and medical treatment.

4. The features described here (hypertension, hypokalaemia and altered serum phosphate) are due to primary hyperaldosteronism which implies excess production of aldosterone, independent of renin-angiotensin system. More than 50% of these cases are due to unilateral adrenocortical adenoma (i.e. Conn's syndrome).

Investigations include serum electrolytes, increased aldosterone and decreased renin, CT/MR1 of abdomen for localizing the tumour. Treatment is by surgery (spironolactone is given for 4 weeks pre-operatively as 300 mg/24 hours).

Theme 16: Diagnosis of thyroid disease

1. Symptoms of hyperthyroidism or thyrotoxicosis include:

   Weight loss despite increase in appetite, heat intolerance, sweating, diarrhoea, tremors irritability, emotional lability, psychosis, oligomenorrhoea and infertility.

   Signs include tachycardia, warm peripheries, fine tremors, goitre, hair thinning, palmar erythema and lid lag.

   Grave's disease is an autoimmune disorder due to antibodies against TSH receptors. It is especially common in women 30–50 years of age. Additional signs in Graves' disease include exophthalmos, ophthalmoplegia, thyroid bruit, vitiligo, pretibial myxoedema and thyroid acropachy.

   There is an increase in T_3 and T_4 and decrease in TSH levels.

   Immediate symptomatic control is achieved by propranolol. Antithyroid drugs used are carbimazole or propylthiouracil. Partial thyroidectomy or radio-iodine (I^{131}) may be required in some.

2. Symptoms of hypothyroidism include tiredness, lethargy, weight gain, constipation, cold intolerance, menorrhagia, hoarse voice, depression, dementia and myalgia. Clinical signs are bradycardia, dry skin and hair, goitre, slowly relaxing reflexes (hung-up reflexes), non pitting oedema, toad-like facies, pericardial effusion, CCF, peripheral neuropathy and cerebellar ataxia.

   Investigations show decreased T_4 and increased TSH (in thyroid failure). In secondary hypothyroidism due to decreased TSH from pituitary, TSH is normal or decreased

   Treat with thyroxine if TSH 10, or thyroid autoantibodies are positive, or previous Graves' disease, otherwise monitor TSH annually.

3. Amiodarone is a class III anti-arrhythmic drug. Its effects on the thyroid are complex and

variable. It commonly causes a rise in free T_4, and a fall in free T_3. But clinically the patient may remain euthyroid. Amiodarone contains significant amounts of iodine. In some patients, it causes a thyroiditis-like picture and mild transient hyperthyroidism. But in those with thyroid autonomy, severe thyrotoxicosis may be precipitated and may even persist for upto 6 months after the drug has been stopped due to its slow release from the adipose tissue.
- Antithyroid drug is given as long as amiodarone is prescribed.

4. Hard, fixed thyroid swelling is suggestive of anaplastic (undifferentiated) carcinoma. Local infiltration is an early feature of these tumours which spreads by both lymphatics and by blood stream. They are more common in elderly women, and are extremely lethal. Survival for more than 1–2 years after presentation is unusual.

Treatment is either palliative (radiotherapy or combination chemotherapy) or surgical. Curative resection is justified only if there is no infiltration through the thyroid capsule and no metastasis.

Theme 17: Prenatal screening: Diagnosis

1. Down's syndrome is a genetic disorder caused due to non disjunction leading to trisomy of chromosome 21. Maternal serum AFP, unconjugated oestriol and total human chorionic gonadotropin are assessed, (the 'Triple test') in relation to maternal age, weight and gestation to estimate the risk of Down's syndrome. In an affected pregnancy, level of AFP and unconjugated oestriol tend to be low while that of HCG is high. A child with Down's syndrome will have a flat facial profile, abundant neck skin, dysplastic ears, muscle hypotonia, dysplastic pelvis (evident on X-rays), round head, protuding tongue, Brushfield's spots, short broad hands with single palmar crease, widely spaced 1st and 2nd toes a high arched palate. Patients with Down's syndrome are associated with duodenal atresia, VSD, patent ductus, ASD, low IQ and a small stature.

2. Raised AFP levels are found in: open neural tube defects, multiple pregnancy, Intra-uterine fetal death, anterior abdominal wall defects and renal anomalies in the fetus. Spina bifida which implies an incomplete vertebral arch is a myelodysplasia (neural tube defect). Babies born with spina bifida often have a small skin covered lesion (a meningococele). A maternal serum α fetoprotein level of > 90 U/ml at 18 weeks detects almost 80% of open spina bifidas. In mothers who already have an affected baby, folic acid 5 mg/day should be given before conception (as the neural tube is formed by 4 weeks, i.e. before pregnancy may even be recognized). If there is no past history of neural tube defects, 0.4 mg of folic acid is recommended before conception to 13 weeks after. Many surgeries may be needed to rectify spina bifida.

3. Duchenne's muscular dystrophy, presents in boys between 1–6 years of age. They have

waddling, clumsy gait. Selective washing causes calf pseudohypertrophy. Later wheelchairs are needed. Aim is to keep the boy walking with the help of knee–ankle–foot orthoses. Creatine kinase is raised and muscle biopsy shows abnormal fibres surrounded by the fat and fibrous tissue. Spinal fixation with Luque operation or bracing helps scoliosis. But there is no specific treatment and genetic counselling is important.

4. In mothers who already have an affected baby, folic acid 5 mg/day should be given before conception as the neural tube is formed by 4 weeks, i.e. before pregnancy may even be recognized. If there is no past history of neural tube defects, 0.4 mg of folic acid is recommended before conception to 13 weeks after.

5. Alzheimer's dementia is the most common form of dementia in UK. Suspect AD in any enduring, acquired deficit of memory and cognition. Onset may be from 40 years though it may be seen earlier in patients suffering from Down's syndrome. On histological examination plaques with neurofibrillary tangles and cortical β-amyloid protein are found. On MRI an increased cortical atrophy in the medial temporal lobe can be seen. In stage I of AD there is falling memory and spatial disorientation. In stage II the personality disintegrates and in stage III the patient is apathetic, wasted and bedridden.

6. Cystic fibrosis is an autosomal recessive condition caused by mutation in cystic fibrosis transmembrane conductance regulator (CFTR) gene on chromosome 7. It leads to defective chloride secretion and increased sodium absorption across the epithelium. The changes in the composition of airway surface liquid predisposes the lung to chronic pulmonary infections and bronchiectasis. At present prenatal diagnosis is offered only to parents who are known carriers, usually because they have an affected child already. Screening can be done using fetal DNA from amniotic fluid cells or from chorionic villous sampling. Clinical features include failure to thrive, meconium ileus in neonates, cough, wheeze, recurrent chest infections, bronchiectasis, haemoptysis, respiratory failure, pancreatic insufficiency (diabetes mellitus, steatorrhoea), distal intestinal obstruction, gallstones, cirrhosis, sinusitis, nasal polyps, male infertility, etc.

Sweat test is positive in cystic fibrosis; Na > 60 mmol/L and sweat Cl > 70 mmol/L on two occasions. Management is symptomatic.

Theme 18: CT findings in hearing loss: Diagnosis

1. Cholesteatoma develops as a complication of chronic suppurative otitis media. It is defined as the presence of keratinising squamous epithelium in the middle ear or mastoid antrum. Once cholesteatoma enters the middle ear cleft, it invades the surrounding structures by enzymatic bone destruction. It has the property to destroy bone due to enzymes, such as collagenase, acid phosphatase and proteolytic enzymes. Thus, it may cause destruction of ear ossicles, erosion of the bony labyrinth, etc. It presents as a white mass in the middle ear and causes conductive hearing loss.

2. Otitis media with effusion is also known as serous or secretory otitis media, or glue ear. The following points favour this diagnosis here:
   i. It is common in school-going children (3–12 years).
   ii. There is accumulation of non-purulent effusion in the middle ear cleft.
   iii. There is no destruction of bones.
   iv. There is clouding of mastoid air cells due to fluid (seen in X-ray of mastoids).

   It presents with a conductive hearing loss and delayed speech in children.

   On otoscopy tympanic membrane appears dull and retracted. Fluid level and air bubbles may be seen through the tympanic membrane.

   Treatment includes decongestants, antihistaminics (antiallergic), middle ear aeration (valsalva manoeuvre). Surgical treatment is with myringotomy and aspiration of fluid. In recurrent cases, a grommet insertion may be required.

3. Otosclerosis or otospongiosis is an autosomal dominant hereditary disorder. It consists of foci of irregularly laid spongy bone which replaces normal dense enchondral layers of bony otic capsule. It most commonly affects the stapes, but may also involve the cochlea. Half of the patients have a family history of the disorder. It is more common in females. Deafness usually starts between 20–30 years of age. It may involve the cochlea and cause sensorineural hearing loss. Hearing loss is conductive and often bilateral. Paracusis willisii i.e. patient hears better in noisy than quiet surroundings, is often seen. Symptoms are usually excacerbated due to pregnancy, menstruation and menopause.

   On otoscopy, reddish hue may be seen through the tympanic membrane (Schwartz's sign). In pure tone audiometry, there is a dip in bone conduction curve called the Carhart's notch (maximum at 2000 Hz).

   Sodium fluoride has been tried as a mode of treatment. Stapedectomy is the treatment of choice.

4. The physiological aging process is associated with sensorineural hearing loss called presbyacusis. This occurs due degeneration of the organ of corti. Higher frequencies are affected. There is difficulty in hearing in the presence of background noise and recruitment phenomenon is positive in which all sounds suddenly become intolerable when volume is raised. CT scan will be normal in these cases.

Theme 19: Causes of epistaxis

1. Orf is caused by DNA viruses belonging to pox virus family. It is a zoonotic disease transmitted from sheep, and may cause epistaxis.
2. Trauma inflicted on the nose from the front, side or below can result in injuries to the septum. Septal injuries with mucosal tears cause profuse epistaxis (while those with intact mucosa cause a septal haematoma, which causes absorption of the septal cartilage and saddle nose deformity). Air passing through a septal perforation will also produce a gurgling sound.
3. Exposure to nickel and chromium predisposes to development of cancer of paranasal sinuses. Chromium is also known to be a causative factor in the development of nasopharyngeal carcinoma which can cause epistaxis.
4. Hypertension is the most common cause of epistaxis in the elderly. It mostly causes posterior epistaxis from the postero-superior part of the nasal cavity. Bleeding may be severe. If there is no active bleed, treatment would consist of observation with control of hypertension.
5. Coagulopathies are known to be more common in young girls. Persistent bleeding (e.g. after dental extraction) is caused by coagulation disorders or coagulopathies.

Theme 20: ENT: Diagnosis

1. Carcinoma maxillary sinus is more common in men aged 40–60 years. Early features include nasal stuffiness, blood stained nasal discharge, headache, facial paraesthesia and epiphora. Further, spread to the nasal cavity can cause nasal obstruction and epistaxis. Anterior spread causes swelling of the cheek and invasion of facial skin. It may also spread superiorly and inferiorly causing proptosis, diplopia, ocular pain, epiphora, dental pain, loosening of teeth, ulceration of the gingiva etc. X-ray of the sinus may show clouding. Treatment consists of combination of radio-therapy and surgery.
2. Nasal polypi are non-neoplastic masses of oedematous nasal or sinus mucosa. They are mostly seen in cases of allergic or vasomotor rhinitis. Nasal polyps are of 2 types:
   i. Bilateral multiple ethmoidal polyps.
   ii. Single unilateral antrochoanal polyps.
   Clinical features include nasal stuffiness leading to total nasal obstruction, loss of sense of smell, watery discharge, sneezing, mass protruding from the nose and hyponasality of voice. Polypectomy is done generally by endoscopy.

Theme 21: Diagnosis of GI conditions

1. *H. Pylori* is the most common cause of chronic gastritis. *H. Pylori* or Helicobacter pylori is a spiral organism which exclusively colonises gastric epithelium (found in duodenum only in the patches of gastric metaplasia). It is capable of producing urease which converts urea to ammonia and hence buffers gastric acidity. It is a motile organism, and is associated with duodenal ulcers most strongly. It is also associated with gastric ulcers, gastric cancer, gastric B cell lymphomas and rarely, non-ulcer dyspepsia. The ^{13}C–urea breath is the best noninvasive test for detecting *H. pylori*. *H pylori* eradication requires 'triple therapy' with lansoprazole, clarithromycin, amoxicillin/metronidazole, all given for 1 week.

2. Change of lower oesophageal epithelium from squamous to columnar is known as Barrett's oesophagus (this option was not given in the question paper). Barrett's oesophagus occurs as a consequence of chronic gastro-oesophageal reflux disease (GORD). It is recognised endoscopically as areas of pink, gastric like mucosa extending from the cardia into the oesophagus.

   Risk of adenocarcinoma of oesophagus is increased 40 fold in Barrett's oesophagus therefore regular endoscopy and biopsy are required for early diagnosis of the malignancy.

3. Duodenal ulcers are the more common form of peptic ulcers. These present with epigastric pain typically occurring before meals, worse at night and relieved by eating or drinking milk. 50% are asymptomatic. The rest present with recurrent episodes of above mentioned symptoms. They have a strong association with *H.pylori*.

   Duodenal ulcers are diagnosed by upper G.I. endoscopy.

   Treatment consists of life-style modification and *H. pylori* eradication.

Theme 22: Upper GI bleeding

1. Primary biliary cirrhosis is characterized by damage of inter lobular bile ducts by chronic granulomatous inflammation causing progressive cholestasis, cirrhosis and portal hypertension. It is most probably an autoimmune disorder. 90% of patients are women. Peak age at presentation is 40–60 years.

   It presents with pruritis, jaundice, skin pigmentation, xanthelasma, hepatomegaly and splenomegaly. Upper GI bleeding may occur secondary to portal hypertension leading to lower oesophageal variceal haemorrhage.

   Diagnosis is established by increased hepatic enzymes (alkaline phosphate and γ GT especially) and presence of antimitochondrial antibodies (positive in 98%).

2. 80–90% of the patients with peptic ulcer have *H. pylori* infection. Patients with peptic ulcer may present with complications such as haematemesis. *H. pylori* eradication in such patients is imperative for definitive treatment. *H. pylori* eradication is done by 'triple therapy' which includes Lansoprazole 30 mg 12 hourly with Clarithromycin 500 mg 12 hourly with Amoxicillin 1 gm 12 hourly (or Metronidazole 40 mg 12 hourly). All these drugs are given for 1 week.

3. The mention of evidence of spiral forms in microscopy suggests that endoscopy with biopsy has already been done and *H. pylori* presence has been confirmed on microscopy. Once bleeding has stopped, the diagnosis of the cause of bleeding should be sought after. Diagnostic procedures should be done within 24 hours of bleeding because erosions and tears can heal rapidly. GI endoscopy and barium meal are two favoured investigations in cases of upper GI bleed. Since endoscopy has already been done, barium meal examination should be done now.

4. Upper GI bleed with retching and vomiting is due to oesophagitis. On endoscopy, it appears as a range of findings, from mild redness to severe, bleeding ulceration with stricture formation. Management comprises lifestyle changes and antacids. H_2-receptor antagonists help relieve the symptoms without healing oesophagitis. Proton pump inhibitors are the treatment of choice: Symptoms resolve and oesophagitis heals in majority of patients.

5. This is a case of NSAID associated peptic ulcer with erosion which has led to bleeding and hence tarry stools. The 1st step in the management in such patient is to stop NSAIDs if possible. Or else H_2-receptor antagonists (e.g. cimetidine, ranitidine), proton pump inhibitors (e.g. lansoprazole) or misoprostol can be used.

Theme 23: Pre-operative investigation

1. An irregular pulse is suggestive of atrial fibrillation or heart block. ECG is indicated pre-operatively in all patients above 65 years of age, with poor exercise tolerance, with history of MI, hypertension, rheumatic fever or other heart diseases.

2. Hepatitis B, C, D and GB can spread through blood products and via IV drug abusers. Such patients are also at a risk of HIV. As a part of pre-operative management, such patients must be screened for HIV and hepatitis viruses, after appropriate counselling and consent.

3. U & E, full blood count and blood glucose are tested in most patients pre-operatively. As in this case the GMC has mentioned that the patient is fit we presume that the history, examination and baseline investigations of the patients have not revealed any abnormality. Therefore nothing needs to be done for this patient.

4. Sickle test is performed pre-operatively in all patients from Africa, West Indies and Mediterranean region. Sickle test is also done in patients whose origins are in malarial endemic areas (including most of India).

5. The mention of fever with history of dental extraction makes it necessary to rule out infective endocarditis in this patient. Golden rule: fever with a new murmur implies endocarditis until proved otherwise. Any cause of bacteraemia (e.g. dental extraction) predisposes valves to the risk of bacterial colonization. Echocardiography should be done in this patient to rule out any valvular vegetations. Transthoracic echocardiography may show vegetations > 2 mm size. Transoesophageal echocardiography is more sensitive and better for visualizing mitral valve lesions.

Theme 24: Palliative care/analgesia

1. Supplementary O_2 or morphine should be considered in patients having malignancy and presenting with breathlessness. Benzodiazepines and relaxation techniques are usually sufficient as the cause of breathlessness is mostly anxiety. Since morphine has its own side effects such as nausea, benzodiazepines would be a better choice in this patient. Moreover since the patient is suffering from anorexia, oral route is not indicated and hence benzodiazepines need to be given by the intravenous route.

2. The analgesic 'ladder' consists broadly of three steps. Step I includes non-opioid analgesics like aspirin, paracetamol and NSAIDs. Step II includes weak opioids such as codeine, dihydrocodeine and dextropropoxyphene. Step III includes strong opioids such as morphine, diamorphine and hydromorphine. The presentation in the patient is suggestive of bony metastasis in which even strong opioids are usually ineffective for pain relief. Radiotherapy is the mainstay in such patients for pain relief. 8–30 Gy dosage is delivered in 1, 2, 5 or 10 fractions.

3. The analgesic 'ladder' consists broadly of three steps. Step I includes non-opioid analgesics like aspirin, paracetamol and NSAIDs. Step II includes weak opioids such as codeine, dihydrocodeine and dextropropoxyphene. Step III includes strong opioids such as morphine, diamorphine and hydromorphine. Most ductal carcinomas of the pancreas present with metastasis. Most patients with disabling pain respond either to strong opioid analgesia or radiotherapy. As IV morphine has not been able to help, radiotherapy must be given to the patient.

4. This is another case of metastatic carcinoma. Such patients usually require the analgesia falling on the step III of the analgesic 'ladder'.

Patients are started on oral morphine initially. Patients not responding may be either given a higher dosage or given via a parenteral route or given a still stronger opioid.

5. The patient in this case is not responding to oral morphine and hence either the dose should be increased or the route be changed. Giving morphine SC via a syringe driver would have the advantage of a stable drug concentration in the blood and may alleviate pain on a lesser dosage itself.

6. As explained in the second question.

Theme 25: Management of chronic renal failure

1. Management of pulmonary oedema in renal failure includes high flow O_2, venous vasodilators and intravenous diuretics e.g. frusemide. Venesection (100–200 ml) should be considered in patient in extremis. If no response, urgent haemodialysis is necessary. Other indications for haemodialysis in renal failure include persistent hyperkalaemia (K^+ ≥ 7 mmol/L), severe or worsening metabolic acidosis (pH < 7.2 or base excess < − 10), uraemic pericarditis and uraemic encephalopathy.

2. Hyperkalaemia may cause arrhythmias or cardiac arrest. ECG shows tall 'tented' T waves, small or absent P waves, increased PR interval, widened QRS complex. Its treatment requires (i) 10 ml 10% calcium gluconate IV over 1 minute repeated till ECG improves (ii) IV insulin with glucose. Calcium resonium PO or PR can also be considered. Haemodialysis is indicated if K ≥ 7 mmol/L. Other indications for haemodialysis include severe or worsening metabolic acidosis (pH < 7.2 or base excess < −10), refractory pulmonary oedema, uraemic pericarditis and uraemic encephalopathy.

3. End stage renal failure implies the degree of renal failure that, without renal replacement therapy, would lead to death. A full blood count in a patient with renal failure shows a normocytic normochromic anaemia. The anaemia of renal failure is partly due to erythropoietin deficiency. Once other causes of anaemia e.g. iron deficiency, infections etc. have been ruled out, recombinant erythropoietin can be administered to maintain Hb > 10 g/dL. The maintenance dose of erythropoietin is 50–150 units/kg twice weekly.

4. Adult polycystic kidney disease is an autosomal dominant condition with genes on chromosomes 16 & 4. Patients present with renal enlargement with cysts, abdominal pain, haematuria, UTI, renal calculi, hypertension or renal failure. An abdominal USG is sufficient to diagnose.

Even a small drop in blood pressure may help in saving significant renal function in patients with renal failure. ACE inhibitors such as captopril can decrease rate of loss of function even if blood pressure is within normal range. Note: There is little evidence of benefit due to ACE inhibitors in patient of hypertension due to polycystic kidney disease.

Theme 26: Urological investigations

1. Hypercalcaemia and hypercalciuria are predisposing risk factors for recurrent renal stones. Causes of hypercalcaemia include malignancy, Hyperparathyroidism, sarcoidosis, vitamin D intoxication, Addison's disease, Cushing's syndrome, lithium etc. Out of the options given in the theme parathormone needs to be measured. It will not only diagnosis the condition as hyperparathyroidism but will also diagnosis the subtype. Hypercalcaemia with increase in PTH is seen in primary and tertiary hyperparathyroidism. Hypocalcaemia with increase in PTH is seen in secondary hyperparathyroidism. Hypercalcaemia with decrease in PTH seen in malignant hyperparathyroidism. Hypercalcaemia with normal PTH level is seen in primary hyperparathyroidism.

2. Renal calculi is a possibility in patients with prostatic carcinoma as it a cause of hypercalcaemia which itself is a risk factor for renal calculus. The fact that X-rays do not reveal anything almost rules out obstruction due to calculi. This is most probably a case of extramural obstruction due to impinging prostatic carcinoma over the urethra causing bilateral hydronephrosis. Bilateral obstruction carriers a poor prognosis unless treated urgently. Urethral or suprapubic catheter are used for treating lower tract obstruction but since it is not mentioned in the options, nephrostomy which is done to relieve acute upper tract obstruction, needs to be done here.

3. This is a case of urinary tract infection due to obstruction. The presentation of patient with loin pain, fever and hydronephrosis is suggestive of acute pyelonephritis. To facilitate visualization of a suspected lesion in a ureter or renal pelvis, retrograde or antegrade urography should be attempted. In fact these studies are preferred over IVU in azotaemic patients. The retrograde approach involves catheterization of involved ureter while antegrade technique necessitates placement of a catheter in the renal pelvis, percutaneously. Since these two are not mentioned in the options, urine culture is performed to know of the organism and its sensitivity pattern. Cefuroxime 1.5 gm 8 hourly or Trimethoprim or Cephalexin are generally given post operative for 10–14 days in patients with acute pyelonephritis.

4. As the patient has been operated for carcinoma cervix the cause of obstruction and hence anuria and bilateral hydronephrosis, most likely is ligation of, or injury to the ureters during the surgery. Such patients would require an IVU to accurately localize the site and degree of obstruction.

Theme 27: Red eye: Investigations

1. The area of occupation in this case is suggestive of foreign body in the eye. Remember that one should have a low threshold for diagnosing an intraocular foreign body and help. X-ray of the orbit is a must in all suspected cases of foreign body. Orbital ultrasound may be required for suspected high velocity foreign bodies.

2. This is a case of corneal abrasion possibly due to a twig. Such lesions may cause intense pain and hence blepharospasm. A drop of local anaesthetic e.g. 1% tetracaine should be applied before examination. Corneal lesions stain green with fluorescein stain which helps in the diagnosis. The fluorescein drops are orange and turn yellow on contact with the eye. Such abrasions usually heal within 48 hours with gentamicin eye ointment and padding.

3. Ophthalmic shingles implies zoster of 1st (ophthalmic) branch of the trigeminal nerve. Pain, tingling or numbness around the eye may be seen before the appearance of a blistering rash. In this patient the mention of 'symptoms of conjunctivitis' suggests that one should rule out anterior uveitis. All patients with ophthalmic shingles with nose-tip involvement (Hutchinson's sign) and red eye should be referred to an ophthalmologist to rule out anterior uveitis with a slit lamp.

4. Purulent conjunctivitis can be due to viral or bacterial causes. Adenovirus infection causes small lymphoid aggregates which appear as follicles on conjunctiva. Purulent discharge is more prominent in bacterial conjunctivitis. Purulent discharge may stick the eyes together. Conjunctival swabs are taken in such patients to diagnose and appropriately treat them.

5. Acute closed angle glaucoma is usually seen in the middle aged or elderly. The acute uniocular attack is preceded by blurring of vision or haloes around lights. It is caused due to blockage of drainage of aqueous from anterior chamber via canal of Schlemm. Intraocular pressures rise upto 60–70 mm Hg (Normal value 15–20 mm Hg). Patients may present with ocular pain, headache, diminished vision, corneal oedema, circumcorneal redness, dilated and fixed pupil and a hard eye. Patients must be admitted and intraocular pressures must be monitored.

Theme 28: Poisoning: Diagnosis

1. Opiate overdose may be deliberate or accidental, in combination with alcohol and benzodiazepines or due to use of heroin of unexpected purity. Opiates may cause coma, respiratory depression, pinpoint pupils, hypotension and constipation. Naloxone is the specific antidote.

2. As such there are no clear cut interaction patterns between tricyclics and diazepam but diazepam in hypnotic doses can cause dizziness, vertigo, ataxia, disorientation, amnesia and prolongation of reaction time. Tricyclics on the other hand, potentiate CNS depressants e.g. alcohol and antihistaminics.

3. Digoxin toxicity can cause yellow green visual haloes, arrhythmias, nausea, anorexia and poor cognition. Digoxin-specific antibody fragments are given to such patients as an antidote.

4. Metoclopramide is an antiemetic. Its toxicity can cause sedation, diarrhoea and muscle dystonias. Long term use can lead to parkinsonism, galactorrhoea and gynaecomastia.

5. More than 150 mg/kg or 12 gm of paracetamol in adults can be fatal. Prompt treatment can prevent liver failure and death. Patients with paracetamol toxicity may present with vomiting, RUQ pain, and anorexia in the first 24 hours. Liver damage is detectable only after 18 hours of ingestion of the drug. Maximum liver damage occurs 72–96 hours after ingestion. Liver damage can be assessed by plasma ALT and AST or prothrombin time. Hepatic failure, manifest as jaundice and encephalopathy, may be seen between 3rd and 5th day. Methionine and N–acetylcysteine are antidotes in paracetamol poisoning.

Theme 29: Drugs reactions and toxicity

1. In prolonged vitamin B_{12} deficiency there may be megaloblastic anaemia or neurological degeneration or both. Vitamin B_{12} is required for the integrity of myelin. In severe disease there is diffuse and uneven demyelination. It may manifest as peripheral neuropathy or spinal cord degeneration or cerebral manifestations (resembling dementia) or optic atrophy.

2. The dose of lithium given should aim to achieve a plasma level of ~0.7–1.0 mmol/L. Early signs of toxicity can be seen at plasma levels of ~1.5 mmol/L of lithium. Features of lithium toxicity include blurred vision, diarrhoea and vomiting, hypokalaemia, drowsiness, ataxia, coarse tremors, dysarthria, hyperextension, seizures, psychosis, coma and shock.

3. Metoclopramide is an antiemetic. Its toxicity can cause sedation, diarrhoea and muscle dystonias. Long term use can lead to parkinsonism, galactorrhoea and gynaecomastia.

4. Therapeutic range of carbamazepine is 20–50 mmol/L in the plasma. It is a first line drug for partial seizures and second line drug for generalized seizures. It is also useful in post-herpetic neuralgia. The drug should be started as 100 mg 12 hourly PO. Toxic effects of the drug include rash, nausea, diplopia, dizziness, ataxia, nystagmus, fluid retention, hyponatraemia and blood dyscrasias.

5. Patients with herpes who develop herpetic neuralgia require oral analgesics or low dose amitriptyline for control of pain. Pain in a dermatomal distribution precedes malaise and fever by a few days. Thoracic dermatomes and the ophthalmic division of trigeminal nerve are most vulnerable. In this case one should try to control pain with oral analgesics such as paracetamol or other NSAIDs.

6. β-blockers block β-adrenoceptors. β_1 blocking causes negatively inotropic and chronotropic effect. β_2 blocking causes peripheral

vasoconstriction and bronchoconstriction. β blockers are used in patients of angina, hypertension, post MI and heart failure. They are contraindicated in patients of Asthma, PVD and heart block. Side effects include lethargy, impotence, nightmares and headache. Severe bradycardia and hypotension can be seen at toxic levels.

Theme 30: Treatment of STDs

1. Gonorrhoea is due to Neisseria gonorrhoea infection. Females affected with the organism may be either asymptomatic or present with vaginal discharge, dysuria, proctitis. Males generally present with purulent urethral discharge, dysuria, proctitis and tenesmus. Ophthalmia neonatorum is an obstetric complication which presents as a purulent discharge from the eye of a neonate less than 21 days old. Treatment is with a single dose of Amoxicillin 3 gm PO with probenecid 1 gm PO. Ofloxacin or ciprofloxacin PO are used if penicillin allergy/resistance or with pharyngeal infection.

2. Chlamydia trachomatis is the commonest bacterial sexually transmitted infection in industrialized countries. Highest prevalence is noted in women under 25 years of age. In men it is most common cause of non gonococcal urethritis. In women it causes cervicitis and PID. ELISA, PCR, ligase chain reaction (LCR) and direct fluorescent antibody (DFA) tests can be used for diagnosis. Uncomplicated cases can be treated by doxycycline 100 mg twice daily for 1 week. For pregnant patients, erythromycin 500 mg twice daily for 2 weeks or azithromycin 1 gm single dose can be given.

3. As explained above.

4. Thrush (candida albicans) is the most common cause of vaginal discharge which is typically white curds. Pregnancy, immunodeficiencies, diabetes, the pill and antibiotics are known risk factors. Strings of mycelium and oval spores can be seen on microscopy. Treatment is with a single imidazole pessary e.g. Clotrimazole 500 mg and cream application for the vulva.

5. Bacterial vaginosis presents with a fishy smelling discharge. Vaginal pH is > 5.5. Causative organisms include Gardnerella vaginalis, Mycoplasma hominis, Peptostreptococci and Bacteroides species. There is increased risk

of preterm labour and amniotic infection in pregnant women. Stippled vaginal epithelial 'clue cells' are seen on wet microscopy. Treatment is with metronidazole 400 mg 12 hourly PO for 5 days or 2 gm PO or PV gel or clindamycin 2% vaginal cream application at night PV for 7 times.

Theme 31: Gynaecology: Next step of management

1. Cervical cancer has a pre invasive phase—CIN i.e. Cervical Intraepithelial Neoplasia. Papanicolaou smears identify women who need cervical biopsy. Papanicolaou smears can show dyskaryosis which reflects CIN. The main cause of cervical cancer is Human Papilloma virus (HPV 16, 18 and 33). Prolonged usage of OCPs has been implicated as an important co-factor. Patients with smears suggestive of CIN II or III will undergo colposcopy while those with minor changes as mild atypia or inflammation will have a repeat smear.

2. As explained above.

3. The mention of post menopausal dyspareunia is suggestive of atrophic vaginitis. Vaginal dryness due to fallen oestrogen levels, can lead to vaginal and urinary infections, dyspareunia, traumatic bleeding, stress incontinence and prolapse. But always remember the golden rule: all postmenopausal bleeding must be investigated to rule out endometrial carcinoma. Postmenopausal bleeding is an early sign in endometrial carcinoma. Diagnosis is made by uterine sampling or curettage. All parts of the uterine cavity must be sampled.

4. Cervical ectropion also known as erosion is a normal phenomenon. It is seen temporarily due to hormonal influence during puberty, with the use of OCPs (as in this patient) or during pregnancy. As columnar epithelium is soft and glandular, it is prone to bleeding, excess mucus production and to infection. Treatment is with cautery if the condition is very disturbing otherwise no treatment is required.

Theme 32: Gynaecological diagnosis

1. In stress incontinence small quantities of urine escape if intra-abdominal pressure rise e.g. sneezing, laughing etc. It is commonly seen in multiparous women. A prolapse or incontinence may be seen on examination. Mild cases respond to pelvic floor exercises or physiotherapy. Severe cases require operations such as urethroplasty or trans-abdominal colposuspension. In patients with mixed stress and urge incontinence, detrusor instability should be treated first as this can be made worse by operations for stress incontinence.

2. The bladder is unstable in urge incontinence with high detrusor muscle activity. It is seen in both nulliparous and parous women. No organic cause is found in most cases. The condition improves with 'bladder training' i.e. gradually increasing the time interval between voiding.

3. Urinary tract infection implies presence of a pure growth of $> 10^5$ colony forming units/mL. *E. coli* is the most common organism causing UTI. Patients may present with features of cystitis e.g. frequency, dysuria, urgency, strangury, haematuria, suprapubic pain or acute pyelonephritis e.g. fever, rigors, vomiting, loin pain and tenderness. Trimethoprim 200 mg 12 hourly PO for 3 days is given for cystitis. Cefuroxime 1.5 gm 8 hourly IV for 10–14 days is given for acute pyelonephritis.

Theme 33: Treatment in skin lesions

1. Eczema can be either atopic (most common form), allergic or caused by irritants or venous stasis. Atopic eczema is usually multifactorial with a genetic predisposition. Staphylococcus aureus colonises lesions and toxins act as a superantigen. Patients with atopic eczema have a low threshold for itching with dry and lined skin. The papules that develop are scratched, become exudative and secondary infection associated with lymphadenopathy ensues. Emollients are essential for dry skin. Topical steroids are applied to areas of active eczema usually twice daily. 1–2.5% hydrocortisone is applied on face and flexures. Strength of steroid depends upon severity, site and age of the patient.

2. The presentation of the child in this case is suggestive of superadded bacterial infection. Secondary infection is very common and vigorous treatment of infection is justified. Antibiotics should be given according to sensitivities of bacteria from time to time. Erythromycin is especially valuable; mupirocin, topically is as effective.

3. As explained in first question.

4. Herpetic whitlow is an occupational disease usually affecting the medical personnel, dentists, nurses and physiotherapists. In children, whitlows can result from autoinoculation. The whitlow is extremely painful. The digits swell, become red and may be accompanied by painful lymphadenopathy and high fever. A day or two later the typical vesicle develops with clear fluid which evolves into a cloudy fluid and then into a yellow crusted lesion. Medical and nursing staff should wear gloves if they are likely to come into contact with lesions or bodily secretions. Likewise medical personnel who have herpetic whitlows should not handle patients. Aciclovir should be given as early as possible i.e. 800 mg 5 times daily PO for 5 days.

5. All patients of Herpes who have ophthalmic involvement, motor involvement, are aged above 50 years and who are immuno-compromised require treatment. Aciclovir should be started immediately 800 mg 5 times daily PO is given for 5 days. 10 mg/kg 8 hourly by slow IV is given for 10 days in immuno-compromised patients.

6. As explained above.

7. Patients with herpes who develop herpetic neuralgia require oral analgesics or low dose amitriptyline for control of pain. Patients with post herpetic neuralgia may require carbamazepine, phenytoin or capsaicin cream.

8. 90 percent of adults in the UK are immune to chicken pox. Shingles is a reactivation that can occur during pregnancy. Diagnosis can be confirmed by electron microscopy and culture of vesicle fluid. Pregnant women are more vulnerable to chicken pox and may develop pneumonitis which can be fatal. Early administration of IV aciclovir may ameliorate the severity but intensive care support may be needed. Varicella zoster can affect fetus in two ways. (i) If infection occurs prior to 20 weeks of gestation, there is a 1% risk of congenital varicella syndrome. (ii) Neonatal chicken pox can occur if mother presents with infection, two days before to five days after delivery.

Theme 34: Convulsions in a child: Management.

1. This seems to be a case of febrile convulsion and hence measures to bring down the fever will prevent further attacks. But since the child is convulsing, immediate IV benzodiazepines are needed to abort the attack. Lorazepam 50–100 μg/kg should be given intravenously.

2. A febrile convulsion is diagnosed if the following occur together. (i) a tonic-clonic, symmetrical generalized seizure (ii) occurring as the temperature rises rapidly (iii) child is aged between 6 months to 5 years (iv) no signs of CNS infection or previous history of convulsion (v) number of seizures is < 3, each lasting < 5 min. 30% of children have recurrences. Parents of such children should be taught to use rectal diazepam with a tube.

3. The presentation of child with fever, rash and convulsions is suggestive of meningococcal meningitis. Diagnosis is made by visualization of gram negative cocci in pairs. Any rash with signs of meningism is to be treated as meningococcal until proved otherwise. Lumbar puncture is crucial for diagnosing meningitis and should be performed until contraindications to the procedure are present. Contraindications for LP include (i) bleeding diathesis (ii) cardiorespiratory compromise (iii) infection at the site of needle insertion (iv) raised intracranial pressure.

4. The mention of obesity of the patient in this case is suggesting an altered metabolism of the drug. Valproate is 90% bound to plasma proteins and is completely metabolised in liver by oxidation and gluconoride conjugation. Drug serum levels should be checked in this case and dose adjusted so that it falls in the therapeutic range.

5. Electroencephalography is useful for distinguishing the various types of seizures. For example, there may be confusion between

disturbances of consciousness due to typical absences, and disturbances due to complex partial seizures. The distinction is important not only for the right therapy to be given, but also has prognostic value.

Theme 35: Epidemiology in psychiatric disorders.

1. Four criteria are typically used for defining anorexia nervosa.
   i. The person choses not to eat, leading to dangerous weight loss.
   ii. The person has intense fear of becoming obese, despite being underweight.
   iii. The person has disturbance in weight perception.
   iv. Amenorrhoea is noted in women.
      It is 20 times more common in females than males. It is the third commonest chronic illness in teenage girls. Cognitive behavioural therapy is used in such cases.
2. Drug addiction is seen more commonly in the younger age group and its incidence decreases with age. The drugs usually involved in addiction are opiates, amphetamines, cocaine, lysergic acid, hydrocarbons ('glue sniffing'), barbiturates and cannabis. Opiate withdrawal can be helped by methadone. Barbiturate withdrawal should be after admission as it may cause seizures and death.
3. Patients with anxiety usually present with tension, agitation, feelings of impending doom, trembling, insomnia, poor concentration, hyperventilation, 'goose flesh', headaches, palpitations, poor appetite and nausea. It may be due to stress e.g. at work or life events or due to genetic predisposition, faulty learning or secondary gain. Anxiolytics, cognitive behavioural therapy, SSRI, hypnosis and progressive relaxation training are different modes of management in such patients.
4. Patients with depression often have somatic symptoms with or without anxiety. Patients may have low mood, loss of interest, socially withdrawn, poor self-esteem, tearfulness, guilt, psychomotor retardation. Management includes addressing the source of distress, psychological interventions and drugs e.g.

fluoxetine, tricyclics. It is seen more commonly in women than in men. Its incidence increases with age.

5. As explained above.

6. Schizophrenia is a common mental disorder which typically presents in adulthood with delusions, hallucinations and disordered thought. The 1st rank symptoms seen in ~70% of patients are (i) Thought insertion (as in this patient) (ii) Thought broadcast (iii) Thought withdrawal (iv) Passivity (v) Hearing voices commenting on the actions of the patients (vi) Primary delusions (vii) Somatic hallucinations.

Theme 36: Neurological diagnosis.

1. Space-occupying lesions in the brain present with features of raised intracranial pressure i.e. headache, vomiting, papilloedema and seizures. Patients may have evolving focal neurological deficit depending upon the site of the lesion. CT & MRI are used for locating the cause. LP is contraindicated. Complete removal of gliomas is difficult as resection margins are rarely clear but surgery does give a tissue diagnosis and allows debulking before radiotherapy can be given.

2. Strokes result from ischaemic infarction or bleeding in brain manifested by acute focal CNS signs and symptoms. Stroke may be due to thrombosis in situ, atherothromboembolism, heart emboli, aneurysmal rupture or trauma. Patients may present with features depending upon the affected site:

    i. In cerebral hemispheric infarcts, patients may present with contralateral hemiplegia which is initially flaccid then becomes spastic, contralateral sensory loss, homonymous hemianopia, dysphasia.

    ii. In brainstem infarct patients may present with quadriplegia, disturbances of gaze and vision, locked in syndrome.

    iii. Patients with lacunar infarcts may have pure motor, pulse sensory, mixed motor and sensory signs or ataxia.

3. Motor neurone disease is caused by degeneration of neurons in motor cortex, cranial nerve nuclei and anterior horn cells. There is no sensory loss in MND as compared to Multiple sclerosis and polyneuropathies. Golden rule: think of MND in those > 40 years of age presenting with foot drop, spastic gait, weak grip or aspiration pneumonia. Patients with upper motor neurone disease present with weakness, spasticity, brisk reflexes, plantars upgoing. Patients with lower motor neurone disease present with weakness, wasting, fasci-

culation of tongue, abdomen, back or thighs. Treatment is essentially symptomatic.

4. Multiple sclerosis is a chronic disorder which consists of plaques of demyelination and axon loss at sites throughout the CNS. Patients may present with unilateral optic neuritis– pain on eye movements and rapid deterioration in central vision, nystagmus, fatigue, weakness or spasticity in limbs, constipation, frequency and urgency, impotence, ataxia, dementia, vertigo, even depression. No test is pathognomic and diagnosis is essentially clinical. Symptoms may worsen by heat or exercise. There is no cure but methylprednisolone shortens relapse and β interferon decreases relapse rate.

5. Alzheimer's dementia is the most common form of dementia in UK. Suspect AD in any enduring, acquired deficit of memory and cognition. Onset may be from 40 years though it may be seen earlier in patients suffering from Down's syndrome. On histological examination plaques with neurofibrillary tangles and cortical β-amyloid protein are found. On MRI an increased cortical atrophy in the medial temporal lobe can be seen. In stage I of AD there is falling memory and spatial disorientation. In stage II the personality disintegrates and in stage III the patient is apathetic, wasted and bedridden.

Theme 37: Causes of confusion

1. Hypoglycaemia is the most common endocrine emergency. Plasma glucose < 2.5 mmol/L is defined as hypoglycaemia. Patients may present with sweating, hunger, tremors, drowsiness, seizure, loss of consciousness and rarely focal symptoms. Treatment in this case would require giving glucose 25–50 gm IV bolus or glucagon 0.5–1.0 mg subcutaneously.

2. Following points favour the diagnosis of subdural haematoma : (i) more common in elderly as brain shrinkage makes bridging veins more vulnerable (ii) mostly results due to trauma which may have been mild e.g. recurrent falls (iii) presents with fluctuating level of consciousness. CT. Scan of the head shows a concave or crescent shaped hyperdense clot with or without midline shift. Treatment is with evacuation via burr holes.

3. Alzheimer's dementia is the most common form of dementia in UK. Suspect AD in any enduring, acquired deficit of memory and cognition. Onset may be from 40 years though it may be seen earlier in patients suffering from Down's syndrome. On histological examination plaques with neurofibrillary tangles and cortical β-amyloid protein are found. On MRI an increased cortical atrophy in the medial temporal lobe can be seen. In stage I of AD there is falling memory and spatial disorientation. In stage II the personality disintegrates and in stage III the patient is apathetic, wasted and bedridden.

4. Urinary tract infection implies presence of a pure growth of more than 10^5 colony forming units/mL. Infection may occur at the bladder (cystitis), prostate (prostatitis) or kidney (pyelonephritis). Female sex, sexual intercourse, diabetes, immunocompromised status, pregnancy, menopause, urinary tract obstruction and renal stones are some of the risk factors. Patients may present with

frequency, dysuria, urgency, haematuria, fever, vomiting, loin pain, ARF, low backache. *E. coli* is the most common organism causing UTI. Treatment is with trimethoprim 200 mg 12 hourly PO for 3 days in patients with cystitis. Cefuroxime is given in cases of pyelonephritis and ciprofloxacin for prostatitis.

5. Low basal metabolic rate is seen in hypothyroidism. Patients with hypothyroidism may also present with tiredness, lethargy, weight gain, constipation, depression, menorrhagia, bradycardia, dry skin, non pitting oedema, pericardial effusion, cerebellar ataxia, peripheral neuropathy. Treatment in hypothyroidism includes thyroxine, the dose of which is adjusted to normalize TSH.

Theme 38: Psychiatry.

1. The signs of alcohol withdrawal i.e. delirium tremens, include tachycardia, hypotension, tremors, seizures, visual or tactile hallucinations. The symptoms of nausea, sweating, mood changes, vomiting etc. usually appear within 6 hours of stopping alcohol. The symptoms fluctuate but peak on 3rd to 4th day of withdrawal and subside over a week. Such patients need to be admitted and given generous amounts (e.g. 10 mg 6 hourly) of diazepam in initial 3 days. Thereafter the doses are tapered off.

2. As explained above.

3. The mention of tremors before exams is suggestive of anxiety with hyperstimulated state. The student must be staying awake for long study hours by large amounts of consumption of coffee. The consumption of coffee should be brought down.

4. Starvation can be due to (i) decreased diet intake (ii) decreased assimilation of the diet. A decrease in diet intake could be due to poverty, chronic alcoholism, anorexia nervosa, severe depression neurodegenerative dementias of aging, anorexia associated with AIDS, disseminated malignancy or renal failure. Decreased assimilation of the diet may be due to benign or malignant oesophageal, gastric or intestinal obstruction, due to pancreatic insufficiency, coeliac disease. Starvation decreases the size of all body compartments. During prolonged starvation, metabolism is supported by stores of body fat. Normal-weight individuals can sustain fasting for 2 months but obese individuals can fast for as long as 12 months! Starvation leads to malnutrition and can lead to various vitamin and mineral deficiencies.

5. Patients who wish to stay away from alcohol can be given group psychotherapy in self-help organizations such as alcoholics anonymous.

Disulfiram, which produces an unpleasant reaction if alcohol is taken, can be tried as 800 mg stat and then decreased to 100–200 mg/day PO over 5 days. Naltrexone can reduce the pleasure that alcohol brings and hence decreases craving. Acamprosate decreases craving in alcoholics and can treble abstinence rates. Acamprosate is given as 666 mg 8 hourly PO.

6. Methadone is a synthetic opiate with an action lasting more than a day. In UK, it is available as a coloured syrup as an oral preparation. Dose-assessment is recommended. Most patients are found to required a daily stabilization dose of ≤ 60 mg of methadone. Inpatient dose reduction of methadone can be done over 1–5 days. Outpatient dose reduction may require 2–4 weeks.

Theme 39: Chest pain: Diagnosis.

1. Pericarditis can be present in post MI patients as such and also as a part of Dressler's syndrome which includes recurrent pericarditis, pleural effusions, fever, anaemia and raised ESR. Patients with pericarditis complain of central chest pain relieved by sitting forwards. Their ECG will show a saddle shaped ST elevation and treatment is with NSAIDs.

2. Angina is due to myocardial ischaemia and presents as central chest heaviness, tightness or pain which is brought on by exertion. It may also be precipitated by emotion, cold weather and heavy meals. Stable angina is induced by exertion and relieved by rest. Unstable i.e. crescendo angina is of increasing frequency or severity and occurs with minimal exertion or even at rest as in this patient.

Theme 40: Miscellaneous

1. Hypercalcaemia affects 10–20% of patients with cancer and 40% of patients with myeloma. Patients present with anorexia, lethargy, nausea, polydipsia, polyuria, constipation, dehydration, confusion and weakness. These are most obvious when serum calcium levels are higher than 3 mmol/L. Such patients require rehydration with 0.9% saline and IV biphosphonates. Calcitonin can be used in resistant hypercalcaemia.

2. Malignant mesothelioma is a tumour of mesothelial cells occurring usually in the pleura. It is associated with occupational exposure to asbestos. The latent period between the development of tumour and exposure may be as high as 45 years. Patients present with chest pain, dyspnoea, weight loss, finger clubbing and recurrent pleural effusions. CT scan shows a pleural thickening and effusion. Diagnosis can be made by pleural biopsy using an Abram's needle and thoracoscopy.

3. Tuberculosis is a chronic granulomatous disease of humans caused by a group of closely related obligate pathogens, the mycobacterium tuberculosis complex. In clinical specimens, the tubercle bacilli occur in small clumps and in early cultures they appear as rope-like microcolonies termed 'serpentine cords'. In all suspected cases, the relevant clinical samples e.g. sputum, pleural fluid, pleura, urine, pus, ascites, peritoneum or CSF, should be obtained for culture, to establish the diagnosis. Auramine or Ziehl–Nielsen (ZN) staining reveal acid fast bacilli. Radiography shows consolidation, cavitation, fibrosis and calcification. Immunological tests include tuberculin skin test, Mantoux test, Heaf and Tine tests. Initial phase of the treatment includes 8 weeks of administration of rifampicin, isoniazid, pyrazinamide, ethambutol or streptomycin. Continuation phase requires 2 drugs administered for 4 months viz. rifampicin and isoniazid.

Three

July 2003
Question Paper

Theme 1: Perianal diagnosis

Options:

a. Proctalgia fugax
b. Perianal warts
c. Rectal carcinoma
d. Prolapsed rectum
e. Anal haematoma
f. Pilonidal sinus
g. Fissure in ano
h. Haemorrhoids
i. Crohn's disease

For each presentation below, choose the SINGLE most appropriate diagnosis from the above list of options. Each option may be used once, more than once, or not at all.

1. A patient with fecal shooting and sudden and deep pain in the anal region.
2. A patient complains of severe pain in anus when defecating. Pain is so severe that he cannot undergo anal examination.
3. A patient with very severe anal pain and purple swelling in the anus.
4. A patient with rectal bleeding, weight loss, abdominal pain and anal tags.
5. A patient with weight loss and change in bowel habit. Rigid sigmoidoscopy shows an ulcer.

Theme 2: Abdominal pain

Options:

a. Cholecystitis
b. UTI
c. Renal colic
d. Mesenteric thrombosis
e. Appendicitis
f. Acute gastroenteritis
g. Peptic ulcer perforation
h. Ectopic pregnancy
i. Torsion ovarian cyst
j. Strangulated hernia
k. Ulcerative colitis

For each presentation below, choose the SINGLE most appropriate diagnosis from the above list of options. Each option may be used once, more than once, or not at all.

1 A 20 year old man with abdominal pain which soon radiates to right lower quadrant.
2. After 8 weeks of amenorrhoea a woman presents with abdominal pain and bleeding.
3. A patient presents with pain in the loin which is radiating to the groin.
4. A patient with chronic peptic ulcer develops haematemesis.
5. A 40 year old obese woman with upper abdominal pain and vomiting, develops generalized tenderness in the abdomen.

Theme 3: Mechanism of action of contraception

Options:

a. Inhibits transplantation
b. Disruption of corpus luteum
c. Inhibits implantation
d. Inhibits ovulation
e. Spermicidal
f. Hostile to cervical mucus

For each contraceptive below, choose the SINGLE most appropriate mechanism of action from the above list of options. Each option may be used once, more than once, or not at all.

1. OCPs.
2. POP.
3. IUCDs.
4. Mirena Coil.
5. Sponge.
6. Morning after pill.

Theme 4 : Upper GI conditions

Options:

a. Oesophagitis
b. Lansoprazole
c. X-ray abdomen
d. Triple therapy
e. Biopsy
f. Barium swallow
g. Upper GI endoscopy
h. Erect CXR
i. Sucralfate with H_2 blockers

For each presentation below, choose the SINGLE most appropriate investigation/ management from the above list of options. Each option may be used once, more than once, or not at all.

1. A patient presents with dyspeptic symptoms and on endoscopy *H. pylori* was found.
2. A patient presents with multiple superficial ulcers in stomach two days after a fire accident .
3. A patient with dyspeptic symptoms after long term use of NSAIDs.
4. A patient with symptoms of reflux. In upper GI endoscopy, no sign of stricture was found.
5. A 55 year old man presents with weight loss and in upper GI endoscopy a tumor is shown in the antrum.
6. A patient with several ulcers seen on endoscopy has a tumour in pancreas on USG. He has tried other treatments already.

Theme 5: Treatment of hypertension

Options:

a. Methyldopa
b. Admit and observe
c. Labetalol
d. IV frusemide
e. Surgery
f. IV MgSO4
g. ACE inhibitor

For each presentation below, choose the SINGLE most appropriate treatment from the above list of options. Each option may be used once, more than once, or not at all.

1. An asthmatic woman in her first trimester presents with hypertension.
2. A man having hypertension was normal two weeks ago in his job. Investigations reveal a high aldosterone level and low renin level.
3. A woman has hypertension in her third trimester of pregnancy.
4. A multipara at 28 weeks of gestation presents with headache. Her BP is 150/96 with hyper-reflexia and three beats of ankle clonus.

Theme 6: Treatment in head trauma

Options:

a. Assess adequacy of breathing
b. Intubate the patient
c. Monitor ICP
d. Pronounce the patient dead
e. CT and observe
f. Shift to operation theatre
g. Observe for 6 hours
h. Burr hole
i. Discharge with advice

For each presentation below, choose the SINGLE most appropriate management from the above list of options. Each option may be used once, more than once, or not at all.

1. A child after head trauma presents with some small bruising on the scalp. Otherwise the child is normal.
2. A patient with small skull fracture presents with GCS 15 and no other neurological signs.
3. An alcoholic patient after head trauma presents with GCS 14 and normal neurological signs.
4. A patient after head trauma presents with GCS 15 but GCS deteriorating rapidly.
5. A patient presents with head trauma. CT shows cerebral oedema.
6. A patient presents with head trauma and depressed fracture.

Theme 7: Diagnosing infectious diseases

Options:

a. Varicella
b. Syphilis
c. Falciparum malaria
d. Pneumonia
e. Bronchial carcinoma
f. Lymphoma
g. Sarcoidosis
h. Brucellosis
i. Measles
j. Scabies
k. TB
l. Rabies

For each presentation below, choose the SINGLE most appropriate diagnosis from the above list of options. Each option may be used once, more than once, or not at all.

1. A patient coming back from South America and presents with night sweats and fevers. In CXR there is upper zone shadowing.
2. A patient coming back from holiday in a farm. He presents with malaise, fevers and spleno-megaly.
3. A patient coming back from Africa with fevers and seizures.
4. A patient presents with fever, malaise and lymphadenopathy. He gives no history of travel.
5. A patient with haemoptysis and cough story like TB but chronic without travel history. He seems to have lost weight in recent months.

Theme 8: Basic sciences: Diagnosis

Options:

a. NIDDM
b. Peptic ulcer
c. Conn's syndrome
d. IDDM
e. Alcoholism
f. Sleep apnoea syndrome
g. UTI
h. Pneumonia
i. Cushing's disease

For each presentation below, choose the SINGLE most appropriate diagnosis from the above list of options. Each option may be used once, more than once, or not at all.

1. A change in diet may relieve all symptoms of this receptor mediated disease.
2. All symptoms of this disease like obesity will resolve after curative surgery.
3. All symptoms of this disease like sleepiness during days will resolve after treatment.
4. Treatment helps vitamin deficiency.

Theme 9: HRT

Options:

a. Local oestrogens
b. Continuous
c. Biphosphonates
d. Non continuous
e. Subcutaneous oestrogen implantation

For each presentation below, choose the SINGLE most appropriate method of HRT from the above list of options. Each option may be used once, more than once, or not at all.

1. A 48 year old woman presents with flushing and needs HRT.
2. A 54 year old woman who is two years post menopausal needs HRT.
3. A woman presenting after hysterosalpingo-oophorectomy.
4. A woman presents with post-menopausal dyspareunia.
5. A woman with osteoporosis needs treatment.

Theme 10: Investigations in medical conditions

Options:

a. Urethral swab
b. EMG
c. S. bilirubin
d. Blood urea
e. Arteriography
f. Rheumatoid factor
g. CXR
h. EEG
i. Blood sugar

For each presentation below, choose the SINGLE most appropriate investigation from the above list of options. Each option may be used once, more than once, or not at all.

1. A patient presents with symptoms of Gono-coccal urethritis.
2. A patient presents with weight loss and polyuria.
3. A patient presents with pulse delay in legs as compared to the arm.
4. A patient presents with migrant polyarthritis and early morning stiffness.
5. A young patient presents with very severe occipital headache.

Theme 11: Accidental injuries in children

Options:

a. Sickle cell anaemia
b. ITP
c. Osteogenesis imperfecta
d. Normal finding
e. Accidental injury
f. HSP
g. Child neglect
h. NAI
i. Coeliac disease

For each presentation below, choose the SINGLE most appropriate diagnosis from the above list of options. Each option may be used once, more than once, or not at all.

1. A child presents with bruises on wrists and ankles.
2. A child with pharyngitis and purpuras on the back of his thigh and buttock.
3. A child presents with swelling on wrist after injury.
4. A child from black and white parents presents with Mongolian spots.

Theme 12 : Diagnosis of psychiatric disorders

Options:

a. Schizophrenia
b. Obsessive compulsive disease
c. Gilles de la Tourette syndrome
d. Senile dementia
e. Depression
f. Agoraphobia
g. Parkinson's disease
h. Life events
i. Korsakoff's psychosis
j. Alcoholic hallucination

For each presentation below, choose the SINGLE most appropriate diagnosis from the above list of options. Each option may be used once, more than once, or not at all.

1. A young patient presents with auditory hallucinations.
2. An alcoholic patient presents with hallucinations alone.
3. A patient with some symptoms of parkinson's claims that some people are in his home and is afraid of going home.
4. A woman presents with low mood. She sleeps too much and denies to eat.
5. A 68 year old man, chronic alcoholic and continues to drink is now having confusion.
6. A young boy irritable, and brought to psychiatrist for shouting obscenities at school.

Theme 13: Investigation in medical conditions

Options:

a. S. bilirubin
b USG abdomen
c. Occult blood test-stool
d. CXR
e. Prolactin levels
f. TFTs
g. S. triglycerides
h. Electrolytes
i. GGT
j. LP

For each presentation below, choose the SINGLE most appropriate investigation from the above list of options. Each option may be used once, more than once, or not at all.

1. A patient is going to start lithium therapy.
2. A patient presents with photophobia, neck stiffness, fever and headache. No sign of raised ICP.
3. A patient with anorexia nervosa develops confusion and seizures.
4. An alcoholic is giving up. He needs lab test to evaluate his addiction.
5. A patient using phenothiazines develops galactorrhoea.

Theme 14: Prostate conditions

Options:

a. Bone survey
b. PSA
c. TURP
d. USG pelvis
e. S. calcium
f. Transrectal USG and biopsy
g. α blockers

For each presentation below, choose the SINGLE most appropriate management from the above list of options. Each option may be used once, more than once, or not at all.

1. A patient with benign prostatic hypertrophy refuses surgery.
2. A patient with benign prostatic hypertrophy and obstruction.
3. A patient is concerned about having prostate cancer.
4. A patient with prostatic symptoms and nodule in PR.
5. Having prostate cancer, a patient develops femoral lesion.

Theme 15: Fractures: Diagnosis

Options:

a. Navicular facture
b. Calcaneal fracture
c. Colle's fracture
d. Greenstick fracture
e. Supracondylar fracture humerus
f. Humeral shaft fracture
g. Ulnar fracture
h. Scaphoid fracture

For each presentation below, choose the SINGLE most appropriate diagnosis from the above list of options. Each option may be used once, more than once, or not at all.

1. A child falls on an outstretched hand and has wrist drop.
2. A young man injures his wrist while playing football. There is tenderness distal to the wrist.
3. A rugby player presents with painful forearm with deformation after protecting himself from hitting while playing.
4. A 6 year old girl falls on her outstretched arm and sustains an injury. She is able to extend her fingers on flexing her wrist.

Theme 16: Poisoning in children

Options:

a. Urea and creatinine
b. Blood sugar
c. ECG
d. Check ferrous levels
e. Check oestrogen levels
f. Observation only
g. Electrolytes
h. Liver function tests
i. Arterial blood gases

For each presentation below, choose the SINGLE most appropriate investigation from the above list of options. Each option may be used once, more than once, or not at all.

1. A baby was found playing with Aspirin pills some hours ago.
2. A baby swallowed some OCPs.
3. A baby swallowed some red tablets of his pregnant mother.
4. A baby swallowed some TCAs.
5. A boy drinks Vodka and is unconscious.

Theme 17: Testicular swelling

Options:

a. Orchidectomy
b. Biopsy
c. Surgical exploration
d. Sonography
e. FNAC
f. Chemotherapy
g. Radiotherapy

For each presentation below, choose the SINGLE most appropriate management/ investigation from the above list of options. Each option may be used once, more than once, or not at all.

1. A 30 year old patient has a testicular swelling for the past 3 years.
2. A 40 year old patient has a testicular swelling for the past 3 years.
3. A young man has testicular swelling for the past 2 months.
4. A young man with sudden onset severe testicular pain.

Theme 18: Neurological conditions

Options:

a. Vertebrobasilar ischaemia
b. SAH
c. Alzheimer's disease
d. Multiple sclerosis
e. Plummer vinson syndrome
f. Stroke
g. Motor neurone disease
h. Lewy body dementia

For each presentation below, choose the SINGLE most appropriate diagnosis from the above list of options. Each option may be used once, more than once, or not at all.

1. A patient presents with dysarthria, headache and dysphagia.
2. A patient presents with hoarseness and dysphagia develops paresis of the lower limb.
3. A patient who is confined to the wheelchairs and has some neurological problems, develops blurred vision leading to blindness soon.
4. A patient is confined to the bed. He has got increasingly forgetful within the last few years.
5. A patient presents with ori creases and dysphagia.
6. A patient always looks right when walking.

Theme 19: Diagnosis of skin disorders

Options:

a. Erythema multiforme
b. Pyoderma gangrenosum
c. SLE
d. Melanoma
e. Psoriasis
f. Diabetic ulcer
g. Lichen sclerosis
h. Basal cell carcinoma
i. Squamous cell carcinoma

For each presentation below, choose the SINGLE most appropriate diagnosis from the above list of options. Each option may be used once, more than once, or not at all.

1. A patient with a pigmented lesion with an ulcerated center.
2. An obese patient with neuropathic symptoms develops ulcer on the leg.
3. A patient presents with skin manifestations of Crohn's disease.

Theme 20: Diagnosing emergencies

Options:

a. Pulmonary contusion
b. Pulmonary embolism
c. Aortic dissection
d. MI
e. Pneumonia
f. Oesophageal rupture
g. Acute renal failure
h. Tension pneumothorax

For each presentation below, choose the SINGLE most appropriate diagnosis from the above list of options. Each option may be used once, more than once, or not at all.

1. A patient whose pulse rate is 92, BP is 120/80, temperature is 37°C. JVP is raised and inverted T in one lead.
2. A patient whose pulse rate is 72, BP is 132/86, Temperature 37 CXR is normal and ECG shows Q waves in leads V 1, 2 & 3.
3. A patient whose pulse rate is 95, BP is 142/82, temperature is 39°C. CXR shows mid zone consolidation and ECG is normal.
4. A patient whose pulse rate is 85, BP is 139/86, temperature is 37°C. CXR shows absence of vascular markings over the right lung field and ECG is normal.
5. A patient has temperature 37°C, JVP normal and effusion and pneumo-mediastinum in CXR.

Theme 21: Treatment of psychiatric disorders

Options:

a. TCAs
b. Play therapy
c. Behavioural therapy
d. Fluoxetine
e. Haloperidol
f. ECT
g. Lithium
h. Psychotherapy

For each presentation below, choose the SINGLE most appropriate treatment from the above list of options. Each option may be used once, more than once, or not at all.

1. A nurse that recently washes and cleans everything more than usual.
2. An old lady with depression having suicidal risk and does not eat.
3. A patient requires treatment for postnatal depression.
4. A patient with moderate depression stabilized by some medication and now has MI and getting treated for CCF.

Theme 22: Diagnosis of gynaecological conditions

Options:

a. Thrush
b. Herpes
c. Gonorrhoea
d. Lichen sclerosis
e. Syphilis
f. Vulval carcinoma
g. L. inguinale
h. E. vermicularis
i. Cervical carcinoma
j. Vaginal carcinoma

For each presentation below, choose the SINGLE most appropriate diagnosis from the above list of options. Each option may be used once, more than once, or not at all.

1. A diabetic woman presents with white itchy plaques on vagina.
2. An elderly woman presents with pigmented itchy shiny vulva.
3. An elderly woman presents with itchy vulva that has an ulcer on examination.
4. A woman presents with ulcer over the vulva and lymphadenopathy.
5. A female has dysuria and has vesicles in the vaginal area.

Theme 23: Management in trauma

Options:

a. High flow O$_2$
b. Admit and observe
c. MRI thoracic spine
d. Intubate
e. Chest strapping
f. Shift to OT immediately
g. IV fluids: 1 litre in 30 min
h. Analgesics

For each presentation below, choose the SINGLE most appropriate management from the above list of options. Each option may be used once, more than once, or not at all.

1. A patient presents with fracture of one rib.
2. A woman presents with compressed fracture of thoracic vertebra on X-ray.
3. A patient presents with sternum fracture.
4. A patient with blunt trauma to the abdomen is stable but suddenly deteriorates and BP and pulse rate changes.
5. A patient presenting with abdominal trauma, has haematoma in spleen.

Theme 24: Management of thyroid disorders

Options:

a. Propranolol
b. Thyroidectomy
c. Thyroxine
d. Radiotherapy
e. Propylthiouracil
f. Carbimazole

For each presentation below, choose the SINGLE most appropriate treatment from the above list of options. Each option may be used once, more than once, or not at all.

1. A patient with hyperthyroidism is going to have an operation. He needs to relieve his symptoms.
2. A patient with hyperthyroidism is sensitive to carbimazole and had developed rash.
3. A patient has symptoms of hyperthyroidism.
4. A patient wants to increase basal metabolism.

Theme 25: Diagnosis of epilepsy

Options:

a. EEG
b. Tonic clonic seizure
c. 24 hour telemonitoring
d. Petitmal seizure
e. Vasomotor
f. Febrile seizure
g. CT head
h. Jacksonian seizure

For each presentation below, choose the SINGLE most appropriate diagnosis/ investigation from the above list of options. Each option may be used once, more than once, or not at all.

1. A girl has symptoms of epilepsy without lack of consciousness and it always occurs when people are around her.
2. A child that misses some sentences and then is back again.
3. A patient with jerking of all limbs followed by loss of consciousness and incontinence.
4. A girl falls during morning school in the yard and was pale.
5. A child has seizure when having URTI.

Theme 26: Cause of renal stone

Options:

a. Renal tubular acidosis
b. Beryllium exposure
c. Small intestinal resection
d. Hypercalcaemia
e. Idiopathic
f. Dehydration
g. Triamterine
h. Infection

For each presentation below, choose the SINGLE most appropriate cause from the above list of options. Each option may be used once, more than once, or not at all.

1. A marathon runner develops renal colic.
2. A patient with chronic UTI develops stones in kidney.
3. A middle-aged develops stone without any background.
4. A patient has a big renal stone with features of obstruction.

Theme 27: Management of ear conditions

Options:

a. By hooks or suction
b. Discharge with advice
c. Under LA
d. Antibiotics
e. Myringotomy
f. Olive oil then syringing
g. Under GA

For each presentation below, choose the SINGLE most appropriate management from the above list of options. Each option may be used once, more than once, or not at all.

1. A mentally retarded enters an elastic bead in the ear which is obstructing meatus.
2. A child comes with swelling and her carer remembers that she entered a plastic bead in her ear some days ago.
3. A foreign body in the ear causing partial obstruction.
4. A man wakes up with tinnitus and feeling of something in his ear.
5. A child with otitis media and fever.

Theme 28: Eye conditions: Diagnosis

Options:

a. Migraine
b. Conjunctivitis
c. Optic neuritis
d. Cataract
e. Iritis
f. Dacrocystitis
g. Retinal detachment
h. Secondary glaucoma
i. Acute glaucoma

For each presentation below, choose the SINGLE most appropriate diagnosis from the above list of options. Each option may be used once, more than once, or not at all.

1. A patient presents with blurred vision day after a blunt trauma to the eye with raised ICP.
2. A 20 year old man presents with redness that is limited to medial aspect of the eye.
3. A patient presents with headache and blurred vision. His pupil is fixed and dilated.
4. A patient with spondylitis develops eyeache and redness.

Theme 29: Abdominal pain in children

Options:

a. Gastroenteritis
b. USG abdomen
c. Intussusception
d. Hirschprung's disease
e. Barium enema
f. Jejunal biopsy
g. Testicular torsion
h. Appendicitis

For each presentation below, choose the SINGLE most appropriate diagnosis from the above list of options. Each option may be used once, more than once, or not at all.

1. A child with intermittent abdominal pain and mass palpable in the right quadrant.
2. A 2 year girl with failure to thrive and other symptoms of coeliac disease.
3. A child with abdominal pain and rice water stools.
4. One young infant has constipation and on PR examination was found to have pellet like faeces which come out with a gush.

Theme 30: Pre-operative investigation

Options:

a. ECG
b. TFTs
c. LFTs
d. APTT
e. U & E
f. Bronchoscopy
g. INR
h. CXR
i. S. amylase
j. Drug levels

For each presentation below, choose the SINGLE most appropriate investigation from the above list of options. Each option may be used once, more than once, or not at all.

1. A patient using frusemide is going to have surgery.
2. A patient with COPD is to undergo a surgery.
3. A patient is going to have surgery. He is under treatment with warfarin.

Theme 31: Pre-operative medication

Options:

a. Subcutaneous heparin
b. Laxatives
c. Stop smoking
d. Stop alcohol
e. Antibiotics

For each presentation below, choose the SINGLE most appropriate management from the above list of options. Each option may be used once, more than once, or not at all.

1. A patient is using stocking socks and is due for surgery.
2. A patient going to have femoral neck replacement, is obese.
3. A patient with an unstable angina is going to have a surgery.
4. A patient is going to have an abortion.
5. A patient with incisional hernia, drinks 20 units alcohol/week and 40 cigarettes/day.
6. A patient who is to be operated for thyroid, drinks 30 units alcohol per week.
7. A man who drinks 20 units a week and smokes 20 cigarettes a day for the last 5 years needs to undergo an operation which will last for 2 hours.

Theme 32: Treatment of emergencies

Options:

a. Inhaled β agonists
b. NSAIDs
c. Intubation
d. Antibiotics
e. Apomorphine
f. Antihistaminics
g. Thoracotomy
h. Adrenaline

For each presentation below, choose the SINGLE most appropriate treatment from the above list of options. Each option may be used once, more than once, or not at all.

1. A patient having pneumothorax is not responding to chest drain.
2. A patient with chest pain since ½ hr radiating to back. His ECG shows ST elevation.
3. A patient with sudden onset blue lips and breathlessness.
4. A patient with breathlessness, fever and shadowing on CXR.

Theme 33: Asthma in children

Options:

a. Oral theophylline
b. Antihistaminics
c. Adrenaline
d. Antibiotics
e. Inhaled sodium chromoglycate
f. Short acting β agonist
g. O_2
h. Nebulized salbutamol

For each presentation below, choose the SINGLE most appropriate treatment from the above list of options. Each option may be used once, more than once, or not at all.

1. A patient that is not answering to short acting β agonists and refuses using cortons.
2. A child has dyspnoea in playing football.
3. A child is not answering to beta agonists.
4. A child is in severe attack.

Theme 34: Bleeding disorders

Options:

a. Bone marrow biopsy
b. Full blood count
c. Vitamin K
d. Coagulation factors
e. DIC
f. FFP and vitamin K

For each presentation below, choose the SINGLE most appropriate investigation/ management from the above list of options. Each option may be used once, more than once, or not at all.

1. A child presents with prolonged bleeding. He has been on warfarin for some time now.
2. A child presents with haemarthrosis.
3. A child presents with symptoms of sickle cell anaemia.
4. A patient presents with severe bleeding from different organs.
5. A patient on coagulation therapy now presents with bleeding.

Theme 35: Diagnosing emergencies

Options:

a. Myocardial infarction
b. Aortic aneurysm
c. Frusemide
d. Anaphylaxis
e. Cardiac valve
f. Pneumothorax
g. Respiratory failure
h. Lung contusion

For each presentation below, choose the SINGLE most appropriate diagnosis from the above list of options. Each option may be used once, more than once, or not at all.

1. A patient presents with breathlessness and tracheal deviation to one side.
2. A patient presents with severe chest pain radiating to the back. His ECG is normal.
3. A patient with breathlessness and has abnormal sound in the apex.
4. A patient presents with hydropneumothorax and surgical emphysema after an RTA.
5. A patient with signs of severe pulmonary oedema and basal crepitations.

Theme 36: Renal problems

Options:

a. Renal artery stenosis
b. Sarcoidosis
c. IgA nephropathy
d. Papillary necrosis
e. Adult polycystic kidney disease
f. Haemorrhagic cystitis
g. Renal calculus
h. Urethral calculus
i. CRF

For each presentation below, choose the SINGLE most appropriate diagnosis from the above list of options. Each option may be used once, more than once, or not at all.

1. A patient with pallor, dry skin, lethargy and anuria.
2. A patient that has renal stones and hypercalcaemia.
3. A woman having fullness in loin. No other complaints.
4. A patient using NSAIDs presents with renal problems.
5. A patient presents with a picture like that of Henoch–Schönlein purpura.
6. Patient had recurrent urinary infection, now anuric, and complaining of severe pain in the scrotum.

Theme 37: Diagnosing genetical disorders

Options:

a. Y linked
b. X linked
c. Autosomal dominant
d. Autosomal recessive
e. Multigenic
f. No genetic association

For each presentation below, choose the SINGLE most appropriate mode of inheritance from the above list of options. Each option may be used once, more than once, or not at all.

1. A boy has the disease that was present in his grandfather and father.
2. A 6 month old girl whose father is checking regularly his full blood count and mother regularly receives blood transfusion.
3. A boy presents with painful swollen knee after minor trauma.
4. An elderly man with diabetes mellitus.
5. An elderly man with otosclerosis.

Theme 38: Medical diagnosis

Options:

a. Pseudogout
b. Osteoarthritis
c. Psoriatic arthritis
d. Rheumatoid arthritis
e. Multiple myeloma
f. Gout
g. Ankylosing spondylitis

For each presentation below, choose the SINGLE most appropriate diagnosis from the above list of options. Each option may be used once, more than once, or not at all.

1. A patient who is on antihypertensives presents with swelling in PIP and knee and bifringate in tap.
2. A patient presents with bone pain and malaise and abnormal proteins in urine.
3. A young man with complaints of morning stiffness in the back. His HLA B27 was found to be positive.

Theme 39: Incontinence

Options:

a. Catheter culture
b. IVU
c. X ray KUB
d. Pelvic USG

For each presentation below, choose the SINGLE most appropriate investigation from the above list of options. Each option may be used once, more than once, or not at all.

1. A child presents with recurrent infection and was catheterized. Now the child has again presented with incontinence.

Three

July 2003 Answers

Theme 1: Perianal diagnosis

1. (a) Proctalgia fugax
2. (g) Fissure in ano
3. (e) Anal haematoma
4. (i) Crohn's disease
5. (c) Rectal carcinoma

Theme 2: Abdominal pain

1. (e) Appendicitis
2. (h) Ectopic pregnancy
3. (c) Renal colic
4. (g) Peptic ulcer perforation
5. (g) Peptic ulcer perforation

Theme 3: Mechanism of action of contraception

1. (d) Inhibits ovulation
2. (f) Hostile to cervical mucus
3. (c) Inhibits implantation
4. (c) Inhibits implantation
5. (e) Spermicidal
6. (b) Disruption of corpus luteum

Theme 4 : Upper GI conditions

1. (d) Triple therapy
2. (i) Sucralfate with H_2 blockers
3. (g) Upper GI endoscopy
4. (a) Oesophagitis
5. (e) Biopsy
6. (b) Lansoprazole

Theme 5: Treatment of hypertension

1. (a) Methyldopa
2. (e) Surgery
3. (b) Admit and observe
4. (f) IV $MgSO_4$

Theme 6: Treatment in head trauma

1. (i) Discharge with advice
2. (g) Observe for 6 hours
3. (e) CT and observe
4. (h) Burr hole
5. (c) Monitor ICP
6. (f) Shift to operation theatre

Theme 7: Diagnosing infectious diseases

1. (k) TB
2. (h) Brucellosis
3. (c) Falciparum malaria
4. (f) Lymphoma
5. (e) Bronchial carcinoma

Theme 8: Basic sciences: Diagnosis

1. **(a)** NIDDM
2. **(i)** Cushing's disease
3. **(f)** Sleep apnoea syndrome
4. **(e)** Alcoholism

Theme 9: HRT

1. **(d)** Non continuous
2. **(b)** Continuous
3. **(e)** Subcutaneous oestrogen implantation
4. **(a)** Local oestrogens
5. **(c)** Biphosphonates

Theme 10: Investigation in medical conditions

1. **(a)** Urethral swab
2. **(i)** Blood sugar
3. **(g)** CXR
4. **(f)** Rheumatoid factor
5. **(e)** Arteriography

Theme 11: Accidental injuries in children

1. **(h)** NAI
2. **(f)** HSP
3. **(e)** Accidental injury
4. **(d)** Normal finding

Theme 12: Diagnosis of psychiatric disorders

1. **(a)** Schizophrenia
2. **(j)** Alcoholic hallucination
3. **(g)** Parkinson's disease
4. **(e)** Depression
5. **(i)** Korsakoff's psychosis
6. **(c)** Gilles de la Tourette syndrome

Theme 13: Investigation in medical conditions

1. **(f)** TFTs

2. **(j)** LP
3. **(h)** Electrolytes
4. **(i)** GGT
5. **(e)** Prolactin levels

Theme 14: Prostate conditions

1. **(g)** α blockers
2. **(c)** TURP
3. **(b)** PSA
4. **(f)** Transrectal USG and biopsy
5. **(a)** Bone survey

Theme 15: Fractures: Diagnosis

1. **(f)** Humeral shaft fracture
2. **(h)** Scaphoid fracture
3. **(g)** Ulnar fracture
4. **(e)** Supracondylar fracture humerus

Theme 16: Poisoning in children

1. **(f)** Observation only
2. **(e)** Check oestrogen levels
3. **(d)** Check ferrous levels
4. **(c)** ECG
5. **(b)** Blood sugar

Theme 17: Testicular swelling

1. **(a)** Orchidectomy
2. **(g)** Radiotherapy
3. **(d)** Sonography
4. **(c)** Surgical exploration

Theme 18: Neurological conditions

1. **(f)** Stroke
2. **(g)** Motor neurone disease
3. **(d)** Multiple sclerosis
4. **(c)** Alzheimer's disease
5. **(e)** Plummer vinson syndrome
6. **(a)** Vertebrobasilar ischaemia

Theme 19: Diagnosis of skin disorders

1. **(d)** Melanoma
2. **(f)** Diabetic ulcer
3. **(b)** Pyoderma gangrenosum

Theme 20: Diagnosing emergencies

1. **(h)** Tension pneumothorax
2. **(d)** MI
3. **(e)** Pneumonia
4. **(b)** Pulmonary embolism
5. **(f)** Oesophageal rupture

Theme 21: Treatment of psychiatric disorders

1. **(c)** Behavioural therapy
2. **(f)** ECT
3. **(d)** Fluoxetine
4. **(d)** Fluoxetine

Theme 22: Diagnosis of gynaecological conditions

1. **(a)** Thrush
2. **(d)** Lichen sclerosis
3. **(f)** Vulval carcinoma
4. **(g)** L. inguinale
5. **(b)** Herpes

Theme 23: Management in trauma

1. **(h)** Analgesics
2. **(c)** MRI thoracic spine
3. **(e)** Chest strapping
4. **(g)** IV fluids: 1 litre in 30 min
5. **(b)** Admit and observe

Theme 24: Management of thyroid disorders

1. **(a)** Propranolol
2. **(e)** Propylthiouracil
3. **(f)** Carbimazole
4. **(c)** Thyroxine

Theme 25: Diagnosis of epilepsy

1. **(c)** 24 hour telemonitoring
2. **(d)** Petitmal seizure
3. **(b)** Tonic clonic seizure
4. **(e)** Vasomotor
5. **(f)** Febrile seizure

Theme 26: Cause of renal stone

1. **(f)** Dehydration
2. **(h)** Infection
3. **(e)** Idiopathic
4. **(h)** Infection

Theme 27: Management of ear conditions

1. **(a)** By hooks or suction
2. **(g)** Under GA
3. **(a)** By hooks or suction
4. **(f)** Olive oil then syringing
5. **(d)** Antibiotics

Theme 28: Eye conditions: Diagnosis

1. **(h)** Secondary glaucoma
2. **(f)** Dacrocystitis
3. **(i)** Acute glaucoma
4. **(e)** Iritis

Theme 29: Abdominal pain in children

1. **(c)** Intussusception
2. **(f)** Jejunal biopsy
3. **(a)** Gastroenteritis
4. **(d)** Hirschprung's disease

Theme 30: Pre-operative investigation

1. **(e)** U & E
2. **(h)** CXR
3. **(g)** INR

192

Plab Part I

Theme 31: Pre-operative medication

1. **(a)** Subcutaneous heparin
2. **(a)** Subcutaneous heparin
3. **(a)** Subcutaneous heparin
4. **(e)** Antibiotics
5. **(c)** Stop smoking
6. **(d)** Stop alcohol
7. **(c)** Stop smoking

Theme 32: Treatment of emergencies

1. **(g)** Thoracotomy
2. **(e)** Apomorphine
3. **(h)** Adrenaline
4. **(d)** Antibiotics

Theme 33: Asthma in children

1. **(a)** Oral theophylline
2. **(f)** Short acting β agonist
3. **(e)** Inhaled sodium cromoglycate
4. **(h)** Nebulized salbutamol

Theme 34: Bleeding disorders

1. **(f)** FFP and vitamin K
2. **(d)** Coagulation factors
3. **(b)** Full blood count
4. **(e)** DIC
5. **(c)** Vitamin K

Theme 35: Diagnosing emergencies

1. **(f)** Pneumothorax
2. **(b)** Aortic aneurysm
3. **(e)** Cardiac valve
4. **(h)** Lung contusion
5. **(c)** Frusemide

Theme 36: Renal problems

1. **(i)** CRF
2. **(b)** Sarcoidosis
3. **(e)** Adult polycystic kidney disease
4. **(d)** Papillary necrosis
5. **(c)** IgA nephropathy
6. **(h)** Urethral calculus

Theme 37: Diagnosing genetical disorders

1. **(a)** Y linked
2. **(b)** X linked
3. **(b)** X linked
4. **(e)** Multigenic
5. **(c)** Autosomal dominant

Theme 38: Medical diagnosis

1. **(f)** Gout
2. **(e)** Multiple myeloma
3. **(g)** Ankylosing spondylitis

Theme 39: Incontinence

1. **(a)** Catheter culture

Three

July 2003
Explanation

Theme 1: Perianal diagnosis

1. Proctalgia fugax is a disease characterized by attacks of severe idiopathic pain arising in the rectum. The pain is described as stabbing cramp-like. It often occurs when the patient is in bed at night. It seems to occur commonly in patients suffering from anxiety or undue stress and is also said to afflict young doctors! It is probably due to segmental cramp in the pubococcygeus muscle. It is unpleasant, incurable but fortunately harmless.

2. Anal fissure or Fissure-in-ano, is a midline longitudinal split in squamous lining of the lower anus often present with a mucosal tag at the external aspect–'the sentinel pile'. Mostly it is due to hard faeces or constipation. Defecation or PR examination is very painful, as in this patient.

3. The presentation of severe pain in the anal region along with a purple swelling in the anus are sufficient enough to diagnose this as anal haematoma. Moreover there is no mention of bleeding per rectum which further supports the diagnosis.

4. Crohn's disease is an inflammatory GI condition characterized by transmural granulomatous inflammation. Mostly seen in the terminal ileum and proximal colon with skin lesions in between. Smoking increases the risk 3–4 folds. Patients present with abdominal pain, weight loss, diarrhoea, aphthous ulcers, abdominal tenderness, RIF mass and perianal abscesses or tags. Small intestinal obstruction or toxic dilatation can occur as complications. One must investigate by sigmoidoscopy, rectal biopsy and barium enema which may show cobble stoning, 'rose thorn' ulcers. Prednisolone is used for mild attacks. For severe attacks, patient needs to be admitted and given IV hydrocortisone $\pm$ metronidazole $\pm$ rectal hydrocortisone.

5. Rectal carcinoma is the 4th most common malignancy in women. Local spread occurs circumferentially and within 2 years complete encirclement would have taken place. Spread via the venous system occurs late. Patients present with bleeding which is the earliest and most common symptom alongwith a sense of incomplete defecation (tenesmus). Alteration in the bowel habit, weight loss and pain abdomen at a later stage are also seen. 90% of all neoplasms can be felt digitally. Proctosigmoidoscopy will always show the carcinoma. A histological examination will not only confirm the diagnosis but also stage it. A

sphincter saving operation (anterior resection) is usually done for tumours of upper 2/3rd of the rectum. For tumours involving the lower 1/3rd of the rectum, a permanent colostomy (abdominoperineal excision) is often required.

Theme 2: Abdominal pain

1. This is case of acute appendicitis. It is the most common surgical emergency. As inflammation begins, patients complaints of central abdominal pain. Once the peritoneum is inflamed the pain shifts to the right lower quadrant as seen in this patient. Patients typically present with anorexia, fever, tachycardia, tenderness, guarding and rebound tenderness in right iliac fossa. Rovsing's sign (see notes) is positive. Treatment is with prompt appendicectomy with pre operative metronidazole and cefuroxime.

2. This is a case of ectopic pregnancy. Golden role: Always think of an ectopic in a sexually active woman with abdominal pain or bleeding. There is usually ~ 8 weeks of amenorrhea in patients of ectopic pregnancy. Abdominal pain is caused due to tubal colic which is later followed by vaginal bleeding.

3. This is a patient with renal colic. Patients generally present with pain in the loin radiating to the groin. Pain is usually intermittent and associated with vomiting. It requires further investigations to rule out nephrolithiasis. Treatment includes IV fluids, analgesics and antiemetics. Antibiotics are given if there is evidence of infection.

4. Haematemesis means vomiting of blood. It may be bright red in colour or may look like coffee grounds. It may be due to duodenal or gastric ulcer, due to Mallory–Weiss tear, oesophageal varices, malignancy, bleeding disorder or drug induced. Supra-umbilical laparotomy or minimal access surgery is required in this patient to close the hole with an omental plug.

5. Although the presentation of the patient in this case is not typical but peptic ulcer perforation would be the best bet. The site of pain is in the upper abdomen which is also the site in peptic ulcer disease. Vomiting can occur especially in cases of GI perforation and finally but most

importantly the sign of generalized tenderness suggest the presence of peritonitis which is almost always seen in GI perforation.

Theme 3: Mechanism of contraception

1. Chief mechanism of action of combined OCPs is inhibition of ovulation. Both oestrogen and progesterone act synergistically on the hypothalamo-pituitary axis and prevent the release of GnRH from the hypothalamus through a negative feedback mechanism. Thus, there is no peak release of FSH and LH from the anterior pituitary. So, follicular growth is either not initiated or if initiated, ovulation does not occur.

2. Progesterone only pill (minipill) works mainly by making cervical mucus thick and viscous thus preventing sperm penetration. It has to be taken daily from the first day of the cycle. Chief advantage of POP is that it has no adverse effect on lactation. Also, the side effects due to oestrogen in the combined pills are totally avoided.

3. IUCDs (Intra Uterine Contraceptive Devices) induce histological and biochemical changes in the endometrium by causing a non-specific inflammatory reaction. They also increase tubal motility, which results in quick migration of the fertilized ovum into the uterine cavity before the endometrium is receptive. Both these processes result in failure of implantation.

4. Mirena coil is an IUCD which carries levonor-gestrel. IUCDs (Intra Uterine Contraceptive Devices) induce histological and biochemical changes in the endometrium by causing a non-specific inflammatory reaction. They also increase tubal motility, which results in quick migration of the fertilized ovum into the uterine cavity before the endometrium is receptive. Both these processes result in failure of implantation.

5. Vaginal sponge is made of synthetic polyurethane impregnated with non oxynol-9 as spermicide. It acts as a surfactant which either immobilises or kills the sperms. The sponge is inserted immediately before the

coitus into the vagina to cover the cervix. It should not be removed for 6 hours after intercourse. The sponge is for single use only over a 24 hour period.

6. Levonorgestrel with or without ethinyl oestradiol is used as morning-after pill. It is to be initiated within 72 hours of unprotected intercourse. The earlier it is taken after unprotected intercourse, the fewer are the chances of pregnancy. The mechanism of action is not exactly known but it probably involves disruption of ovulation or corpus luteal function depending upon the time in the menstrual cycle when it is taken.

Theme 4: Upper GI conditions

1. *H. Pylori* is the most common cause of chronic gastritis. *H. Pylori* or Helicobacter pylori is a spiral organism which exclusively colonises gastric epithelium (found in duodenum only in the patches of gastric metaplasia). It is capable of producing urease which converts urea to ammonia and hence buffers gastric acidity. It is a motile organism, and is associated with duodenal ulcers most strongly. It is also associated with gastric ulcers, gastric cancer, gastric B cell lymphomas and rarely, non-ulcer dyspepsia. The ^{13}C–urea breath is the best noninvasive test for detecting *H. pylori*. *H pylori* eradication requires 'triple therapy' with lansoprazole, clarithromycin, amoxicillin/metronidazole, all given for 1 week.

2. This is a patient with Curling's ulcer which may be present in the gastric or duodenal regions. They are typically present in association with burns. The treatment for such ulcers remains the same as that of peptic ulcers.

3. This is a patient of drug induced gastritis. As the presentation is acute, one has to rule out perforation. Therefore an upper GI endoscopy is a must. Endoscopy is advised in patients of dyspepsia if there are 'alarm' symptoms e.g. > 45 years of age, weight loss, vomiting, haematemesis, anaemia and dysphagia. Moreover endoscopy should be done if despite conservative treatment with antacids, symptoms recur and *H. pylori* status is found to be negative.

4. This is a patient of GORD i.e. Gastro Oesophageal Reflex Disease which is due to dysfunction of the lower oesophageal sphincter. If reflux is of chronic duration, as must have been in this case, it may cause oesophagitis or benign oesophageal stricture. As the presence of stricture has been ruled out on endoscopy, patient must be suffering from oesophagitis.

5. Carcinoma stomach is associated with blood group A, *H. pylori* infection, smoking, atrophic gastritis and adenomatous polyps. The adenocarcinoma may be polypoid, ulcerating or leather bottle type (linitis plastica). Patients generally present with dyspepsia, weight loss, vomiting, dysphagia, hepatomegaly. Troissier's sign is positive and acanthosis nigricans is noted. All gastric ulcers should be biopsied to rule out malignancy as even malignant ulcers may appear to heal on drug treatment. Wide excision of the tumour is required as the curative surgery.

6. The GMC in this question seems to be looking for a treatment for the ulcers rather than the pancreatic carcinoma. Therefore lansoprazole which is a proton pump inhibitor, is the right answer.

Theme 5: Treatment of hypertension

1. Pre-eclampsia is pregnancy induced hypertension with proteinuria with or without oedema. It develops after 20 weeks of pregnancy and usually resolves within 10 days of delivery. Patients may present with headache, epigastric pain, vomiting and tachycardia. In all asymptomatic patients, hypertension may be treated with methyldopa under supervision in a hospital. If signs worsen deliver the baby as delivery is the only cure.

2. Primary hyperaldosteronism is excess production of aldosterone, independent of renin-angiotensin system. More than half the cases are due to unilateral adrenocortical adenoma (Conn's syndrome). Investigations reveal increased aldosterone and decreased renin levels. A normal or high renin level excludes the diagnosis. Surgery is the treatment of choice with spironolactone given upto 300 mg/day PO for 4 weeks pre-operatively.

3. This is another case of pre-eclampsia. Patients need to be admitted and kept under observation if their BP rises by > 30/20 mmHg over their booking BP or if BP $\geq$ 160/100 or if BP $\geq$ 140/90 with proteinuria or if there is growth restriction. BP is monitored 2–4 hourly.

4. This is a case of impending eclampsia. Therefore needs to be given IV Mg SO_4. Therapeutic range of Mg^{2+} levels is 2–4 mmol/L. It should be stopped if respiratory rate < 14/min. The 1st seizure is managed with 4 gm $MgSO_4$ in 0.9% saline. Repeated seizure required 2 gm $MgSO_4$ as IV bolus.

Theme 6: Treatment in head trauma

1. This is a case of trivial head injury in which the GCS is 15 and no earlier loss of consciousness or post traumatic amnesia. Such patients may be discharged home after careful clinical examination. Indications to keep the patient under observations and reasses after 6 hours is if the patient complains of headache, dizziness or vomiting.

2. CT scan head is only required for minor head injury if (i) Glasgow coma scale < 15, two hours post injury (ii) suspected open or depressed fracture (iii) any sign of basal skull fracture (iv) amnesia before impact of > 30 min (v) dangerous way of injury. As none of the above are mentioned in the question, CT is not required and the patient can be sent home after observation for 6 hours.

3. As the patient in this question is an alcoholic. We can suspect recurrent head injuries in the past. Such recurrent head injuries can cause a subdural haematoma. We must do a CT head and observe the patient for some time to rule out a subdural haematoma.

4. This is a case of extradural haematoma as the deterioration in the GCS score is rapid. Extradural haemorrhage is generally due to fracture of temporal or parietal bone causing laceration of the middle meningeal artery and vein. The lucid interval is typical of extradural haemorrhage. CT would show a haematoma which is often biconvex (lens) shaped. Urgent evacuation of the clot through multiple burr holes may be necessary before the patient can be transferred to higher centres.

5. Cerebral oedema is of 3 types (a) vasogenic (b) cytotoxic (c) interstitial. Normal ICP is 0–10 mmHg. The oedema due to severe head injury is possibly both cytotoxic and vasogenic. Patients generally present with headache, drowsiness, vomiting, seizures, falling pulse with rising BP (Cushing's response), Cheyne–stokes respiration and pupil changes. As in this case no such features have been mentioned, we assume the ICP is still under normal limit. Therefore patient needs to be kept under observation and his ICP monitored.

6. Since it is a case of depressed fracture, neurosurgery is required to prevent neurological loss. Therefore out of the given options above, shifting the patient to the operation theatre is the right management strategy.

Theme 7: Diagnosing infectious disease

1. The presentation of the patient with night sweats, fever and upper zone shadowing on CXR along with the fact that patient has recent history of travel to South America suggests tuberculosis.

   Tuberculosis is a chronic granulomatous disease of humans caused by a group of closely related obligate pathogens, the mycobacterium tuberculosis complex. In clinical specimens, the tubercle bacilli occur in small clumps and in early cultures they appear as rope-like microcolonies termed 'serpentine cords'. In all suspected cases, the relevant clinical samples e.g. sputum, pleural fluid, pleura, urine, pus, ascites, peritoneum or CSF, should be obtained for culture, to establish the diagnosis. Auramine or Ziehl–Nielsen (ZN) staining reveal acid fast bacilli. Radiography shows consolidation, cavitation, fibrosis and calcification. Immunological tests include tuberculin skin test, Mantoux test, Heaf and Tine tests. Initial phase of the treatment includes 8 weeks of administration of rifampicin, isoniazid, pyrazinamide, ethambutol or streptomycin. Continuation phase requires 2 drugs administered for 4 months viz. rifampicin and isoniazid.

2. Brucellosis is a zoonosis common in Middle–east and typically affects the farmers or vets. It may present as fever, sweats, malaise, anorexia, vomiting, weight loss, hepatosplenomegaly, diarrhoea, backache, rash, orchitis or myalgia. Diagnosis is by blood culture and serology. Treatment is by doxycycline and streptomycin.

3. The history of travel to Africa (an endemic area for malaria) along with the presenting features of rigors and fever suggests the diagnosis of malaria. The mention of seizures in the question points towards cerebral malaria which is a complication seen in plasmodium falciparum infection. Diagnosis requires serial thin and thick blood films which are taken at the time of fever. Thick films help in rapid detection of malarial parasites, while thin film helps in identification of the plasmodium subtype. Treatment is with quinine and tetracycline/doxycycline/clindamycin.

4. Lymphomas are malignant proliferation of lymphocytes. They are histologically divided into Hodgkins and Non Hodgkins lymphomas. In both the types, patients present with fever, malaise, lymphadenopathy, weight loss and night sweats. Rarely alcohol induced pain may also be noted. Reed–Sternberg cells are characteristically seen in Hodgkins lymphoma. Lymph node biopsy is diagnostic. Radiotherapy and/or chemotherapy are the mainstay in the treatment.

5. This is a patient with carcinoma bronchus. Cigarette smoking, old age, asbestos inhalation and radiation are important risk factors. The patient typically presents with cough, haemoptysis, dyspnoea, chest pain and weight loss. It can cause recurrent laryngeal nerve palsy, SIADH, SVC obstruction and Horner's syndrome. On CXR, circular opacity, hilar enlargement, consolidation may be seen. Diagnosis is by bronchoscopy and biopsy for histological evaluation. Treatment is by excision for peripheral tumours and chemotherapy for small cell tumours.

Theme 8: Basic sciences: Diagnosis

1. Type II DM or NIDDM is seen in older age group patients especially who are obese. Obesity probably causes insulin resistance by the associated increased rate of release of non esterified fatty acids causing post receptor defects in insulin's action. The first step in the management of NIDDM is weight loss and exercise.

2. Cushing's disease is treated by selective removal of pituitary adenoma via a trans-sphenoidal or very rarely transfrontal approach. Cushing's disease is due to adrenal hyperplasia due to excess ACTH from pituitary tumour. 90% of pituitary causes are microadenomas. Cushing's disease is commoner in women with a peak age incidence at 30–50 years.

3. Weight reduction is the first step in the management of obstructive sleep apnoea syndrome which is characterized by intermittent closure or collapse of the pharyngeal airway which causes apnoeic episodes during sleep. The typical patient is a fat, middle aged man with complaints of snoring, daytime somnolence, morning headache or poor sleep quality.

4. Weight loss and vitamin B deficiency are well known facts which occur due to alcoholism. Alcoholism can cause fatty liver, hepatitis, cirrhosis, Korsakoff's psychosis ± Wernicke's encephalopathy. Alcohol withdrawal with the help of benzodiazepines and multiple high potency vitamins given IM may reverse the effects caused due to alcoholism.

Theme 9: HRT

1. Non continuous HRT is indicated in this patient as the patient has not yet achieved menopause. She has started having symptoms of flushing which need to be managed. Therefore non continuous HRT is indicated.

2. In this patient it has been clearly mentioned that the patient is 2 years post menopausal. Around 80% of the UK women at the age of 50 retain their uterus. In our patient also there is no mention of hysterectomy being done. She needs to have continuous or cyclic progestogen along with oestrogen given orally or via transdermal therapy.

3. Subcutaneous oestrogen implantation is restricted in UK to patients who have undergone hysterectomy with or without oophorectomy. It involves positioning of a pellet of oestradiol in the subcutaneous tissue, usually in the lower abdomen. Such implants are reviewed at 6 monthly intervals and are generally well tolerated. This mode of treatment successfully treats menopausal symptoms and also protects against bone loss.

4. This is a case of atrophic vaginitis. Creams, pessaries and rings are useful for such cases. Oestriol preparations are applied PV daily for 3 weeks and then twice weekly. If creams are unacceptable, oestrogen containing vaginal ring, which is replaced every 3 months, can be used for upto 2 years.

5. Osteoporosis means decreased bone density. Exercise, calcium rich diet, avoiding smoking and excess alcohol all help in the management of osteoporosis. HRT decreases the risk of fracture if given for 5–10 years post menopausally. This patient has already been diagnosed with osteoporosis, therefore Biphosphonates are the definitive treatment. It is used both for treating and preventing osteoporosis. It also decreases fracture rate. Alendronate is licensed for osteoporosis treatment in UK. They inhibit osteoclast activity and so bone resorption.

Theme 10: Investigation in medical conditions

1. Gonococcal urethritis is a sexually transmitted disease caused by Neisseria gonorrhoea. Incubation period is 2–10 days. Patients present with purulent urethral discharge with or without dysuria. Women with gonococcal urethritis may present with vaginal discharge and dysuria. Diagnosis is by urethral swab and treatment is with amoxicilin and probenecid.

2. This is a suspected case of diabetes mellitus. Diabetes mellitus is due to lack or diminished effectiveness of endogenous insulin and is characterized by hyperglycaemia. For diagnosis of DM, fasting venous plasma glucose level should be ≥ 7 mmol/L. If in doubt an oral glucose tolerance test should be performed and a value above 11.1 mmol/L is diagnostic of DM. In case the patient comes without any preparation and wishes to know whether he is a diabetic, a random blood glucose level can be checked in which a value ≥ 11.1 mmol/L would be diagnostic of DM.

3. This is a patient with coarctation of aorta. Headache, epistaxis, cold extremities and claudication with exercise may be seen in such patients. Hypertension in upper limbs and delayed pulsation in the femoral arteries is detected. A CXR may show a dilated left subclavian artery and a dilated descending aorta. Indentation of the aorta at the site of coarctation and pre and post stenotic dilatation (the 'Z' sign) is pathognomic of the entity. Notching of the ribs may also be seen which is due to erosion by dilated collateral vessels.

4. This is a case of rheumatoid arthritis for which rheumatoid factor (an anti IgG antibody) estimation in the blood is required. Rheumatoid arthritis is a persistent, symmetrical, deforming arthropathy with peak onset in 5th decade and a M : F ratio of 3 : 1. Patients typically present with swollen, painful and stiff hands and feet especially in the morning. Patients have sausage shaped fingers and MCP joint swellings which later become Boutonniere and swan neck deformities of the fingers. It is associated with carpal tunnel syndrome, keratoconjunctivitis sicca, osteoporosis and amyloidosis. Treatment is with exercise, physiotherapy, intralesional steroids and NSAIDs.

5. This is a case of subarachnoid haemorrhage which is mostly due to rupture of saccular aneurysm. Patients typically present with very severe headache especially in the occiput. Kernig's sign is positive and it takes around 6 hours to develop. CT head shows subarachnoid or ventricular blood. CSF examination shows xanthochromia. But as in this patient neither are in the options so we must choose arteriography to visualize the saccular aneurysm.

Theme 11: Accidental injuries in children

1. Bruises over wrist and ankle are suggestive that the child has been tied at the wrists and ankle joints.
2. Henoch–Schönlein (anaphylactoid) purpura generally presents with purple spots or nodules which do not disappear on pressure i.e. intradermal bleeding. They are generally seen over buttocks and extensor surfaces. It may follow a respiratory infection. It may present with nephritis, joint involvement, abdominal pain and intussusception.
3. This is a simple case of accidental injury.
4. Mongolian spots are bluish, well demarcated spots on the buttocks and trunk. The name is a misnomer as these are not related to Down's syndrome. They usually disappear by 1st birthday.

Theme 12: Diagnosis of psychiatric disorders

1. Schizophrenia is a common mental disorder which typically presents in adulthood with delusions, hallucinations and disordered thought. The 1st rank symptoms seen in ~70% of patients are (i) Thought insertion (as in this patient) (ii) Thought broadcast (iii) Thought withdrawal (iv) Passivity (v) Hearing voices commenting on the actions of the patients (vi) Primary delusions (vii) Somatic hallucinations.
2. This seems to be a patient with alcohol withdrawal signs. In delirium tremens there is tachycardia, hypotension, tremors, fits, visual or tactile hallucinations e.g. animals crawling all over the body. It is treated with benzo-diazepines given in generous doses and then tapering them off.
3. This looks like a patient of Parkinson's disease which is one of the causes of parkinsonism. It is due to degeneration of substantia nigra dopaminergic neurons along with the pathological hallmark Lewy bodies in this area. Patients may present with tremors, rigidity, bradykinesis and difficulty in stopping and starting walking. Tremors are most marked at rest. It is a typical 'pill rolling' of thumb over fingers. Patients may also have expressionless face, dribbling and festinant gait. Treatment is with dopamine agonists e.g. L-dopa.
4. In clinical depression, low mood occurs with sleep difficulty, change in appetite, hopelessness, pessimism and suicidal thoughts. Patients with major depression may present with anhedonia, poor appetite, weight loss, early waking, psychomotor retardation/agitation, decrease in sexual drive, decrease ability to concentrate, feeling of worthlessness, inappropriate guilt with recurrent thoughts of suicide. Treatment has to be multipronged with psychological cognitive therapy, antidepressants or even ECT.

5. This is a patients of Korsakoff's psychosis. Weight loss and vitamin B deficiency are well known facts which occur due to alcoholism. Alcoholism can cause fatty liver, hepatitis, cirrhosis, Korsakoff's psychosis ± Wernicke's encephalopathy. Alcohol withdrawal with the help of benzodiazepines and multiple high potency vitamins given IM may reverse the effects caused due to alcoholism.

6. This is a patients of Gilles de la Tourette syndrome. Mean age of onset is 6½ years. The child presents with blinking, nodding, explosive, occasionally obscene verbal ejaculations or gestures with or without anger control problems and attention deficit disorder. Haloperidol sulpiride or clonidine are useful in treatment.

Theme 13: Investigation in medical conditions

1. Lithium carbonate is advised to patients with psychosis. Intracellular levels take time to build up. The dose is adjusted so that a plasma level of 0.7–1.0 mmol/L of Li^+ is achieved. This is measured in 4th–7th day of the start of the treatment. Lithium levels are further checked weekly then monthly and then every 3 months. Lithium affects thyroid and can cause hypothyroidism. Plasma TSH levels need to be checked every 6 months and T_4 levels are checked before starting the treatment.

2. This is a patient of meningitis. Meningitis is inflammation of the meninges. It is most commonly due to bacterial, viral, fungal or other infections. As in this case there is no feature suggestive of any aetiological organism, a CSF examination needs to be done to find the cause. Therefore a lumbar puncture is required for CSF examination. As it is mentioned in the question that there are no signs of raised ICP, LP can be safely done.

3. As the patient is of anorexia nervosa we suspect that the patient has not taken anything orally for some time. His presentation of confusion and seizures can be either due to hypoglycaemia or deranged electrolytes especially sodium. But as hypoglycaemia is not in the options we chose S. electrolytes. Both hypernatraemia and hyponatraemia can present as confusion and seizures.

4. Gamma–Glutamyl Transpeptidase (GGT or γGT) levels in the serum are measured in liver diseases especially alcohol induced damage, due to cholestasis and drugs. It is normally 11–51 IU/L in males and 7–33 IU/L in females.

5. Phenothiazines are antipsychotic drugs which are used to treat schzophrenia and mania. Their mechanism of action is by blocking the central dopamine receptors. Their side effects include

impotence, extrapyramidal effects, gynaecomastia and galactorrhoea (due to increased S. prolactin levels). Therefore his S. prolactin levels need to be measured.

Theme 14: Prostatic conditions

1. Benign prostatic hypertrophy is a common problem. Decrease in urinary flow is associated with increased frequency, urgency and voiding difficulty. Treatment involved is mainly surgical and in some cases medical. In this case as the patient refuses surgery, medical treatment with α blockers like terazocin and indoramin are the drugs of choice. Finasteride, an 5α–reductase inhibitor can also be used.

2. TURP i.e. transurethral resection of prostate remains the most common surgical option for patients of BPH with voiding difficulties. Perioperative antibiotics e.g cefuroxime needs to be given. 1/5th all TURP's need redoing within 10 years.

3. Prostatic carcinoma is the 2nd most common malignancy in men. Incidence increases with age and is associated with increased levels of testosterone and a positive family history. Patients may present with nocturia, hesitancy, poor stream or urinary obstruction. Weight loss and bone pain are suggestive of metastasis. PR examination may reveal hard, irregular prostate gland. Diagnosis is by measuring serum prostate specific antigen levels and doing transrectal USG and biopsy. As the patient in this case does not have prostatic symptoms, a serum PSA level is sufficient to rule out prostatic carcinoma.

4. Prostatic carcinoma is the 2nd most common malignancy in men. Incidence increases with age and is associated with increased levels of testosterone and a positive family history. Patients may present with nocturia, hesitancy, poor stream or urinary obstruction. Weight loss and bone pain are suggestive of metastasis. PR examination may reveal hard, irregular prostate gland. Diagnosis is by measuring serum prostate specific antigen levels and doing transrectal USG and biopsy. As the patient in this case does have prostatic symptoms, a

transrectal USG and biopsy needs to be done for confirmed diagnosis.

5. Patients with prostatic cancer are suspected to have metastasis if they present with weight loss and bone pains. As in this case the patient has developed a femoral lesion, a bone scan needs to be done to localize other bony lesions and hence the extent of metastasis.

Theme 15: Fractures: Diagnosis

1. Fracture of the shaft of the humerus is often caused by a fall on an outstreched arm. Radial nerve may be injured. Radial nerve (C5–T1) is the nerve of extension of the elbow, wrist and fingers. Its injury will produce wrist drop. Splinting and support from the wrist to the neck (Collar & Cuff sling) usually gives satisfactory reduction. Immobilization should be for 8 to12 weeks.

2. Scaphoid fractures usually result from falls on the hand. Patients present with swelling, pain and tenderness 2 cm distal to Lister's tubercle of the radius. These fractures are easily missed on radiography and oblique 'scaphoid' view radiographs are required. Non-displaced fractures are often treated with immobilization in a long-arm thumb-spica cast for several weeks and then in a short-arm thumb-spica cast until union occurs. Avascular necrosis of the proximal fragment may be a complication in some cases.

3. A fracture of the radius or ulna, without angulation, may occur as a consequence of a blow applied directly to the forearm. The presence of fracture of one forearm bone should always raise the suspicion that the inferior or superior radio-ulnar joint has been dislocated as well. The fracture requires immobilization in an above-elbow plaster for 6 weeks in an adult and 3 weeks in a child.

4. Volkmann's ischaemic contracture can occur following interruption of the brachial artery near the elbow. It is seen commonly after a supracondylar fracture of the humerus. Keeping the elbow in extension after the injury prevents brachial artery damage. Muscle necrosis of flexor pollicis longus and flexor digitorum profundus results in contraction and fibrosis. This further causes a flexion deformity at wrist and elbow with forearm pronation, wrist flexion, thumb flexion and adduction,

MCP joint extension and interphalangeal joint flexion. Treatment involves removal of constricting splints. For contractures, release of compressed nerves and tendon lengthening and transfers can be tried.

Theme 16: Poisoning in children

1. Effects of aspirin poisoning are dose-related and potentially fatal. Mild degrees of toxicity can be seen at 150 mg/kg of consumption, moderate at 250 mg/kg and severe toxicity at > 500 mg/kg. Features of aspirin poisoning are seen early as compared to paracetamol poisoning. Vomiting, dehydration, hyper-ventilation, tinnitus, vertigo, seizures, hypotension, heart block, pulmonary oedema and hyperthermia are some of the features of aspirin poisoning. Since it has been mentioned that the child was found with aspirin tablets some hours ago, the features of poisoning should have been evident by now had the child consumed aspirin. Therefore no active intervention is required and simply observing the child for sometime would suffice.

2. Oral contraceptive pills contain oestrogens e.g. ethinylestradiol, with a progestogen. The hormones in the pills are either in a fixed ratio or vary through the month (phased). Since it has been clearly mentioned that the child has consumed OCPs, the hormonal levels in the blood should be measured.

   Note: Side effects of OCPs over a period of time include venous thromboembolism, breast cancer, depression, headaches, loss of libido, nausea, weight gain, cholestatic jaundice, gall stones, vaginal discharge, breast pain, chloasma and leg cramps.

3. Pregnancy increases iron needs by 700–1400 mg per pregnancy. But along with it rises pregnancy induced iron absorption by upto 9 times. Iron and folate supplements are recommended in pregnancy. The tablets consumed by the child in this case must be the iron tablets. Therefore ferrous levels should be checked in the blood. If serum iron concentration exceeds predicted normal iron binding capacity (usually > 90 μmol/L) free iron is circulating and treatment is needed.

Toxic features are unlikely unless more than 60 mg of elemental iron/kg body weight has been ingested. Features of poisoning may include nausea, vomiting, abdominal pain, diarrhoea, polymorph leucocytosis, hyper-glycaemia, hypotension, coma and shock.

4. Adverse effects due to tricyclic antidepressants include dry mouth, tachycardia, blurred vision, glaucoma, constipation, urinary retention, drowsiness, weight gain, cardiac conduction defects, cardiac arrhythmias and seizures. Cardiotoxicity is their most serious side-effect which is due to their membrane stabilizing action. Cardiotoxicity can be seen in ingestion of even 1 gm of TCAs. An ECG is required in all cases of TCA overdose to monitor the cardiac status.

5. The clinical features of alcohol intoxication are related to blood concentrations. Mild intoxication can produce emotional lability, slight impairment of visual acuity and muscular co-ordination. Moderate intoxication produces visual impairment, sensory loss, slowed reaction time and slurred speech. Severe intoxication can produce marked muscular inco-ordination, blurred vision, stupor, hypothermia, hypoglycaemia and seizures. Severe hypoglycaemia results from inhibition of gluconeogenesis. It is more common in children than adults and typically occurs within 6–36 hours of moderate to large amounts of alcohol consumption. Intravenous glucose should be given since hypoglycaemia is usually unresponsive to glucagon.

Theme 17: Testicular swelling

1. Testicular tumours are the most common malignancy in males between the ages 15–44 years. Generally seminomas present between 30–40 years of age and teratoma present between 20–30 years of age. They typically present as painless lump, noticed after trauma or infection. The presentation of the patient in this case along with the age of presentation suggests teratoma. The treatment in such patients is orchidectomy.

2. Testicular tumours are the most common malignancy in males between the ages 15–44 years. Generally seminomas present between 30–40 years of age and teratoma present between 20–30 years of age. They typically present as painless lump, noticed after trauma or infection. The presentation of the patient in this case along with his age at presentation is suggestive of seminoma. Seminomas are exquisitely radiosensitive therefore radiotherapy remains the mainstay of the treatment along with orchidectomy.

3. In this case the details about the swelling have not been provided by the GMC. Therefore one cannot be sure whether this is an epididymal cyst, hydrocele, tumour, orchitis or granuloma. In such cases ultrasound may help in sorting out testicular tumours from other lumps.

4. Painful testis may be due to torsion of testis, epididymitis, tumour, trauma and acute hydrocele. This is a patient with torsion of the testis. Patients generally present with sudden onset pain in one testes along with pain in the abdomen, nausea and vomiting. Patients have hot, tender and swollen testis. Prompt surgery can save testes which may include a possible orchidectomy along with bilateral fixation of testes. The testis is exposed at surgery and untwisted.

Theme 18: Neurological conditions

1. Strokes result from ischaemic infarction or bleeding in brain manifested by acute focal CNS signs and symptoms. Stroke may be due to thrombosis in situ, atherothromboembolism, heart emboli, aneurysmal rupture or trauma. Patients may present with features depending upon the affected site:

   i. In cerebral hemispheric infarcts, patients may present with contralateral hemiplegia which is initially flaccid then becomes spastic, contralateral sensory loss, homonymous hemianopia, dysphasia.

   ii. In brainstem infarct patients may present with quadriplegia, disturbances of gaze and vision, locked in syndrome.

   iii. Patients with lacunar infarcts may have pure motor, pulse sensory, mixed motor and sensory signs or ataxia.

2. Motor neurone disease is caused by degeneration of neurons in motor cortex, cranial nerve nuclei and anterior horn cells. There is no sensory loss in MND as compared to Multiple sclerosis and polyneuropathies. Golden rule: think of MND in those > 40 years of age presenting with foot drop, spastic gait, weak grip or aspiration pneumonia. Patients with upper motor neurone disease present with weakness, spasticity, brisk reflexes, plantars upgoing. Patients with lower motor neurone disease present with weakness, wasting, fasciculation of tongue, abdomen, back or thighs. Treatment is essentially symptomatic.

3. Multiple sclerosis is a chronic disorder which consists of plaques of demyelination and axon loss at sites throughout the CNS. Patients may present with unilateral optic neuritis– pain on eye movements and rapid deterioration in central vision, nystagmus, fatigue, weakness or spasticity in limbs, constipation, frequency and urgency, impotence, ataxia, dementia, vertigo, even depression. No test is pathognomic and diagnosis is essentially clinical. Symptoms may worsen by heat or exercise. There is no cure but methylprednisolone shortens relapse and β interferon decreases relapse rate.

4. Alzheimer's dementia is the most common form of dementia in UK. Suspect AD in any enduring, acquired deficit of memory and cognition. Onset may be from 40 years though it may be seen earlier in patients suffering from Down's syndrome. On histological examination plaques with neurofibrillary tangles and cortical β-amyloid protein are found. On MRI an increased cortical atrophy in the medial temporal lobe can be seen. In stage I of AD there is falling memory and spatial disorientation. In stage II the personality disintegrates and in stage III the patient is apathetic, wasted and bedridden.

5. Plummer vinson syndrome is also known as Paterson–Brown–Kelly syndrome. Patients typically present with dysphagia and iron deficiency anaemia. Dysphagia may be due to an post cricoid oesophageal web. This is a premalignant condition that may occur in the absence of anaemia, usually in middle aged women.

6. This is a patient of lateral medullary syndrome. It is due to infarction of the lateral medulla and the inferior surface of the cerebellum. Patients generally present with vertigo, vomiting, dysphagia, nystagmus, ipsilateral ataxia, paralysis of soft palate, ipsilateral Horner's syndrome, analgesia to pinprick on ipsilateral face and contralateral trunk and limbs.

Theme 19: Diagnosis of skin disorders

1. Melanoma is a dermatological malignancy caused due to excessive UV exposure. The 'Glasgow 7': major include change in (i) size (ii) shape (iii) colour, minor include (iv) inflammation (v) bleeding/oozing (vi) diameter of the lesion > 7 mm (vii) itching. Prevention includes avoiding excessive sun exposure, wearing sun protective clothing and use of broad-spectrum SPF sunscreens. Melanoma must be completely excised with 1 cm of normal skin around the lesion for every millimeter of depth, upto 3 cms.

2. Skin manifestations in diabetes mellitus include infection, ulcers, necrobiosis lipoidica (shiny areas on shin with yellow skin) and granuloma annulare. Neuropathy in diabetes puts the patient at high risk of foot ulceration. In this case the patient must be a non insulin dependent diabetic where the patients are generally of the older age group and often obese.

3. Pyoderma gangrenosum implies recurring nodulopustular ulcers around 10 cm wide, with tender red/blue overhanging edges. They are seen in patients with Crohn's disease. These ulcers heal with cribriform scars and are seen on legs, abdomen and face. Saline cleansing with high dose oral or intralesional steroids are required.

Theme 20: Diagnosing emergencies

1. This is a patient with tension pneumothorax. The mediastinum is pushed over into the contralateral hemithorax. Patients present with dyspnoea, tachycardia, hypotension, raised JVP, tracheal deviation away from the side of pneumothorax, increased percussion note, decreased air entry on the affected side. Unless the air is rapidly removed, cardio-respiratory arrest will occur. Emergency treatment consists of removal of air by inserting a large-bore needle with syringe into the second intercostal space in the mid clavicular line. Next step after that would be to insert a chest drain.

2. In patients with MI, CXR will show no abnormality. The ECG changes in patients with MI include (i) Hyperacute T waves and ST elevation within hours of acute Q wave infarction (ii) T wave inversion and resolution of ST segment is noted within 1 day (iii) Pathological Q waves begin to form within few days (iv) In non Q wave i.e. subendocardial infarction ECG may show T wave inversion with ST depression.
Note: In 1/5th of patients with MI, ECG may be normal initially.

3. A midzone consolidation noted on the CXR with a normal ECG and raised temperature are suggestive of pneumonia. Patients present with fever, cyanosis, tachycardia, hypotension, signs of consolidation like decreased expansion, dull percussion note, increased tactile vocal fremitus, bronchial breathing and pleural rub. Treatment is with oxygen, antibiotics and IV fluids.

4. Pulmonary embolism usually arises from a venous thrombus in the pelvis or legs. Risk factors include history of DVT, OCPs, immobility and hypercoagulability. Patients may present with breathlessness, pleuritic chest pain, fever, haemoptysis, tachycardia,

gallop rhythm, hypotension, raised JVP and pleural rub. ECG may be normal. CXR may show oligaemia of the affected segment, dilated pulmonary artery. The investigation of choice is CT pulmonary angiography. If unavailable V/Q scan should be done. Low molecular weight heparin is used to anti-coagulate.

5. Perforation of the oesophagus can result from inexpert use of an oesophagoscope. The most frequent cause of oesophageal perforation is a sharp foreign body plus instrumentation to remove it. Patients may present with distress, dysphagia and dyspnoea. A CXR may disclose the presence of air in the mediastinum, pleural cavity or in the neck which may be palpable (surgical emphysema). In mid or lower oesophageal ruptures, urgent thoracotomy under antibiotic cover is performed. In small oesophageal perforations with no evidence of perforation on CXR, massive antibiotic treatment with parenteral feeding may suffice.

Theme 21: Treatment of psychiatric disorders

1. This is a patient of obsessive-compulsive disorder. Compulsions are repeated and senseless rituals whereas obsessions are stereotyped, purposeless words or ideas that come to the mind. The treatment is essentially with behavioural therapy. Treatment includes repeated exposure to the stimulus while encouraging avoiding the ritual. The therapist shows what the patient is supposed to do.

2. Electroconvulsive therapy is instituted in (i) depression if (a) patient is not responding to the antidepressant (b) with psychotic features (c) need to control speedily e.g. postpartum, with suicidal risk. (ii) Schizo affective depression (iii) Mania not responding to drugs.

3. Postnatal depression is a common problem. Most postnatal depression resolves within 6 months. It may be due to social, genetic or hormonal causes. Fluoxetine is as effective as cognitive behavioural therapy in short term. Lithium may be additionally helpful. Transdermal oestrogen is partly effective in severe postnatal depression.

4. Postural hypotension due to inhibition of cardiovascular reflexes and α_1 blockade, and cardiac arrhythmias with T wave suppression or inversion are common side-effects of TCAs. Fluoxetine is a prototype of newer SSRIs which is devoid of anticholinergic, sedative and hypotensive side effects. It also does not prolong cardiac conduction time or lower seizure threshold and hence is safer in overdose. Elevation of mood and increased work capacity is reported even in apparently non depressed patients e.g. post myocardial infarction.

Theme 22: Diagnosis of gynaecological conditions

1. Candidiasis (Thrush) is the most common cause of vaginal discharge which is classically white curds. Pregnancy, OCPs, steroids, immunodeficiency, antibiotics and diabetes are important predisposing factors. Diagnosis is by microscopy which shows mycelia and spores. Treatment is by a single clotrimazole pessary.

2. Lichen sclerosis is the commonest condition found in elderly women complaining of vulval itching. It is commonly associated with autoimmune disorders. It is due to elastic tissue turning into collagen after middle age. The vulva gradually becomes white, flat and shiny. There may be an hourglass shape around the vulva and anus. If the patient has been scratching the area the skin may become thickened (litchenified). Treatment is with 0.1% betamethasone valerate cream. Vulval ablation may be needed to relieve the itch.

3. Like the cervical carcinoma, vulval carcinoma also has a pre–invasive phase, the vulval intra-epithelial neoplasia which may be itchy. 95% of the cases are squamous cell. They occur mostly in the elderly. Treatment is by wide local excision or laser ablation.

4. Lymphogranuloma may be due to lympho-granuloma venerum, chancroid or granuloma inguinale. Lymphogranuloma may present with inguinal lymphadenopathy and ulceration. Granuloma inguinale may cause extensive, painless, red genital ulcers and pseudobuboes i.e. abscesses near inguinal nodes. Diagnosis is by visualization of 'closed safety-pin' inclusion bodies in the cytoplasm of histiocytes. Treatment is with tetracycline given for more than 2 weeks.

5. The presentation of dysuria and vesicles in the vaginal area is suggestive of herpes. Herpes type II is sexually acquired and classically causes genital infection. The vulva is ulcerated and very painful. Treatment includes topical aciclovir, strong analgesia, lidocaine gel and salt baths.

Theme 23: Management in trauma

1. A simple rib fracture may be serious in elderly patients or those with chronic lung diseases who have little pulmonary reserve. Uncomplicated fractures require sufficient analgesia to encourage a normal respiratory pattern and effective coughing. Oral analgesia may suffice. Chest strapping or bed rest are no longer advised. Early ambulation with vigorous physiotherapy help. A CXR is taken to exclude an underlying pneumothorax.

2. The thoracic spine may be injured as a component of multiple injury or in isolation. Damage to the thoracic spine is likely to be associated with injuries to other thoracic viscera. All vertebral injuries are to be considered unstable until proved otherwise. Patients with dorsal and lumbar spine injuries should not be moved, except by at least three attendants. Simple examination of the sensory, motor and reflex function usually indicates the site of the lesion. An MRI displays non invasively and without radiation, the extraspinal soft tissues, the vertebral column and the spinal cord. Extradural haematomas, disc and bone fragments, cord contusion and oedema can all be identified in the acute stages of the injury.

3. Fractures of the sternum are usually seen as a result of deceleration on to seat belts. The injury is very painful even in mild cases where only the external plate of the sternum is fractured. There is an increased risk of underlying myocardial damage in sternal fractures and the patient should be admitted with constant ECG monitoring, analgesia and serial cardiac enzymes. Most cases do not need any specific treatment but paradoxical movement or instability of the chest may require chest strapping or surgical fixation.

4. Abdomen and chest may be the sites of hidden blood loss after a blunt abdominal injury. Intra-abdominal bleeding or pelvic fracture should always be considered if patient has hypotension and no source of loss is found. Ruptured spleen may present with shock, abdominal tenderness and distension, left shoulder-tip pain or overlying rib fracture. Visceral injury may cause bruising in the flanks with absent bowel sounds and muscular spasm. Haematuria may be seen in injury to the genitourinary system. Laparotomy is indicated in patients with hypotension, GI, GU or PR bleeding, evisceration, a positive ultrasound or peritoneal lavage. Shock must be managed with IV fluids preferably Haemaccel. If the patient does not respond, exploratory laparotomy should be performed.

5. Ruptured spleen in a patient is suggested by shock, abdominal tenderness and distension, left shoulder tip pain and overlying rib fractures. Management in such patients include maintaining airway, high flow O_2, treating shock, crossmatching blood and a prompt exploratory laparotomy. Since the patient in this condition is not bleeding and has no mention of shock or hypotension, admitting the patient and simple observation for any ominous signs is all that is required.

Theme 24: Management of thyroid disorders

1. Indications for thyroid surgery include pressure symptoms, hyperthyroidism, carcinoma and cosmetic reasons. All patients must be rendered euthyroid pre-operatively by antithyroid drugs and/or propranolol.

2. This is a case of hyperthyroidism. Patients generally present with weight loss, palpitations and diarrhoea. Other presentations include increased appetite, heat intolerance, sweating, tremors, irritability, emotional lability, oligomenorrhoea, tachycardia, lid lag. Tests reveal decrease in TSH and increased T_4 and T_3. Treatment includes propranolol for immediate symptomatic relief and carbimazole to actually normalize the TFT levels. Other modalities of treatment include partial thyroidectomy and radioiodine I^{131} therapy. As in this case the patient is allergic to carbimazole, propylthiouracil is the next alternative.

3. This is a case of hyperthyroidism. Patients generally present with weight loss, palpitations and diarrhoea. Other presentations include increased appetite, heat intolerance, sweating, tremors, irritability, emotional lability, oligomenorrhoea, tachycardia, lid lag. Tests reveal decrease in TSH and increased T_4 and T_3. Treatment includes propranolol for immediate symptomatic relief and carbimazole to actually normalize the TFT levels. Other modalities of treatment include partial thyroidectomy and radioiodine I^{131} therapy.

4. Low basal metabolic rate is seen in hypothyroidism. Patients with hypothyroidism may also present with tiredness, lethargy, weight gain, constipation, depression, menorrhagia, bradycardia, dry skin, non pitting oedema, pericardial effusion, cerebellar ataxia, peripheral neuropathy. Treatment in hypothyroidism includes thyroxine, the dose of which is adjusted to normalize TSH.

Theme 25: Diagnosis of epilepsy

1. The mention of occurrence of attacks of seizures only when people are around her are suggestive of conversion disorder. Such patients need to be tele-monitored. But once conversion disorder is suspected organic disorder exclusion must be sought for accompanied by a search for a psychological explanation of the patients symptoms. Admission to hospital may be necessary for further assessment and treatment.

2. Petitmal or Absences are a type of generalized seizures. There are episodes of brief (£ 10 sec) pauses e.g. the patient stops talking in mid-sentence and then carries on where left off. It is generally seen in childhood. Ethosuximide with/without sodium valproate is used in the treatment.

3. Tonic clonic or classical grand mal are a type of generalized seizures. They are sudden in onset with loss of consciousness. The limbs initially stiffen (tonic phase) then jerk (clonic phase); although the patient may have either of the phases singly as well. Patients are drowsy after the attack. The tongue is usually bitten at the onset of the seizure. Sodium valproate is the first line drug therapy; carbamazepine is an alternative.

4. This is a case of vasovagal syncope. Upright posture is an invariable feature in such patients leading to pooling of 500–1000 ml of blood in lower limbs. Reduced cardiac filling causes baroreceptors to manifest a reflex bradycardia and vasodilatation. Patients may suffer trauma due to fall. Patient may be pale/cyanosed during the attack. Recovery is rapid with no pre-ictal amnesia.

5. This is a case of febrile convulsion. This condition is diagnosed if the following occur together: (a) a tonic/clonic, symmetrical seizure (b) occurring with rising temperature (c) age of child between 6 months and five years. (d)

No signs of CNS infection or previous history of epilepsy (e) number of seizures < 3 and lasting < 5 min. Treatment involves giving diazepam at the time of attack. Otherwise tepid sponging or paracetamol syrup.

Theme 26: Causes of renal stone

1. One of the risk factors for nephrolithiasis is dehydration. This case being a marathon runner, we suspect him to be having dehydration intermittently due to excessive sweating. Stones in the kidney cause loin pain and stones in the ureter cause renal colic. This pain classically radiates from the loin to the groin.

2. Another risk factor for nephrolithiasis is UTI as in this patient. Renal stones may further cause infection which may be acute or chronic or recurrent. It may present with cystitis, pyelonephritis or pyonephrosis. Antibiotics are required for such cases along with IV fluids and symptomatic treatment.

3. This is a case of idiopathic nephrolithiasis. One can also think of idiopathic hypercalciuria as it is one of the risk factors for nephrolithiasis. Genetic factors clearly play a part in the aetiology of idiopathic hypercalciuria which is more common in men than in women suggesting a sex linked inherited component.

4. GMC is possibly referring to the type of stone here. Struvite stones can grow to a large size and fill the renal pelvis and calyces to produce a 'staghorn' appearance. They are radio-opaque with a variable internal density. These stones mainly occur in women or in patients with chronic bladder catheterization and result from urinary tract infection especially with proteus species.

Theme 27: Management of ear conditions

1. Foreign bodies in the ear are common in children and mentally retarded. Organic matter can caused inflammation. For small objects syringing is sufficient. Insects should be killed with oil before removal. Soft objects can be taken out with the help of forceps whereas smooth hard objects should be removed with suction and/hooks. General anaesthesia may be needed in children.

2. As explained above.

3. As explained above.

4. As explained above.

5. Otitis media means inflammation in the middle ear. Acute otitis media presents with rapid onset of pain and fever, often after a viral URTI. Chronic otitis media is also known as serous or secretory otitis media or glue ear, which implies inflammation with middle ear fluid of several months duration. Treatment is with analgesics and appropriate antibiotics e.g. amoxicillin.

Theme 28: Eye conditions: Diagnosis

1. Blunt trauma to the eye can present with primary or secondary haemorrhage. Hyphaema is blood in the anterior chambers. In small amounts it clears spontaneously. Secondary haemorrhage can occur within 5 days of trauma in the form of secondary glaucoma, as must be in this case. It can also present as traumatic mydriasis, vitreous haemorrhage, lens dislocation, tearing of the iris root, splitting of the choroid, detachment of the retina and damage to the optic nerve.

2. Acute dacryocystitis is acute inflammation of the tear sac which is located medially, to the medial canthus. Antibiotics are used to resolve the infection, failure of which may lead to local abscess formation.

3. Fixed dilated pupil may be because of mydriatrics, acute glaucoma, conical i.e. uncal herniation, IIIrd nerve palsy, raised ICP due to any cause e.g. cavernous sinus thrombosis. The presentation of patient in this case is suggestive of acute glaucoma. This is a disease of the middle aged or elderly. The attack is commonly preceded by blurred vision or haloes around lights. It is due to blockage of drainage of aqueous from anterior chamber via the canal of schlemm. IOT may rise to 60–70 mm Hg. Pilocarpine drops and acetazolamide are used in its treatment. Peripheral iridectomy is done after the IOT has been brought under normal range.

4. Acute iritis (Anterior Uveitis) presents with pain of acute onset, photophobia, blurred vision, lacrimation, ciliary congestion and a small pupil. Talbot's test i.e. pain on convergence of eyes, is positive. It is associated with systemic diseases such as ankylosing spondylitis, sarcoidosis. Its treatment is with steroids to decrease inflammation and cyclopentolate to prevent adhesions.

Theme 29: Abdominal pain in children

1. Intussusception presents as severe, colicky, abdominal pain. There is vomiting and stools are blood stained like current jelly. A sausage shaped mass may be palpable in the right lower quadrant. Barium enema shows cupping. It is a surgical emergency, but intussusception of short duration may even be relieved by the hydrostatic pressure of barium enema.

2. Coeliac disease is a condition in which the patient has prolamin intolerance leading to villous atrophy and malabsorption. α-gliadin and anti endomyseal antibodies help the diagnosis. Patient presents with steatorrhoea, abdominal pain, bloating and angular stomatitis. Jejunal biopsy confirms villous atrophy. Management involves gluten free diet. In such patients because of the villous atrophy, iron absorption cannot take place.

3. This is a case of gastroenteritis which is probably due to vibrio cholerae. Other causes of gastroenteritis include campylobacter, staphylococcus, *E. coli*, salmonella, shigella, rotavirus, giardiasis, amoebiasis, cryptosporidium. The big danger is due to dehydration with or without urea and electrolyte imbalance. First treat dehydration with IV or oral rehydration. Milk is to be reintroduced 24 hours later.

4. Hirschprung's disease is congenital absence of ganglia in a segment of colon causing infrequent, narrow stools, GI obstruction and megacolon. This disease is suspected in infants if there is an explosive gush of faeces on withdrawing the finger after a PR examination. It may also present with alternating diarrhoea and constipation with abdominal distension and failure to thrive. Excision of the aganglionic segment is usually needed.

Theme 30: Pre-operative investigation

1. Frusemide is a high ceiling (loop) diuretic which acts by inhibiting $Na^+-K^+-2Cl^-$ cotransport in the thick ascending limb of loop of Henle. IV frusemide causes prompt increase in systemic venous capacitance and decreases left ventricular filling pressure. This is responsible for the quick relief it provides in LVF and pulmonary oedema. It tends to raise blood uric acid levels by decreasing its renal excretion. K^+ excretion is increased mainly due to high Na^+ load reaching the distal tubule. This can cause hypokalaemia. Therefore U&E should be checked pre-operatively in this patient.

2. A pre-operative CXR is required in all those patients with known cardiorespiratory disease, pathology or symptoms or if the patient is > 65 years age.

3. Clotting studies need to be done in liver disease, DIC, massive blood loss and in patients already on warfarin or heparin.

Theme 31: Pre-operative medication

1. This is a patient of DVT. Surgery, past DVT and immobility are risk factors for DVT. Therefore DVT prophylaxis must be instituted in this case. Give heparin 5000 U subcutaneous pre-operatively then every 12 hourly until ambulant.

2. DVT prophylaxis needs to be instituted in this case also as the patient is to undergo an orthopaedic surgery. Give compression hose (not if poor foot pulses) with heparin 5000 U subcutaneously pre-operatively then every 12 hourly until ambulant.

3. The underlying pathology in unsable angina is usually plaque fissuring and rupture, with consequent platelet adhesion and thrombus formation. Since surgery itself predisposes thrombus formation, subcutaneous heparin should be given to the patient.

4. All patients who need to undergo major surgeries require some form of prophylactic antibiotics pre-operatively especially GI and GU surgeries.

5. A person falls under the 'low-risk drinking' category if he consumes ≤ 20 units of alcohol/week (≤ 15 units/week for women). Similarly the number of cigarettes smoked/day should be less than 20. Since the number of cigarettes smoked/day is high in this patient, he should stop smoking.

6. A person falls under the 'low-risk drinking' category if the consumes ≤ 20 units of alcohol/week (≤ 15 units/week for women). Since the patient is consuming much more alcohol than the acceptable range, he should stop taking alcohol.

7. As explained in Question 5.

Theme 32: Treatment of emergencies

1. Surgery is advised if (i) there are bilateral pneumothoraces, (ii) lung fails to expand after intercostal drain insertion, (iii) two or more previous pneumothoraces on the same side (iv) history of pneumothorax on the opposite site (v) in traumatic haemothorax if blood loss is > 200 ml/hour.

2. Myocardial infarction is usually due to occlusion of a coronary artery resulting from rupture of an atheromatous plaque. Patient usually present with acute chest pain lasting > 20 minute. MI is associated with nausea, sweatiness, dyspnoea and palpitations. In elderly or diabetics, MI may also present without chest pain (silent MI). On examination there may be pallor, distress, sweatiness and 4th heart sound. ECG changes—Q waves (as in this case) signify transmural infarction. Hyperacute T waves and ST elevation are also seen. Non Q wave infarct means a sub-endocardial infarct. Other investigations required are cardiac enzymes CK, AST, LDH which are elevated. Troponin T is also elevated. Treatment involves aspirin stat, analgesia with morphine, O_2, thrombolysis with streptokinase or t-PA.

3. Anaphylactic shock is an IgE mediated hypersensitivity reaction. Release of histamine and other agents causes cyanosis, urticaria, capillary leak, wheeze and oedema of larynx, lids, tongue and lips as in this case. Treatment, after securing the airway, is by giving IM adrenaline 0.5 mg i.e. 0.5 ml of 1:1000.

4. The presentation of the patient with fever and basal consolidation on CXR is almost diagnostic of pneumonia. Other features that may be present in patients with pneumonia are malaise, anorexia, cough, purulent sputum, haemoptysis, pleuritic chest pain, tachypnoea, fever, hypotension and signs of consolidation. Investigations required are CXR, sputum for

microscopy and cultures and pleural aspirate (if present) for culture. Treatment involves antibiotics according to sensitivity patterns.

Theme 33: Asthma in children

1. Asthma implies reversible obstruction of the airways. Patient may present with wheeze dyspnoea or cough. It may be life-threatening if peak flow < 33%, presence of cyanosis, silent chest, fatigue or exhausion, agitation, decrease level of consciousness. Steps in management: (i) Try occasional β agonists (ii) Add inhaled steroids or cortons (sodium cromoglycate) (iii) Add inhaled salmeterol or increased dose of steroid (iv) Try oral theophylline/salmeterol or inhaled ipratropium (v) Add prednisolone tablets. In case of severe asthma give high flow 100% O_2 → Nebulized salbutamol→Oral prednisolone→ Amino-phylline→Hydrocortisone with nebulized, ipratropium→Oximetry and CXR→Treat any pneumonia→Repeat nebulizer as needed→ Take to ITU if peak flow continues to fall.

2. As explained above.
3. As explained above.
4. As explained above.

Theme 34: Bleeding disorders

1. In case of major or prolonged bleeding in patients who are already on warfarin, the first step in management is to stop warfarin. Give prothrombin complex concentrate or fresh frozen plasma. Vitamin K 5 mg should be given orally or IV.

2. Episodic bleeding into joints is common in haemophilia. If inadequately treated, it may cause secondary deformity and crippling. The knee ankle and elbow are the most commonly affected. In severe haemophilia spontaneous haemorrhage into joints may take place. Here factor VIII levels are usually < 1 IU/dL i.e. 1% normal. Therefore measurement of the coagulation factor is a must as it also decides upon the treatment plan.

3. Sickle cell anaemia is due to production of abnormal beta peptide chains (Glu → Val at position 6). HbS polymerizes when deoxygenated, causing RBCs to sickle which become fragile and haemolyse. Hb ~6–8 gm/dL with reticulocytes ~10–20% and target cells on blood films. The patient may present simply with anaemia, as in this case or along with sickle cell crises like thrombotic crises or aplastic crises or sequestration crises. Treatment involves giving hydroxyurea if frequent crises or simply blood transfusions to keep HbS level < 30%.

4. Disseminated intravascular coagulation is a pathological activation of coagulation mechanisms due to malignancy, infection, trauma, in pregnancy. Patients may present with extensive bruising, bleeding from old venepuncture sites, renal failure or gangrene. Broken RBCs (schistocytes) can be seen on the blood film. Bleeding can also occur in any of the organs e.g. uterus, lungs or CNS. Platelets are decreased, fibrinogen decreased, PT increased, APTT increased, fibrin degradation products are increased. Treat the cause wherever possible and give FFP and supportive treatment.

5. In case of major or prolonged bleeding in patients who are already on warfarin, the first step in management is to stop warfarin. Give prothrombin complex concentrate or fresh frozen plasma. Vitamin K 5 mg should be given orally or IV. As in this case the bleeding is slight and not profuse, giving vitamin K to the patient would suffice.

Theme 35: Diagnosing emergencies

1. This is a patient with tension pneumothorax. The mediastinum is pushed over into the contralateral hemithorax. Patients present with dyspnoea, tachycardia, hypotension, raised JVP, tracheal deviation away from the side of pneumothorax, increased percussion note, decreased air entry on the affected side. Unless the air is rapidly removed, cardio-respiratory arrest will occur. Emergency treatment consists of removal of air by inserting a large-bore needle with syringe into the second intercostal space in the mid clavicular line. Next step after that would be to insert a chest drain.

2. The most common pathology affecting the aorta is aneurysm formation or dissection. Aneurysms are described as fusiform when the whole circumference is affected or saccular when only a part of the circumference is involved. The most common aetiology is atherosclerosis. Pressure on adjacent structures may cause pain (vertebra), hoarseness (recurrent laryngeal nerve), dysphagia (oesophagus) and respiratory symptoms (left main bronchus). The diagnosis is confirmed by computed tomography or magnetic resonance imaging. Surgical treatment is advised in such cases because without treatment the aneurysm is likely to expand and ultimately rupture.

3. Mitral regurgitation can be due to various causes viz. functional (LV dilatation), annular calcification in the elderly, rheumatic fever, IE, MVP, connective tissue disorders (Ehler–Danlos/Marfan's syndrome), ruptured chordae tendinae, papillary muscle dysfunction or rupture, cardiomyopathy. Patients may present with breathlessness, fatigue, palpitations, displaced hyperdynamic apex, RV heave, soft S1, split S2, loud P2 and a pansystolic murmur at the apex radiating to the axilla. A CXR can show big LA and LV, mitral valve calcification and pulmonary oedema. Echocardiogram can assess LV function and cardiac catheterization can confirm the diagnosis. Surgery is required in patients with deteriorating symptoms by repairing or replacing the valve before irreversible impairment of LV occurs.

4. Lung contusion can be seen in moderate-to-severe blunt thoracic trauma. It usually resolves but lacerations with persistent air leaks may require surgical exploration. Early mobilization prophylactic antibiotics, suction drainage and physiotherapy are important to prevent infection of the underlying lung.

5. This patient is possibly a case of left heart failure. Heart failure implies an inadequate cardiac output and blood pressure for the body's requirement. It can present as left heart failure, right heart failure or together as congestive cardiac failure (CCF).

   Patients with left heart failure present with breathlessness, poor exercise tolerance, fatigue, orthopnoea, paroxysmal nocturnal dyspnoea (PND), nocturnal cough, pink frothy sputum due to pulmonary oedema, wheeze ('cardiac asthma'), nocturia, cold peripheries, weight loss and muscle wasting, resting tachycardia, systolic hypotension, narrow pulse pressure, displaced apex, RV heave, bibasal end-inspiratory crackles, pleural effusions. CXR may reveal cardiomegaly, prominent upper lobe veins, diffuse interstitial or alveolar shadowing, perihilar 'bat's wing' shadowing, pleural effusions and kerley B lines. Echocardiography can indicate the cause and confirm the presence or absence of LV dysfunction. Pharmacological therapy includes diuretics e.g. frusemide, ACE inhibitors, vasodilators, inotropes and β blockers.

Theme 36: Renal problems

1. Chronic renal failure can be graded as mild (GFR 30–50 ml/min), moderate (GFR 10–29 ml/min), severe (GFR <10 ml/min) or end stage (GFR < 5 ml/min). Death ensues in end stage renal failure unless renal replacement therapy is given. Common causes of CRF include glomerulonephritis, pyelonephritis, interstitial nephritis, DM, hypertension, cystic disease, analgesic nephropathy, renal vascular disease and nephrolithiasis. Patients may present with pallor, yellow skin pigmentation, brown nails, purpura, bruising, hypertension, cardiomegaly, pericarditis, pleural effusion, pulmonary or peripheral oedema, retinopathy, arrhythmias, encephalopathy, seizures and coma. Urea, creatinine, phosphate, and alkaline phosphate are raised. Treatment involves treating hypertension with ACE inhibitors, hyperlipidaemia with statins, anaemia with erythropoietin and sodium restriction in diet.

2. Sarcoidosis is a multisystem granulomatous disorder. It commonly affects adults aged 20–40 years. Acute sarcoidosis presents with erythema nodosum and polyarthralgia. Pulmonary manifestations include bilateral hilar lymphadenopathy, fibrosis, pulmonary infiltrates, cough, dyspnoea and chest pain. Non-pulmonary manifestations include lymphadenopathy, hepatosplenomegaly, uveitis, Bell's palsy, neuropathy, SOL, subcutaneous nodules, cardiomyopathy, hypercalcaemia, hypercalciuria, renal stones and pituitary dysfunction. Bone X-rays show 'punched out' lesions in terminal phalanges. Indications for corticosteroid therapy include parenchymal lung disease, uveitis, hypercalcaemia and neurological or cardiac involvement. Prednisolone 40 mg/day PO for 4–6 weeks is given.

3. Adult polycystic kidney disease is an autosomal dominant disorder with genes on chromosome 16 and 4. Patients may have renal enlargement with cysts, abdominal pain, haematuria, UTI, renal calculi, hypertension and renal failure. Extra-renal manifestations include liver cysts, intracranial aneurysms, subarachnoid haemorrhage, MVP and abdominal herniae.

4. Papillary necrosis is a part of the spectrum of pathologies which fall under the term Analgesic Nephropathy. Initially the lesion is confined to the central part of the inner medulla and affects only the interstitial cells, thin ascending limb of Henle's loop and peritubular capillaries. Later necrosis of all medullary elements occur with partial or total papillary separation. Patients may present with proteinuria, haematuria, colic or obstruction giving rise to hydronephrosis or pyonephrosis. Infection in or around necrotic papillae may manifest as acute pyelonephritis or indolent urinary infection. Complete cessation of analgesic consumption is the only specific measure.

5. Henoch–Schönlein purpura (HSP) can be considered a systemic variant of IgA nephropathy. Patients with HSP have flitting polyarthritis of large joints, purpuric rash over extensor surfaces, abdominal symptoms and glomerulonephritis. Diagnosis can be confirmed by finding positive IF for IgA and C3 in skin lesions or renal biopsy.

6. Urethral calculi can arise primarily behind a stricture or in an infected urethral diverticulum. More commonly, the stone is actually a renal calculus that has migrated to the urethra via the bladder. It causes sudden pain in the urethra after an attack of ureteric colic. There is blockage to the flow of urine. It is a painful condition and pain can sometimes be felt radiating to the scrotum. The calculus can be felt sometimes as a hard lump in the urethra.

Theme 37: Diagnosing genetical disorders

1. Disorders determined by mutant genes carried on the X or Y chromosomes are known as sex-linked disorders. As the male passes his Y chromosome only to his sons, Y linked disorders show male-to-male transmission.

2. Since both the parents are affected in this case, the disorder has to be X linked (X chromosome being there in both males (XY) and females (XX). The presentation of the father checking his blood counts and mother receiving regular blood transfusions is suggestive of haemophilia.

3. This is another case of haemophilia. Haemophilia A is due to deficiency of factor VIII. It is inherited as an X-linked recessive disorder. Patients may present early in life or after surgery or trauma as bleeds in joints and muscle, leading to crippling arthropathies and haematomas. Investigations reveal an increased KCCT and decreased factor VIII assays. NSAIDs and IM injections are to be strictly avoided. Minor bleeds may be managed by desmopressin. Major bleeds would require factor VIII levels to increase to 50% of normal. Haemophilia B is also an X-linked recessive disorder due to deficiency of factor IX.

4. Diabetes mellitus results from lack of, or diminished effect of endogenous insulin. It is characterized by hyperglycaemia. Type I (insulin dependent DM) is usually juvenile onset and is characterized by insulin deficiency. Type II (non-insulin dependent DM) is usually seen in the elderly and often obese. NIDDMs may eventually need insulin. Diabetes is a multigenic disorder. Type I DM has > 30% concordance in identical twins and type II DM has ~ 100% concordance in identical twins. Obesity probably causes insulin resistance by increasing the rate of release of non-esterified fatty acids which cause post-receptor defects in insulin's action.

5. Otosclerosis is an autosomal dominant hereditary disorder with incomplete penetration. Half of the patients have a family history of the disease. In this condition the vascular spongy bone replaces the normal lamellar bone of otic capsule origin especially around the oral window which fixes the stapes foot plate. Symptoms are usually seen in adulthood and are exacerbated due to pregnancy, menstruation and menopause. Hearing is often better with background noise. Surgical treatment involves stapedectomy or stapedotomy.

Theme 38: Medical diagnosis

1. The patient in this case is suffering from gout. Points in favour of the diagnosis are (i) the patient is on anti-hypertensive treatment (diuretics) is a precipitating factor for the deposition of sodium monourate crystals in the joint and causes gout. (ii) The patient presents with pain and swelling of the joint which is hot to touch. These presentations are classically seen in the acute stage of gout.

2. Multiple myeloma is a neoplastic proliferation of plasma cell with diffuse bone marrow infiltration and focal osteolytic lesions. Peak age of incidence is 70 years, patients present with bone pain tenderness, pathological fractures, lassitude, pyogenic infection, amyloidosis, neuropathy, signs of hyperviscosity, decreased visual acuity and bleeding. Bence Jones protein may be detectable in urine. Bone radiographs show punched out lesions 'Pepper pot skull'. Treatment includes high fluid intake and melphalan as such or part of ABCM regimen (Adriamycin, Bleomycin, Cyclophosphamide, Melphalan). Biphosphonates are required if hypercalcaemia is present.

3. Patients with ankylosing spondylitis are typically young who present with morning stiffness, backache, sacroiliac pain, progressive loss of spinal movement i.e. spinal ankylosis, neck hyperextension and spino-cranial ankylosis. X-ray of the spine may shows 'bamboo' spine (i.e. squaring of the vertebrae), erosions of apophyseal joints and obliteration of sacroiliac joints. Treatment includes exercise for backache and NSAIDs for pain and stiffness.

Theme 39: Incontinence

1. Urinary tract infection implies presence of a pure growth of more than 10^5 colony forming units/ml. Recurrent infection implies infection with a new organism. Infection may occur at any site in the urinary tract. Infection of the bladder produces cystitis, as in this case. Such patients present with frequency, dysuria, urgency, strangury, haematuria and suprapubic pain. Infection of the prostate may cause prostatitis with 'flu'-like symptoms, low back ache, swollen and tender prostate. Infection at the kidney cause pyelonephritis evident as fever with rigors, vomiting, ARF, loin pain and tenderness. *E. coli* is the most common infecting organism. Since in this case the child has had recurrent infection and was catheterized, catheter should be sent for culture and sensitivity patterns should be sought.

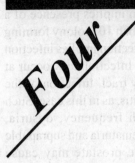

PLAB

Four

March 2003 Question Paper

Theme 1: Management of ophthalmic conditions

Options:

a. Intraocular steroids
b. IV steroids
c. Oral steroids
d. Eye surgery
e. Beta-blockers
f. Laser treatment
g. Systemic antibiotics
h. No treatment is required

For each presentation below, choose the SINGLE most appropriate management from the above list of options. Each option may be used once, more than once, or not at all.

1. A patient presents with sudden loss of vision and history of temporal arteritis.
2. A patient presents with decreased vision on watching TV and gives history of tunnel vision. On examination cupping of disc is seen.
3. Patient with history of SLE develops lens opacities.
4. An diabetic patient develops proliferative diabetic retinopathy.
5. An 80 year old man with marked loss of vision on fundoscopy. Bilateral Macular Degeneration and pigmentation is noted.

Theme 2: Side effect of drugs

Options:

a. Liver failure
b. Bronchiolitis
c. Rash
d. Reye's syndrome
e. Dry mouth
f. Drowsiness
g. Gastric erosion
h. Dilated pupil

For each presentation below, choose the SINGLE most appropriate side effect from the above list of options. Each option may be used once, more than once, or not at all.

1. A child who takes a large amount of paracetamol.
2. A patient on chronic use of Aspirin.
3. A patient taking carbamazepine for some painful problem.
4. A patient with some psychiatric problem on TCA.
5. A patient on chronic use of Ibuprofen.

Theme 3: Involvement of cranial nerve

a. Nerve I
b. Nerve II
c. Nerve III
d. Nerve IV
e. Nerve V
f. Nerve VI
g. Nerve VII
h. Nerve VIII
i. Nerve IX
j. Nerve X
k. Nerve XI
l. Nerve XII

For each presentation below, choose the SINGLE most appropriate involved nerve from the above list of options. Each option may be used once, more than once, or not at all.

1. A patient involved in RTA. Has MRI done which shows longitudinal fracture of temporal petrosal bone of skull and now is unable to perceive smell.
2. A 19 year old patient sustained fracture of base of skull, presents with ptosis, loss of pupillary reflex associated with nystagmus.
3. Patient had trauma to back of skull and since then he cannot shrug his shoulders.
4. A patient cannot move his lower facial muscles but there is sparing of the forehead muscles.
5. A patient had a stroke and has lost the ability to feel taste in the Ant. 2/3 of the tongue.

Theme 4: Diagnosis of anaemia

Options:

a. Pernicious anaemia
b. Aplastic anaemia
c. Iron deficiency anaemia
d. Coeliac disease
e. Anaemia due to iron malabsorption
f. Anaemia due to folate malabsorption
g. Folate deficiency anaemia
h. B_{12} deficiency anaemia

For each presentation below, choose the SINGLE most appropriate cause of anaemia from the above list of options. Each option may be used once, more than once, or not at all.

1. A man on treatment with cyclophosphamide for lung alveolitis develops anaemia.
2. A man with history of gastric erosion develops anaemia.
3. A strict vegetarian develops malnutrition and anaemia.
4. A patient with coeliac disease develops anaemia.

Theme 5: Vaginal conditions in a female child

Options:

a. E. vermicularis
b. Examine under GA
c. Local hygiene
d. Take high vaginal swab
e. Culture and investigate for chlamydia
f. Local nystatin
g. Candidiasis

For each presentation below, choose the SINGLE most appropriate management from the above list of options. Each option may be used once, more than once, or not at all.

1. A child with itching in vulva mostly at night.
2. A child with excoriation and ulceration in the vulval region.
3. Rash is noted in vulva in a diabetic child.
4. A child with some kind of vaginal discharge.
5. Rash in a normal child when nappy removed.

Theme 6: Diagnosis of confusion

Options:

a. Delirium
b. Subdural haemorrhage
c. Extradural haemorrhage
d. Subarachnoid haemorrhage
e. Wernicke's encephalopathy
f. Drug overdose

For each presentation below, choose the SINGLE most appropriate cause of confusion from the above list of options. Each option may be used once, more than once, or not at all.

1. Patient admitted in hospital with some ailment then becomes confused and irritated.
2. A patient is operated, on gaining consciousness becomes confused and disoriented.
3. An alcoholic with history of recurrent falls is confused.
4. A rugby player hit by a ball on head loses consciousness and then become normal. Now he is brought in hospital with detoriating consciousness.

Theme 7: Prevention of heart disease

Options:

a. Statins
b. Reduce weight
c. Stop alcohol and cigarette

For each presentation below, choose the SINGLE most appropriate management from the above list of options. Each option may be used once, more than once, or not at all.

1. A patient presents with hyperlipidaemia develops cardiac problems.
2. A smoker and alcoholic develops cardiac problem.
3. An obese develops cardiac problems.

Theme 8: Investigation in breast lumps

Options:

a. FNAC
b. MRI
c. USG
d. Mammography
e. CXR
f. Stereotactic fine needle biopsy
g. Excisional biopsy
h. Lumpectomy

For each presentation below, choose the SINGLE most appropriate investigation from the above list of options. Each option may be used once, more than once, or not at all.

1. A patient with fibrocystic disease with symptoms related with menses.
2. A patient with breast lump but has morbid fear of needles.
3. A patient with no obvious palpable lump but with axillary lymph nodes.
4. A patient with retraction of nipple.

Theme 9: Investigation in convulsions

Options:

a. EEG
b. CT Scan
c. MRI
d. ECG
e. No investigation required
f. Blood glucose
g. U&E
h. LFTs

For each presentation below, choose the SINGLE most appropriate investigation from the above list of options. Each option may be used once, more than once, or not at all.

1. Mother brings child who had some febrile condition, the child was wrapped in multiple blankets. He had convulsions. When the blanket was removed he was fine and playing happily.
2. A boy with history of convulsions starting with tingling in thumb of one hand.
3. A patient presents with convulsions. An EEG was done which showed firing impulses in the temporal area.
4. A patient had generalized tonic clonic convulsions.

Theme 10: Diagnosis in dementia

Options:

a. Alzheimer's dementia
b. Schizophrenia
c. Pseudodementia
d. Senile dementia
e. Muti-infarct dementia
f. Lewy body dementia
g. Frontal lobe dementia
h. Huntingtons dementia

For each presentation below, choose the SINGLE most appropriate diagnosis from the above list of options. Each option may be used once, more than once, or not at all.

1. A patient had some psychiatric problems with thought insertion.
2. Commonest dementia in UK.
3. Dementia which has neurofibrillary tangles.
4. Patient with cognitive impairment.
5. A hypertensive with dementia.
6. Dementia treated with anti depressants.

Theme 11: Diagnosis of hearing loss

Options:

a. Ménière's disease
b. Wax impaction
c. Acoustic neuroma
d. Acute otitis media
e. Presbyacusis
f. Otosclerosis
g. Viral involvement of nerve
h. Otitis externa

For each presentation below, choose the SINGLE most appropriate cause of hearing loss from the above list of options. Each option may be used once, more than once, or not at all.

1. A patient with intermittent tinnitus, giddiness, and vertigo.
2. A 50 year old man with bilateral deafness, his father also had hearing loss.
3. A brown mass obliterates the tympanic membrane.
4. A woman presents with unilateral conductive hearing loss and pain in the ear after a shower.
5. A patient with tinnitus, vertigo and tingling on one side of face and numbness.

Theme 12: Diagnosis in rheumatology

Options:

a. Chondromalacia patella
b. Rheumatoid arthritis
c. Gout
d. Psoriatic arthritis
e. Enteropathic arthritis
f. Ankylosing spondylitis
g. Septic arthritis
h. Reactive arthritis
i. Pseudogout
j. Gonococcal arthritis.

For each presentation below, choose the SINGLE most appropriate diagnosis from the above list of options. Each option may be used once, more than once, or not at all.

1. A 65 year old man has a swollen left knee joint for ten years with associated swelling but no skin changes. He has no other problems.
2. A 35 year old woman with left knee pain and associated problems, and with nail pitting and discolouration.
3. A 45 year old man on antihypertensive treatment, presents with left knee pain which is swollen and hot to touch.
4. A patient who returned from Thailand develops painful swelling and warm right knee.
5. A female with symmetrical and crippling arthropathy.

Theme 13: Diagnosis of ulcerative colitis

Options:

a. Ulcerative colitis
b. Pseudomembranous colitis
c. Haemorrhoids
d. Anal fissure
e. Crohn's disease

For each presentation below, choose the SINGLE most appropriate diagnosis from the above list of options. Each option may be used once, more than once, or not at all.

1. A patient taking IV antibiotic treatment for some disease develops diarrhoea and bowel changes.
2. A patient has bleeding mixed with stool and also bleeding after passing stool.
3. A patient presents to his GP with complaints of diarrhoea mixed with blood. He also complains of abdominal pain.
4. A patient passes stool with blood streaked on it.

Theme 14: Investigation in lung conditions

Options:

a. CT scan
b. MRI
c. Sputum cytology
d. Sputum culture
e. Lung biopsy

For each presentation below, choose the SINGLE most appropriate investigation from the above list of options. Each option may be used once, more than once, or not at all.

1. Elderly man has lower lobe consolidation and fever, he was treated with antibiotic, which resolved the fever but the consolidation persisted after 4 weeks.
2. A patient with lung affected due to asbestos exposure.

Theme 15: Investigation in haematology

Options:

a. Bleeding time
b. Clotting time
c. Platelet count
d. Von Willebrand
e. INR
f. PTT
g. TT

For each presentation below, choose the SINGLE most appropriate investigation from the above list of options. Each option may be used once, more than once, or not at all.

1. A patient is taking warfarin develops bleeding problems.
2. A female patient with rash and other symptoms of purpura develops haemorrhage.
3. A 16 year old girl is pale and weak presents with menorrhagia and epistaxis. Mother also had similar problems.

Theme 16: Diagnosis of meningitis

Options:

a. Streptococcal meningitis
b. Meningococcal meningitis
c. Viral meningitis
d. Tubercular meningitis
e. Leukaemic infiltration

For each presentation below, choose the SINGLE most appropriate cause of meningitis from the above list of options. Each option may be used once, more than once, or not at all.

1. A 3 year old boy developed URTI and also had recent history of ear discharge. Now presents with neck stiffness.
2. A child is diagnosed with meningitis. His CSF examination shows 10 blood cells with 1-2 lymphocytes, and the glucose level is not too reduced.
3. A child with meningitis, his CSF examination shows presence of gram negative encapsulated diplococci.
4. A child with signs of meningitis and presence of abnormal blood cells in the CSF.

Theme 17: Management of thyroid problems

Options:

a. Propranolol
b. Carbimazole
c. Radioiodine
d. Thyroidectomy
e. Observation only
f. Thyroxine
g. FNAC
h. Auto antibody
i. Thyroid ultrasound
j. MRI

For each presentation below, choose the SINGLE most appropriate management from the above list of options. Each option may be used once, more than once, or not at all.

1. A female patient presents with weight loss, palpitations and diarrhoea.
2. A female patient having previous history of asthma is now complaining of weight loss and diarrhoea.
3. A female patient with diffuse enlargement of thyroid, but otherwise well and asymptomatic.
4. A patient with a solitary thyroid nodule of about 3 cm in size.
5. A woman presents with features of hypo-thyroidism and a tender thyroid.

Theme 18: Management of trauma in children

Options:

a. IV morphine
b. Endotracheal intubation
c. Intraosseous line
d. CV line
e. Oropharyngeal airway
f. Nasopharyngeal airway
g. Dobutamine infusion
h. IV fluids

For each presentation below, choose the SINGLE most appropriate management from the above list of options. Each option may be used once, more than once, or not at all.

1. A 4 year old child presents with 10 % scalds on chest.
2. A 6 year old, intubated after RTA has low BP and high pulse rate.
3. A 2 year old with presents with hypovolaemic shock, unable to get IV access.
4. A 5 year old presents with soot in nostril.
5. A 13 year old in shock, unable to get IV access.

Theme 19: Management of varicella

Options:

a. Oral aciclovir
b. IV aciclovir
c. No treatment required at present
d. Varicella Ig
e. Barrier nursing
f. Quarantine
g. Check immune status
h. Topical aciclovir

For each presentation below, choose the SINGLE most appropriate management from the above list of options. Each option may be used once, more than once, or not at all.

1. A pregnant woman who is in her last trimester of pregnancy, and her husband is infected with varicella.
2. A boy who is taking steroids for asthma gets chicken pox.
3. A child having lymphoma, his father has shingles.
4. A boy has got chicken pox whose sister has just had renal transplant and is returning from the hospital.
5. An 80 year old man develops ophthalmic shingles.
6. A boy has developed vesicles all over the body and also has high fever.
7. A woman with vesicles on small part of the chest.

Theme 20: Diagnosis of acid-base disturbances

Options:

a. Metabolic acidosis
b. Metabolic alkalosis
c. Respiratory acidosis
d. Respiratory alkalosis
e. Hypokalaemia
f. Renal failure
g. Dehydration
h. Fluid overload

For each presentation below, choose the SINGLE most appropriate diagnosis from the above list of options. Each option may be used once, more than once, or not at all.

1. A man having projectile vomiting due to pyloric stenosis presents with hypokalaemia and base excess.
2. A man with villous adenoma of rectum presents with diarrhoea.
3. A man with pulmonary embolism presents with tachycardia, hypotension and breathlessness.
4. A man presents with pallor, dry skin and anuria.
5. A patient with post operative breathlessness, and peripheral oedema.

Theme 21: Psychiatry: Management

Options:

a. Chlorpromazine
b. Clozapine
c. ECT
d. Benzhexol
e. Continue the same drug orally
f. Stop the treatment
g. Hyoscine

For each presentation below, choose the SINGLE most appropriate management from the above list of options. Each option may be used once, more than once, or not at all.

1. A patient after treatment with antipsychotic, develops hypersalivation.
2. A patient after treatment with haloperidol, develops stiffness of limbs.
3. A patient stabbed his father in acute psychosis, and then was treated with antipsychotic. Now he believes himself to have recovered from the illness.
4. A patient who has recurrent hiccups, due to antipsychotic treatment.

Theme 22: Investigation in renal stones

Options:

a. Serum calcium level
b. Plasma urate level
c. Serum alkaline phosphatase, calcium and phosphate level
d. Dietary conditions
e. Urea and electrolytes
f. Urinary calcium
g. USG

For each presentation below, choose the SINGLE most appropriate investigation from the above list of options. Each option may be used once, more than once, or not at all.

1. A 25 year old man presented with recurrent loin pain and stone in the ureter.
2. A 35 year old man presented with loin pain. All serum biochemical investigations were done and are non conclusive.
3. A man with gouty skin changes of the ear pinna.
4. A man with stone in the kidney which is radiolucent.

Theme 23: Investigation of trauma in children

Options:

a. CT scan
b. Barium swallow
c. MRI
d. X-ray abdomen
e. Peritoneal analysis

For each presentation below, choose the SINGLE most appropriate investigation from the above list of options. Each option may be used once, more than once, or not at all.

1. A child with stab wound of abdomen and signs of peritonism and shock.
2. A child involved in RTA was seated in backseat with seat belt on. He presents with pain in left hypochondrium, pallor, low BP and tachycardia.

Theme 24: Investigation in diabetes

Options:

a. Random blood sugar
b. Fasting blood sugar
c. Oral glucose tolerance test
d. Insulin level
e. Urine sugar
f. Blood sugar
g. Post-prandial blood sugar

For each presentation below, choose the SINGLE most appropriate investigation from the above list of options. Each option may be used once, more than once, or not at all.

1. A 25 year old male who is conscious and wants to know immediately whether he is diabetic.
2. A 65 year old male with history of polyuria wants to know about his diabetes.
3. A 20 year old girl presented to you with history of attacks of hypoglycaemia when ever she misses her meal.
4. Mother brings in a child. She is worried if he is diabetic.

Theme 25: Management of ectopic pregnancy

Options:

a. Laparotomy
b. Diagnostic laparoscopy
c. USG
d. 24 hour beta HCG

For each presentation below, choose the SINGLE most appropriate management from the above list of options. Each option may be used once, more than once, or not at all.

1. A 25 year old girl with 8 weeks of amenorrhoea presents with BP 70/50 and pulse 140/min.
2. A 35 year old woman with bleeding per vaginum and USG shows empty uterus.
3. A 28 year old woman presents with 5 weeks amenorrhoea and has history of vaginal bleeding. Her β HCG is 5000.

Theme 26: Control of hypertension

Options:

a. Beta blockers
b. ACE inhibitor
c. Diet control
d. Stop smoking
e. Exercise
f. IV antihypertensive
g. Fish oil

For each presentation below, choose the SINGLE most appropriate management from the above list of options. Each option may be used once, more than once, or not at all.

1. A 30 year old lady presents with a BP of 160/100 recorded on 3 times consecutively. BMI is 27 and drinks 7 units of alcohol and smokes 1 pack cigarettes per day.
2. A 35 year old lady with BMI of 33, drinks 3 units of alcohol/week. And BP recorded is 160/100 three times in a row.
3. A 50 year old with history of hypertension. Not relieved by diuretics.
4. A patient with family history of cardiovascular disorders.

Theme 27: Psychiatry: Management

Options:

a. Oral antipsychotic drug
b. IV antipsychotic drug
c. Stop treatment
d. Continue same treatment
e. Review after 3 months
f. Regular visits to the doctor

For each presentation below, choose the SINGLE most appropriate management from the above list of options. Each option may be used once, more than once, or not at all.

1. A 30 year old with psychiatric problem on oral antipsychotics.
2. Patient who is doing well on antipsychotics, on his regular visit to GP after 3 months.

Theme 28: Diagnosis of cervical pathology

Options:

a. CIN
b. Cervical ectropion
c. Endometrial carcinoma
d. Cervical carcinoma
e. Vaginal carcinoma
f. Atrophic vaginitis
g. Chlamydial infection
h. Cervical smear

For each presentation below, choose the SINGLE most appropriate diagnosis from the above list of options. Each option may be used once, more than once, or not at all.

1. A female presents with a cervical lesion which bleeds to touch, she gives history of multiple sexual partners recently.
2. A female presents with bleeding per vaginum. She is on oral contraceptive pills.
3. A woman with post menopausal bleeding and with endometrial thickening.
4. A woman who has got unpleasant vaginal discharge.
5. A postmenopausal lady presents with post-coital bleeding after having sex for the first time in her life.

Theme 29: Cause of respiratory pathology

Options:

a. Alpha 1 antitrypsin deficiency
b. Chloride channel defect
c. Surfactant deficiency
d. Asthma

For each presentation below, choose the SINGLE most appropriate cause of respiratory pathology from the above list of options. Each option may be used once, more than once, or not at all.

1. A baby who has recurrent pneumonitis.
2. A baby with RDS.
3. A woman who has history of recurrent jaundice as a child and now develops emphysema.
4. A child who develops cough and difficulty in breathing during winter.

Theme 30: Investigation in acid peptic disease

Options:

a. *H. Pylori* serology
b. Oesophageal manometry
c. Endoscopy
d. Faecal occult blood
e. 24 hours ambulatory pH monitoring
f. Barium meal
g. Do nothing

For each presentation below, choose the SINGLE most appropriate investigation from the above list of options. Each option may be used once, more than once, or not at all.

1. A 50 year old obese woman with history of pain in the epigastrium which is present specially at night and after meals, also has water brash.
2. A woman with history of pain in stomach after a fundoplication operation.
3. Woman with long history of peptic ulcer disease with positive *H. pylori* serology comes for re-examination after 4 years.
4. A 36 year old man has been treating himself for dyspeptic symptoms for many years.

Theme 31: Treatment for upper GI conditions

Options:

a. Give antacids
b. Give H_2 blockers
c. Oesophageal dilatation
d. Oesophageal excision
e. Celestin tube
f. Radiotherapy
g. Chemotherapy
h. Endoscopic biopsy

For each presentation below, choose the SINGLE most appropriate treatment from the above list of options. Each option may be used once, more than once, or not at all.

1. A pregnant woman with dyspeptic symptoms since past 4 days.
2. A patient with chronic dyspepsia has developed Barrett's oesophagus.
3. A patient with oesophageal stricture.
4. A patient with a localized oesophageal tumor with no signs of metastasis.
5. Patient with carcinoma of oesophagus and metastases.

Theme 32: Management of injury to upper limb

a. Manipulation
b. Physiotherapy
c. Sling
d. Apply plaster cast
e. Admit for further investigations
f. No treatment required

For each presentation below, choose the SINGLE most appropriate management from the above list of options. Each option may be used once, more than once, or not at all.

1. A child with pulled elbow first presents to A & E.
2. A child with history of fall presents with tenderness and pain below the thumb, X-ray is normal.
3. A child presents with torticollis she has no history of trauma.
4. A child presents to A&E with limping and pain on rotation after playing football.

Theme 33: Management in case of ischaemic limb

Options:

a. Incise the fascia
b. Embolectomy
c. Amputate
d. Arteriovenous grafting

For each presentation below, choose the SINGLE most appropriate management from the above list of options. Each option may be used once, more than once, or not at all.

1. A patient with history of atrial fibrillation presents with a pale, cold, pulseless leg which he can barely move. He has very little perception of touch.
2. A patient with bilateral diabetic lesions on the feet, presents with a foot with multiple malodorous gangrenous lesions on one foot.
3. A patient with trauma to the leg presents with fracture of both the bones, severe pain and a lot of swelling.
4. A diabetic patient with a unilateral ulcer on foot, which has absent pulse. Arteriography shows lack of blood supply.

Theme 34: Management of osteoporosis

Options:

a. HRT
b. Raloxifen
c. Reduce weight
d. Weight bearing exercises
e. Calcium supplement

For each presentation below, choose the SINGLE most appropriate management from the above list of options. Each option may be used once, more than once, or not at all.

1. A woman with high BMI.
2. A 40 year old lady with family history of osteoporosis, comes for advice.
3. A patient who needed dietary calcium.

Theme 35: Head injury: Diagnosis

Options:

a. Mild injury
b. Moderate injury
c. Severe injury
d. Fracture skull
e. Fracture base of skull
f. Extradural haemorrhage
g. Subdural haemorrhage
h. Subarachnoid haemorrhage
i. Coma

For each presentation below, choose the SINGLE most appropriate diagnosis from the above list of options. Each option may be used once, more than once, or not at all.

1. A 45 year old alcoholic with history of recurrent falls was brought to A & E by his wife in a confused state. His GCS is 12.
2. A 7 year old boy with history of fall from cycle. He had lost consciousness initially but is alert and oriented now. Examination reveals no abnormality.
3. A man with head injury who also has haemotympanum.
4. A 23 year old footballer brought to the A & E was talking to the paramedics well after injury but subsequently lost consciousness.
5. A 42 year old man fell down. On examination his GCS is 13.

Theme 36: Diagnosis of drug abuse

Options:

a. Opiate abuse
b. Opiate withdrawal
c. Alcohol withdrawal

For each presentation below, choose the SINGLE most appropriate diagnosis from the above list of options. Each option may be used once, more than once, or not at all.

1. A female patient comes to A&E demanding pain relief.
2. A patient with history of alcohol abuse with signs of alcohol withdrawal.

Theme 37: Analgesia in terminally sick

Options:

a. Patient controlled analgesia
b. NSAIDs
c. Paracetamol
d. Radiotherapy
e. Acupuncture
f. Dihydrocodiene
g. IV opioid
h. TENS

For each presentation below, choose the SINGLE most appropriate analgesia from the above list of options. Each option may be used once, more than once, or not at all.

1. A patient with bladder carcinoma, now presents with metastasis to the spine presents with severe pain in the back.
2. A patient with carcinoma colon has sigmoidectomy done.
3. A woman who has had breast surgery done.
4. A patient with carcinoma rectum presents with severe pain.

Theme 38: Management of cardiac conditions

Options:

a. Verapamil
b. Heparin
c. Amiodarone
d. Beta blocker
e. DC cardioversion
f. Captopril
g. Thiazide diuretic

For each presentation below, choose the SINGLE most appropriate management from the above list of options. Each option may be used once, more than once, or not at all.

1. A pregnant female with tachycardia of 160/minute. She shows no response to Adenosine.
2. A patient with refractory pulmonary oedema and cardiac failure, was prescribed frusemide, but the patient still continues to deteriorate in spite of frusemide therapy.
3. A diabetic patient who develops hypertension.
4. A patient with family history of sudden death, has signs of HOCM.

Theme 39: Diagnosis of respiratory disorders

Options:

a. Bronchiolitis
b. Pericarditis
c. Pneumonia
d. Coarctation of aorta
e. Pneumothorax
f. Sleep apnoea syndrome
g. Bronchiectasis

For each presentation below, choose the SINGLE most appropriate diagnosis from the above list of options. Each option may be used once, more than once, or not at all.

1. An obese male who is tired and lethargic, gives history of repeated awakening during sleep with sweating, palpitations, and tachypnoea.
2. A patient with COPD develops sudden breathlessness and absent respiratory sounds on one side of chest. X-ray shows absent lung shadow in the left upper zone.
3. A tall male develops sudden central chest pain, becomes pale, and tachycardic with difference in pulse.
4. A teenager with fever and cough and pain in left lower side of chest on breathing.
5. A patient with pain in central chest, which is relieved by bending forward, also raised JVP and pericardial rub.
6. A child with cystic fibrosis.

Theme 40: Diagnosis of urinary retention

Options:

a. Clot retention
b. BPH
c. UTI
d. Renal failure
e. Compression of spinal cord
f. Incontinence pants
g. Multiple sclerosis

For each presentation below, choose the SINGLE most appropriate diagnosis from the above list of options. Each option may be used once, more than once, or not at all.

1. An old patient who has been incontinent for a long time now develops signs of dysuria.
2. A patient with carcinoma of prostate, and urinary symptoms, has haematuria and then sudden retention of urine.
3. A patient with history of urinary hesitancy. He has consumed a large amount of alcohol, and then presents with sudden retention of urine.
4. A patient with huge enlargement of prostate, which is even palpable suprapubically. He presents with weakness of feet and retention of urine.
5. A patient with history of recurrent numbness of feet and recurrent focal neurological signs, and retention of urine.

Theme 41: Pre-operative investigations

Options:

a. Exercise ECG
b. Arteriography
c. Spirometry
d. CT scan of the chest
e. Blood sugar
f. EEG
g. Ultrasound abdomen

For each presentation below, choose the SINGLE most appropriate investigation from the above list of options. Each option may be used once, more than once, or not at all.

1. A patient with respiratory problem due for operation.
2. A female on chronic use of OC pills.
3. A patient with history of angina on exertion.

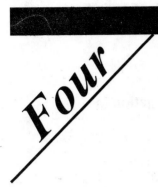

March 2003 Answers

Theme 1: Management of ophthalmic conditions

1. **(c)** Oral steroids
2. **(e)** Beta-blockers
3. **(d)** Eye surgery
4. **(f)** Laser treatment
5. **(h)** No treatment is required

Theme 2: Side effect of drugs

1. **(a)** Liver failure
2. **(d)** Reye's syndrome
3. **(c)** Rash
4. **(e)** Dry mouth
5. **(g)** Gastric erosion

Theme 3: Involvement of cranial nerve

1. **(a)** Nerve I
2. **(c)** Nerve III
3. **(k)** Nerve XI
4. **(g)** Nerve VII
5. **(g)** Nerve VII

Theme 4: Diagnosis of anaemia

1. **(c)** Iron deficiency anaemia
2. **(a)** Pernicious anaemia

3. **(h)** B_{12} deficiency anaemia
4. **(e)** Anaemia due to iron malabsorption

Theme 5: Vaginal conditions in a female child

1. **(a)** E. vermicularis
2. **(b)** Examine under GA
3. **(g)** Candidiasis
4. **(e)** Culture and investigate for chlamydia
5. **(c)** Local hygiene

Theme 6: Diagnosis of confusion

1. **(a)** Delirium
2. **(a)** Delirium
3. **(b)** Subdural haemorrhage
4. **(c)** Extradural haemorrhage

Theme 7: Prevention of heart disease

1. **(a)** Statins
2. **(c)** Stop alcohol and cigarette
3. **(b)** Reduce weight

Theme 8: Investigation in breast lumps

1. **(c)** USG
2. **(d)** Mammography

3. (f) Stereotactic fine needle biopsy
4. (g) Excisional biopsy

Theme 9: Investigation in convulsions

1. (e) No investigation required
2. (a) EEG
3. (c) MRI
4. (a) EEG

Theme 10: Diagnosis in dementia

1. (b) Schizophrenia
2. (a) Alzheimer's dementia
3. (a) Alzheimer's dementia
4. (a) Alzheimer's dementia
5. (e) Multi-infarct dementia
6. (c) Pseudodementia.

Theme 11: Diagnosis of hearing loss

1. (a) Ménière's disease
2. (f) Otosclerosis
3. (b) Wax impaction
4. (b) Wax impaction
5. (c) Acoustic neuroma

Theme 12: Diagnosis in rheumatology

1. (i) Pseudogout
2. (d) Psoriatic arthritis
3. (c) Gout
4. (j) Gonococcal arthritis
5. (b) Rheumatoid arthritis

Theme 13: Diagnosis of ulcerative colitis

1. (b) Pseudomembranous colitis
2. (c) Haemorrhoids
3. (a) Ulcerative colitis
4. (d) Anal fissure

Theme 14: Investigation in lung conditions

1. (e) Lung biopsy
2. (a) CT scan

Theme 15: Investigation in haematology

1. (e) INR
2. (c) Platelet count
3. (d) Von Willebrand

Theme 16: Diagnosis of meningitis

1. (a) Streptococcal meningitis
2. (d) Tubercular meningitis
3. (b) Meningococcal meningitis
4. (e) Leukaemic infiltration

Theme 17: Management of thyroid problems

1. (b) Carbimazole
2. (b) Carbimazole
3. (e) Observation only
4. (g) FNAC
5. (h) Auto antibody

Theme 18: Management of trauma in children

1. (h) IV fluids
2. (g) Dobutamine infusion
3. (c) Intraosseous line
4. (b) Endotracheal intubation
5. (d) CV line

Theme 19: Management of varicella

1. (d) Varicella Ig
2. (a) Oral aciclovir
3. (e) Barrier nursing

4. **(f)** Quarantine
5. **(a)** Oral aciclovir
6. **(b)** IV aciclovir
7. **(h)** Topical aciclovir

Theme 20: Diagnosis of acid-base disturbances

1. **(b)** Metabolic alkalosis
2. **(e)** Hypokalaemia
3. **(c)** Respiratory acidosis
4. **(f)** Renal failure
5. **(h)** Fluid overload

Theme 21: Psychiatry: Management

1. **(g)** Hyoscine
2. **(f)** Stop the treatment
3. **(e)** Continue the same drug orally
4. **(a)** Chlorpromazine

Theme 22: Investigation in renal stones

1. **(c)** Serum alkaline phosphatase, calcium and phosphate level
2. **(g)** USG
3. **(b)** Plasma urate level
4. **(c)** Serum alkaline phosphatase, calcium and phosphate level

Theme 23: Investigation of trauma in children

1. **(a)** CT scan
2. **(a)** CT scan

Theme 24: Investigation in diabetes

1. **(a)** Random blood sugar
2. **(e)** Urine sugar
3. **(b)** Fasting blood sugar
4. **(a)** Random blood sugar

Theme 25: Management of ectopic pregnancy

1. **(a)** Laparotomy
2. **(d)** 24 hour beta HCG
3. **(b)** Diagnostic laparoscopy

Theme 26: Control of hypertension

1. **(a)** Beta blockers
2. **(e)** Exercise
3. **(b)** ACE inhibitors
4. **(c)** Diet control

Theme 27: Psychiatry: Management

1. **(f)** Regular visits to the doctor
2. **(e)** Review after 3 months

Theme 28: Diagnosis of cervical pathology

1. **(a)** CIN
2. **(b)** Cervical ectropion
3. **(c)** Endometrial carcinoma
4. **(g)** Chlamydial infection
5. **(f)** Atrophic vaginitis

Theme 29: Cause of respiratory pathology

1. **(b)** Chloride channel defect
2. **(c)** Surfactant deficiency
3. **(a)** Alpha 1 antitrypsin deficiency
4. **(d)** Asthma

Theme 30: Investigation in acid peptic disease

1. **(c)** Endoscopy
2. **(c)** Endoscopy
3. **(a)** *H. Pylori* serology
4. **(a)** *H. Pylori* serology

Theme 31: Treatment for upper GI conditions

1. (a) Give antacids
2. (h) Endoscopic biopsy
3. (c) Oesophageal dilatation
4. (d) Oesophageal excision
5. (f) Radiotherapy

Theme 32: Management of injury to upper limb

1. (a) Manipulation
2. (d) Apply plaster cast
3. (b) Physiotherapy
4. (e) Admit for further investigations

Theme 33: Management in case of ischaemic limb

1. (b) Embolectomy
2. (c) Amputate
3. (a) Incise the fascia
4. (d) Arteriovenous grafting

Theme 34: Management of osteoporosis

1. (c) Reduce weight
2. (d) Weight bearing exercises
3. (e) Calcium supplement

Theme 35: Head injury: Diagnosis

1. (b) Moderate injury
2. (a) Mild injury
3. (e) Fracture base of skull
4. (f) Extradural haemorrhage
5. (a) Mild injury

Theme 36: Diagnosis of drug abuse

1. (b) Opiate withdrawal
2. (c) Alcohol withdrawal

Theme 37: Analgesia in terminally sick

1. (d) Radiotherapy
2. (a) Patient controlled analgesia
3. (g) IV opioid
4. (g) IV opioid

Theme 38: Management of cardiac conditions

1. (a) Verapamil
2. (g) Thiazide diuretic
3. (f) Captopril
4. (d) Beta blocker

Theme 39: Diagnosis of respiratory disorders

1. (f) Sleep apnoea syndrome
2. (e) Pneumothorax
3. (d) Coarctation of aorta
4. (c) Pneumonia
5. (b) Pericarditis
6. (g) Bronchiectasis

Theme 40: Diagnosis of urinary retention

1. (c) UTI
2. (a) Clot retention
3. (b) BPH
4. (e) Compression of spinal cord
5. (g) Multiple sclerosis

Theme 41: Pre-operative investigations

1. (c) Spirometry
2. (b) Arteriography
3. (a) Exercise ECG

Four March 2003 Explanations

Theme 1: Management of ophthalmic conditions

1. This is a patient of Giant cell arteritis. The typical patient will present with sudden painless loss of vision, malaise, jaw claudication and with tender scalp on temporal arteries. ESR above 40 is suggestive. Temporal artery biopsy report may be false positive in some cases and therefore is not a reliable investigation. Management includes oral prednisolone promptly as the other eye is at risk.

2. This is a case of chronic simple (open angle) glaucoma. Intraocular pressure ≥ 21 mmHg causes optic disc cupping as in this patient. Nerve damage ensues with sausage shaped field defect (scotoma). Nasal and superior fields are lost first and temporal last. High risk group include > 35 years old with positive family history, myopics, diabetic or with thyroid eye disease. Treatment includes beta blocker eye drops, pilocarpine eye drops, carbonic anhydrase inhibitors. If drugs fail surgery is indicated.

3. SLE (systemic lupus erythematosus) is an autoimmune disease in which ANA (antinuclear antibodies) are present. Its treatment invariably requires the use of oral steroids which on long term use can cause cataract, as is mentioned in this patient as lens opacities. The only treatment for cataract is surgery.

4. Proliferative Diabetic Retinopathy is caused due to vascular occlusion which leads to proliferation of new vessels in the retina, optic disc and iris. Patient may have cotton wool spots due to occlusion, vascular leakage, hard exudates, flame shaped haemorrhage, blot haemorrhages and is at increased risk of retinal detachment. Treatment requires good control of diabetes and photocoagulation by laser to treat both maculopathy and proliferative retinopathy.

5. This is a patient with age related macular degeneration. It is the most common cause of registrable blindness in UK. There is a loss of visual acuity, visual fields are unaffected. The disc appears normal but there is pigment, fine exudate and bleeding at the macula. Laser photocoagulation can halt the progress but otherwise there is no treatment as yet available for the condition.

Theme 2: Side effect of drugs

1. Paracetamol poisoning can cause liver failure and hence encephalopathy. Patients may present with vomiting ± RUQ pain and jaundice. Management includes gastric lavage within 2 hours, if > 7.5 gm is taken. Activated charcoal is given within 8 hours of ingestion. N-acetylcysteine given by IV infusion is the antidote of choice in paracetamol poisoning.

2. Aspirin can cause tinnitus, vertigo, dehydration, hyperventilation and Reye's syndrome. Patient with Reye's syndrome presents with vomiting, fever, hypotonia, stupor, liver failure; seen around 1½ year of age. It can also be due to antiemetics or antihistamines.

3. Carbamazepine can cause agranulocytosis and rash. It can also cause neurotoxicity, photosensitivity, lupus like syndrome and aplastic anaemia. Acute intoxication can cause coma and cardiovascular collapse.

4. Tricyclic antidepressants such as amitriptyline, clomipramine, trimipramine can have anticholinergic side effects such as dry mouth, bad taste, constipation, epigastric distress, urinary retention, blurred vision and palpitations. Other adverse effects of TCAs include increased appetite, weight gain, postural hypotension and cardiac arrhythmias.

5. Chronic use of NSAIDs such as salicylates, indomethacin, ibuprofen, diclofenac etc irritate gastric mucosa and can cause gastric erosion, epigastric distress, nausea and vomiting.

Theme 3: Involvement of cranial nerve

1. The patient in this condition is complaining of anosmia. Anosmia is seen in damage to the 1st cranial nerve. i.e. Olfactory nerve. The sites of damage to the olfactory pathway include nasal mucosa, cribriform plate, olfactory tract, temporal lobe due to tumour or trauma as in this case.

2. The IIIrd cranial nerve i.e. the oculomotor nerve supplies the superior rectus, inferior rectus, medial rectus and inferior oblique muscles of the eye and their lesions can cause ptosis, dilatation of the pupil, abduction of the eye and divergent squint respectively.

3. The spinal accessory nerve i.e. the XIth cranial nerve has its nucleus in the nucleus ambiguus (medullary portion) and in C1–5 anterior horn cells (spinal portion). It supplies the pharynx and larynx via Xth cranial nerve. It also supplies the trapezius and sternomastoid muscles. Shrugging the shoulder is done by trapezius muscle and therefore in the involvement of XIth cranial nerve the patient cannot shrug his shoulders, as in this case.

4. The chief function of the VIIth cranial nerve i.e. the facial nerve is the supply of motor fibres to the muscles of facial expression. In Idiopathic (Bell's) palsy, the site of damage to the nerve is probably the labyrinthine portion within the facial canal. Patient can have hyperacusis if nerve to stapedius is involved. LMN lesions, cause loss of frontal wrinkling on ipsilateral side with positive Bell's sign and loss of nasolabial fold. In UMN lesions the function of muscles in upper face are preserved and loss of nasolabial fold is seen in the ipsilateral side with deviation of mouth to the normal side. The chorda tympani fibres are often affected so that taste is impaired on the anterior 2/3rd of the tongue. Treatment requires a short course of dexamethasone and physiotherapy if required.

5. As explained above.

Theme 4: Diagnosis of anaemia

1. Cyclophosphamide is a cytotoxic immuno-suppressant. It has been used in bone marrow transplantation in which a short course is given. Low doses are also used in pemphigus, SLE and ITP. It may cause alopecia and haemorrhagic cystitis due to which there can be chronic blood loss leading to iron deficiency anaemia, as in this case.

2. Patient here has history of gastric erosions which suggests malabsorption of vitamin B_{12}. Pernicious anaemia is due to malabsorption of Vitamin B_{12} resulting from atrophic gastritis and lack of gastric intrinsic factor secretion. Management includes replenishment of stores with hydroxycobalamin given IM on alternate days for 2 weeks.

3. Vitamin B_{12} is present in all foods of animal origin and therefore dietary vitamin B_{12} deficiency is extremely rare and seen only in strict vegetarians as in this case.

4. Coeliac disease is a condition in which the patient has prolamin intolerance leading to villous atrophy and malabsorption. α-gliadin and anti endomyseal antibodies help the diagnosis. Patient presents with steatorrhoea, abdominal pain, bloating and angular stomatitis. Jejunal biopsy confirms villous atrophy. Management involves gluten free diet. In such patients because of the villous atrophy, iron absorption cannot take place.

Theme 5: Vaginal conditions in a female child

1. Enterobius vermicularis (thread worm) causes anal itch as it leaves the bowel to lay eggs on the perineum. Itching is noted mostly in the night. Diagnosis is based on identifying the eggs microscopically. Treatment is with mebendazole and proper hygiene.

2. This child has presented with a vulval ulcer which can be due to syphilis, herpes simplex, lymphogranuloma venereum, Behcet's syndrome, granuloma inguinale. One has to rule out an STD and sexual assault and therefore the child needs to be examined under GA.

3. Candidiasis (Thrush) is the most common cause of vaginal discharge which is classically white curds. Pregnancy, OCPs, steroids, immunodeficiency, antibiotics and diabetes are important predisposing factors. Diagnosis is by microscopy which shows mycelia and spores. Treatment is by a single clotrimazole pessary.

4. In this child the nature of discharge and associated signs and symptoms have not been provided by the GMC. Therefore, to reach a diagnosis, the child needs to be further investigated. The protocol requires a speculum examination and to take endocervical swabs for chlamydia and cervical swabs for gonorrhoea.

5. Nappy rash is a red, desquamating rash, sparing the skin folds. It is due to moisture retention. It requires frequent changes of nappy, careful drying, emollient cream application and most importantly local hygiene. Candida can be isolated from half of all such rashes. Its hallmark is satellite spots beyond the main rash. Such patients require clotrimazole cream application in addition.

Theme 6: Diagnosis of confusion

1. The key feature in delirium is impaired consciousness with onset over hours to days. Patient is likely to be disoriented, sometimes agitated. If there is no past history of psychiatric illness and the patient is in the setting of a general hospital, a confusional state is particularly likely if the symptoms are worse at the end of the day. It can be due to certain drugs such as benzodiazepines, opiates, anticonvulsants, digoxin, surgery or trauma. Management requires finding and treating the cause.

2. As explained above.

3. Subdural haematoma is due to bleeding from bridging veins between the cortex and venous sinuses. The elderly and the alcoholics with frequent falls are more susceptible. Typically the patient will present with fluctuating levels of consciousness and confusion. Patients can also present with sleepiness, headache, personality change, signs of raised ICP and localizing neurological symptoms. Evacuation via burr holes usually leads to full recovery. If untreated, tentorial herniation and coning can take place.

4. The mention of lucid interval in this patient who has history of loss of consciousness and then regained consciousness is almost diagnostic of extradural haematoma. The possibility of extradural haematoma should be considered if after head injury, conscious level falls or is slow to improve. Extradural haemorrhage is commonly due to fractured temporal or parietal bone causing laceration to the middle meningeal vessels. CT scan of the head may show a lens-shaped (biconvex) haematoma. Urgent evacuation of the clot through multiple burr holes may be necessary.

Theme 7: Prevention of heart disease

1. Cholesterol is a major risk factor for coronary heart disease. Statins are the first choice in treating patients who have hyperlipidaemia and have concomitant cardiac problems. They decrease cholesterol synthesis in the liver.

2. Smoking is a chief risk factor for cardiovascular mortality although moderate alcohol drinking may promote cardiovascular health and reduce gastric infection with *H. pylori*, a known risk marker for cardiovascular disease. There is no mention of the amount of alcohol intake patient has, therefore we can easily presume that the amount is more than moderate. Therefore he needs to quit smoking and drinking.

3. In this case there is no mention of the biochemical status of the blood and only obesity is mentioned. Therefore to prevent any further deterioration in his cardiac status the patient needs to lose weight.

Theme 8: Investigation in breast lumps

1. This is a clear cut case of fibrocystic breast disease as the symptom (feeling of lumpiness) is related with the timing of menses. It is one of the benign breast disorders. Only reassurance is needed. But because a mass due to fibrocystic disease is frequently indistinguishable from carcinoma, suspicious lesions should be investigated further. Mammography may be helpful but the breast tissue in young women is usually too radiodense to permit a worthwhile study. Therefore ultrasonography is required to differentiate a cystic from a solid mass.

2. It has been clearly mentioned that the lady has a morbid fear of needles which rules out FNAC as a basic investigation for the lump. The only investigation left to be done now is mammography.

3. The patient in this case has no palpable breast lump but palpable axillary lymph nodes so we must investigate further to rule out any underlying pathology. Lymphatic spread of breast carcinoma primarily occurs to the axillary group of lymph nodes. A fine needle biopsy of the affected lymph nodes would not only help reach a diagnosis but will also help in its staging and act like a marker for the metastatic potential of that tumour.

4. The presenting complaint in about 70% of patients with breast carcinoma is a lump in the breast. Less frequent symptoms are breast pain, nipple discharge, nipple retraction, enlargement/itching of nipples, generalized hardness of breast. In this patient as there is no mention of other complaints related to breast, we presume that there are none. So in this setting the most diagnostic step would be to do an excisional biopsy under LA.

Theme 9: Investigation in convulsions

1. This is a case of febrile convulsion. This condition is diagnosed if the following occur together: (a) a tonic/clonic, symmetrical seizure (b) occurring with rising temperature (c) age of child between 6 months and five years. (d) no signs of CNS infection or previous history of epilepsy (e) number of seizures < 3 and lasting < 5 min. Treatment involves giving diazepam at the time of attack. Otherwise tepid sponging or paracetamol syrup. As in this case the child is presently not convulsing, nothing needs to be done.

2. This is a case of simple partial seizure with somatosensory symptom of tingling in the thumb of one hand and then spreading to the limb or different parts of the body depending upon their cortical representation. EEG is an indispensable investigation as it not only helps differentiate between the types of seizures, helping the management protocols but also helps in localizing the epileptogenic source in evaluating candidates for surgical treatment.

3. In this patient the EEG findings have shown the epileptogenic source as the temporal region which is firing impulses. MRI is indicated for patients with focal neurological symptoms or signs, focal seizures or with EEG findings of a focal disturbance.

4. EEG is an indispensable investigation as it not only helps differentiate between the types of seizures, helping the management protocols but also helps in localizing the epileptogenic source in evaluating candidates for surgical treatment.

Theme 10: Diagnosis in dementia

1. Schizophrenia is a common mental disorder which typically presents in adulthood with delusions, hallucinations and disordered thought. The 1st rank symptoms seen in ~70% of patients are (i) Thought insertion (as in this patient) (ii) Thought broadcast (iii) Thought withdrawal (iv) Passivity (v) Hearing voices commenting on the actions of the patients (vi) Primary delusions (vii) Somatic hallucinations.

2. Alzheimer's dementia is the most common form of dementia in UK. Suspect AD in any enduring, acquired deficit of memory and cognition. Onset may be from 40 years though it may be seen earlier in patients suffering from Down's syndrome. On histological examination plaques with neurofibrillary tangles and cortical β-amyloid protein are found. On MRI an increased cortical atrophy in the medial temporal lobe can be seen. In stage I of AD there is falling memory and spatial disorientation. In stage II the personality disintegrates and in stage III the patient is apathetic, wasted and bedridden.

3. As explained above.

4. As explained above.

5. This is a case of multi infarct or vascular dementia in which hypertension is a risk factor. Such patients are characterized by psychomotor slowing, reduced attention, loss of executive function and personality changes.

6. Pseudodementia is a term applied to patients who are depressed and who apparently are demented. These patients often complain about their memory problems rather them covering them up. Such patients improve dramatically with their improvement in the depressed status.

Theme 11: Diagnosis of hearing loss

1. Ménière's disease is a condition in which there is dilatation of the endolymphatic space of the membranous labyrinth causing vertigo with prostation, nausea, vomiting, tinnitus with/ without progressive sensorineural hearing loss. Treatment of acute vertigo requires cyclizine. Surgical decompression of the endolymphatic sac may relieve vertigo, prevent progress of disease and conserve hearing.

2. Otosclerosis is an autosomal dominant hereditary disorder with incomplete penetration. Half of the patients have a family history of the disorder, as in this patient. In this condition the vascular spongy bone replaces the normal lamellar bone of otic capsule origin especially around the oral window which fixes the stapes foot plate. Symptoms are usually seen in adulthood and are exacerbated due to pregnancy, menstruation and menopause. Hearing is often better with background noise. Surgical treatment involves stapedectomy or stapedotomy.

3. The presentation of a brown mass obliterating the tympanic membrane and without any discharge is almost diagnostic of wax impaction. It is commonly seen in patients with unhygienic life-styles. Patients treatment would include softening the wax with oil drops daily for a week and then syringing the ear or doing suction with the help of a microscope.

4. Unilateral conductive hearing loss in a young woman with no history of discharge suggests wax impaction. It is commonly seen in patients with unhygienic life-style. Patients treatment would include softening the wax with oil drops daily for a week and then syringing the ear or doing suction with the help of a microscope.

5. Acoustic neuromas are slow growing, benign lesions that behave as an SOL. Also known as Vestibular Schwannoma, they cause ipsilateral tinnitus ± sensorineural deafness by

compressing the cochlear nerve. Giddiness is also common. Trigeminal nerve compression may cause tingling and numbness on one side of the face, as in this case. MRI is the best investigation but CT can also show enlargement or erosion of the internal auditory meatus. Surgical treatment is difficult.

Theme 12: Diagnosis in rheumatology

1. This patient is suffering from pseudogout. Points in favour of the condition are (a) his old age as it is a risk factor for pseudogout (b) the affected site is the knee which is the main site affected in pseudogout (c) the chronicity of the illness, as 10 years, which is seen in pseudogout (d) No mention of pain or redness of the skin which is seen in patients of gout rather than pseudogout.

2. The association of nail changes along with arthropathy in this patient supports the diagnosis of psoriatic arthropathy. It is seen in around 7% of patients with psoriasis. Psoriasis is a common chronic inflammatory skin condition with well defined red plaques with silvery scale on extensor aspects of elbows, knees, scalp and sacrum. Nail changes in psoriasis includes onycholysis and pepper pot nail pitting and 'grease spots'.

3. The patient in this case is suffering from gout. Points in favour of the diagnosis are (i) the patient is on antihypertensive treatment (diuretics) is a precipitating factor for the deposition of sodium monourate crystals in the joint and causes gout. (ii) The patient presents with pain and swelling of the joint which is hot to touch. These presentations are classically seen in the acute stage of gout.

4. In this case a history of travel to Thailand is suggestive of an STD which is associated with arthropathy. Hence the diagnosis gonococcal arthritis. The patients may simply have flitting polyarthralgia, although effusions in larger joints are seen. The shoulder, knee, wrist and ankle, followed by the small joints of the hands and feet, are commonly involved often with an associated tenosynovitis.

5. Rheumatoid arthritis is a persistent, symmetrical, deforming arthropathy with peak onset in 5th decade and a M : F ratio of 3 : 1. Patients typically present with swollen painful and stiff

hands and feet especially in the morning. Patients have sausage shaped fingers and MCP joint swellings which later become Boutonniere and swan neck deformities of the fingers. It is associated with carpal tunnel syndrome, keratoconjunctivitis sicca, osteoporosis and amyloidosis. Treatment is with exercise, physiotherapy, intralesional steroids and NSAIDs.

Theme 13: Diagnosis of ulcerative colitis

1. Pseudomembranous colitis is an uncommon cause of diarrhoea due to clostridium difficile toxin. Patients invariably have history of antibiotic therapy. Antimicrobial treatment impairs native resistance to colonization with clostridium difficle. Pseudo membranous colitis is most strongly associated with clindamycin, ampicillin and the cephalosporins, but is not exclusive to them. Low grade fever, abdominal tenderness and a dry furred tongue are commonly noted clinical signs. Signs of dehydration may also be present. Its treatment includes vancomycin or metronidazole.

2. The patient in this case is suffering from haemorrhoids. Constipation with prolonged straining is the key causative factor. As there are no sensory fibres above the dentate line, piles are not painful. Moreover because the bleeding is from the capillaries, it is bright red in colour.

3. Ulcerative colitis is an inflammatory disorder of the colonic mucosa and it never spreads proximal to the ileocaceal valve. It is more common in non smokers than smokers!. Patients typically present with gradual onset of diarrhoea mixed with blood and mucus. It is also associated with aphthous ulcers, erythema nodosum, pyoderma gangrenosum. Conjunctivitis, sacroilitis and cholangiocarcinoma. Toxic dilatation of the colon can occur. Sigmoidoscopy shows inflammed, friable mucosa. Barium enema shows loss of haustra and granular mucosa. Treatment is with prednisolone and sulfasalazine.

4. Fissure in ano, is a midline longitudinal split in the squamous lining of the lower anus, often presents with a mucosal tag at the external aspect, 'the sentinel pile'. Mostly it is due to hard faeces or constipation. Defecation or PR examination is very painful.

Theme 14: Investigation in lung conditions

1. This is a patient with carcinoma bronchus. Cigarette smoking, old age, asbestos inhalation and radiation are important risk factors. The patient typically presents with cough, haemoptysis, dyspnoea, chest pain and weight loss. It can cause recurrent laryngeal nerve palsy, SIADH, SVC obstruction and Horner's syndrome. On CXR circular opacity, hilar enlargement, consolidation may be seen. Diagnosis is by bronchoscopy and biopsy for histological evaluation. Treatment is by excision for peripheral tumours and chemotherapy for small cell tumours.

2. Asbestosis is caused due to inhalation of asbestos fibres. There are 3 types of asbestos fibres (a) chrysolite i.e. white fibres which are least fibrogenic (b) crocidolite i.e. blue fibres which are most fibrogenic (c) Amosite i.e. brown fibres which have intermediate fibrogenic capacity. Patients present with dyspnoea, clubbing, inspiratory crackles. It increases risk of bronchial adenocarcinoma and mesothelioma. CT scan of the thorax is required for diagnosing the condition. Treatment is symptomatic.

Theme 15: Investigation in haematology

1. Prothrombin time is expressed as ratio compared to control. International Normalized Ratio (INR) normally is between 0.9–1.2. It is prolonged by coumarins e.g. Warfarin (as in this case), Vitamin K deficiency and liver diseases. All patients on warfarin must keep a check on the INR status, especially those who develop bleeding problems.

2. Vascular and platelet disorders lead to prolonged bleeding from cuts, purpura and bleeding from mucous membranes. Coagulation disorders on the other hand produce delayed bleeding after injury, into joints, muscles and GI tract. This patient looks like a case of thrombocytopenia as there is presence of purpura along with haemorrhage. Therefore platelet count needs to be done.

3. Von Willebrands factor has 3 roles to play (i) brings platelets into contact with subendothelium (ii) binds platelets together and (iii) binds platelets to factor VIII. Type I (vWD) is autosomal dominant with decreased levels of VW factor. Patients present with bruising, menorrhagia, mucocutaneous bleeding. APTT is typically raised. Treatment requires factor VIII cryoprecipitate and vasopressin.

Theme 16: Diagnosis of meningitis

1. Meningitis is inflammation of the meninges most commonly due to bacterial, viral, fungal or other infections. In this child, there is history of URTI and ear discharge due to infection which we suspect to be streptococcal. Thus, the diagnosis becomes streptococcal meningitis. Its treatment is by Benzylpenicillin 25–50 mg/kg/4 hourly slow IV.

2. The CSF examination in the child suggests the diagnosis of tubercular meningitis.

CSF examination	Pyogenic	Tubercular	Viral (aseptic)
1. Appearance	Turbid	Fibrin web	Clear
2. Predominant cell	Neutrophils	Mono-nuclear	Mono-nuclear
3. Cell counts/mm3	90–1000+	10–1000	50–1000/
4. Glucose	< ½ plasma	<½ plasma	>½ plasma
5. Protein	> 1.5	1–5	< 1

3. The presence of gram negative encapsulated diplococci in the CSF supports the diagnosis of meningococcal meningitis which typically presents in patients with petechiae along with fever, neck stiffness, headache, photophobia, drowsiness and vomiting. LP is critical for diagnosis. Treatment is with Benzylpenicillin. 25–50 mg/kg/4 hourly slow IV.

4. Presence of abnormal blood cells in the CSF shows that this is a case of leukaemic infiltration. Meningeal inflammation can be due to meningeal infiltration by malignant cells as in leukemia, lymphoma and other tumours.

Theme 17: Management of thyroid problems

1. This is a case of hyperthyroidism. Patients generally present with weight loss, palpitations and diarrhoea as in this case. Other presentations include increased appetite, heat intolerance, sweating, tremors, irritability, emotional lability, oligomenorrhoea, tachycardia, lid lag. Tests reveal decrease in TSH and increased T_4 and T_3. Treatment includes propranolol for immediate symptomatic relief and carbimazole to actually normalize the TFT levels. Other modalities of treatment include partial thyroidectomy and radioiodine I^{131} therapy.

2. This is another case of hyperthyroidism but with history of Asthma. Therefore the use of a β blocker, even for symptomatic relief is contraindicated. Here again carbimazole is the treatment of choice.

3. The normal thyroid gland is impalpable. Goitre implies generalized enlargement of the gland. A simple i.e. euthyroid goitre can be either diffuse hyperplastic or multinodular. Diffuse hyperplastic goitre can be seen at puberty when metabolic demands are high. This is known as puberty goitre. If TSH stimulation ceases, the goitre may regress but can recur later at times of stress e.g. pregnancy. Such goitres are soft, diffuse and do not require any other investigation.

4. A single thyroid lump is commonly seen. Only ~10% of such lumps will be malignant. Other causes of such lumps are cyst, adenoma, a discrete nodule in a multinodular goitre. The first step in investigation is to get T_3, T_4 done and then an USG to see whether the lump is cystic or solid. FNA and cytology of the fluid remains the gold standard to finally diagnose the pathology. Malignancy is more likely if the nodule is > 4 cm across. In this patient the nodule is of 3 cm size but one has to rule out malignancy. Therefore an FNAC is a must.

5. This is a patient of Hashimoto's thyroiditis. It is an autoimmune disease in which there is lymphocyte and plasma cell infiltration. It is usually seen in the 7th decade. Patients are often euthyroid but autoantibody titres are raised. Therefore to reach the diagnosis one has to know the level of autoantibody titre, as is required in this patient.

Theme 18: Management of trauma in children

1. Two-thirds of paediatric burns are actually scalds. Due to a larger surface area: volume ratio and fewer thermoregulatory compensatory mechanisms, there is a greater tendency to hypothermia. 'Rule of nines' has been altered in paediatric burn cases due to different body proportions. In children, head and leg burns constitute 14% area each. All paediatric cases who have sustained more than 10% burns should be transferred to burns unit. More than 10% burns in a child and more than 15% burns in adults require IV fluids. The amount of infusion is calculated by Muir and Barclay formula or Parkland formula.

2. The presentation of the child and its association with an RTA is suggestive of hypovolaemic shock due to blood loss. Colloid infusion 60 ml/kg should be started as soon as possible and blood should be sent for crossmatching. If perfusion is still poor or CVP > 10 cm H_2O, dobutamine may be needed.

3. In paediatric and neonatal practice immediate vascular access is required in following circumstances: cardiopulmonary arrest, severe burns, prolonged status epilepticus, hypovolaemic and septic shock. Rapid intravenous access is not easily obtained in many cases and intraosseous infusion may be required. Intraosseous infusion is a relatively safe and effective means of obtaining vascular access. It is recommended for life-threatening paediatric emergencies in which other methods of access have failed. It is contraindicated in osteoporosis, osteogenesis imperfecta, infection or fracture at the site of insertion. Proximal tibia is the best site. Other sites are the distal tibia or distal femur. It should be discontinued as soon as conventional IV access is attained.

4. Singed nostrils or soot in the nostrils are suggestive of inhalation of hot gases which

may cause upper airway obstruction with passage of time. Such patients must be considered for early intubation or surgical airway.

5. Cases presenting with shock should receive 100% O_2 by tight-fitting mask. Colloid 20 ml/kg bolus needs to be given IV. If the child does not respond the dose should be repeated. In case if IV line is not accessible or if the condition worsens, CVP line should be inserted. Intra osseous infusion should be considered if all the above measures of vascular access fail.

Theme 19: Management of varicella

1. Infection with varicella within the first 20 weeks of pregnancy causes congenital varicella in 2% cases. Such infants have cerebral cortical atrophy, cerebellar hypoplasia, microcephaly, convulsions, low IQ, limb hypoplasia and rudimentary digits. Although infection with varicella in pregnancy merits aciclovir therapy, the lady in this case is not yet infected with varicella. 1000 mg intramuscular varicella zoster globulin should be administered as it prevents infection in 50% of susceptible contacts.

2. All patients of herpes who have ophthalmic involvement, motor involvement, are aged above 50 years of age and who are immuno compromised require treatment. Aciclovir should be given as early as possible. Aciclovir is licensed as a 7-day course in chicken pox. Paediatric dose of aciclovir is 20 mg/kg 6 hourly given PO.

3. All patients of herpes who have ophthalmic involvement, motor involvement, are aged above 50 years of age and who are immuno compromised require treatment. Since the child in this case has not yet been infected with the virus and only his father has shingles, barrier nursing is all that is required.

4. All patients of herpes who have ophthalmic involvement, motor involvement, are aged above 50 years of age and who are immuno compromised require treatment. The girl is a susceptible host due to immune-compromised state as she has just had a renal transplant. Since she has not yet been infected, aciclovir is not indicated. Simple quarantine measures to keep her brother away from her would suffice.

5. Ophthalmic herpes is the infection of 1st branch of Trigeminal nerve. Pain, tingling or numbness around the eye may precede a blistering rash. Nose tip involvement means

involvement of the nasociliary branch of trigeminal nerve. This is also known as Hutchinson's sign. Treatment is with Aciclovir 800 mg 5 times daily PO for a week.

6. All patients of herpes who have ophthalmic involvement, motor involvement, are aged above 50 years and who are immuno-compromised require treatment. Aciclovir should be given as early as possible. As the patient is immunocompromised in this case, Aciclovir 10 mg/kg/8 hourly is given IV for 10 days.

7. Eruption of vesicles in Herpes is often preceded by symptoms of burning or itching. Grouped painful vesicles on erythematous base which heal without scarring are noted. Usually no treatment is required in such cases. Topical aciclovir prevents or reduces the severity of recurrences.

Theme 20: Diagnosis of acid base disturbances

1. This is a case of metabolic alkalosis in which there is an increase in the pH along with increase in HCO_3^-. Various causes for metabolic alkalosis include vomiting (especially severe and projectile, as in this patient), hypokalaemia (either due to diuretic use or simply vomiting), burns or due to ingestion of base.

2. Hypokalaemia is defined as K^+ level < 2.5 mmol/L. It presents with muscle weakness, hypotonia, tetany and cardiac arrhythmias. ECG changes include inverted T waves and prominent U waves. The causes of hypo-kalaemia include villous adenoma of rectum and diarrhoea, as in this patient. Other cau-sative factors are diuretics, vomiting, Cushing's syndrome, Conn's syndrome, renal tubular failure and steroid use. Treatment includes oral or IV supplements of potassium and treating the cause.

3. This is a patient with respiratory acidosis in which there is a decrease in the pH along with increase in CO_2 levels. Any lung, neuro-muscular or physical cause of respiratory failure such as pneumonia, pulmonary embo-lism (as in this case), pulmonary oedema, asthma, emphysema, ARDS, Guillian Barrè syndrome, diaphragmatic paralysis etc can cause respiratory acidosis. The PaO_2 levels are generally low and patient would need O_2 therapy. In patients with COPD, O_2 needs to be judiciously given as too much O_2 can make matters worse.

4. The presentation of the patient suggests the diagnosis of renal failure. Most likely this patient suffers from chronic renal failure as the signs of anaemia and dry skin are present in the patient. But the presence of anaemia, decreased calcium or increased phosphates may not help distinguish ARF from CRF, though their absence suggests ARF.

5. Post-operative breathlessness can be due to pneumonia, pulmonary collapse, fluid overload, MI, pulmonary embolism or pneumothorax. The presentation of peripheral oedema along with breathlessness is suggestive of fluid overload in the patient.

Theme 21: Psychiatry: Management

1. Hyoscine is an anticholinergic drug which is less potent and longer acting than atropine. It is used for oesophageal and gastrointestinal spastic conditions. In this case, as the patient has developed hypersalivation, it can be used to correct it as it decreases sweat, salivary, tracheobronchial and lacrimal secretions.

2. Haloperidol is a potent antipsychotic which produces few autonomic effects. It is the preferred drug for acute schizophrenia. In this case, the patient seems to have developed a rare side effect of haloperidol–Neuroleptic malignant syndrome. The drug needs to be stopped immediately.

3. Despite the fact that the patient in this case has a belief that he has recovered completely, the drug should still be continued and tapered off only with the advice of a psychiatrist to avoid a relapse of psychosis.

4. Intractable hiccups may respond to parenteral chlorpromazine.

Theme 22: Investigation in renal stones

1. In this patient, as the diagnosis has already been made as ureteric stone; the next level of investigation must address the cause of stone formation and also the probability of such stone formation in future. Types of renal calculi are calcium oxalate ~40%, calcium oxalate/phosphate ~14%, triple phosphate ~15%, calcium phosphate ~13%, uric acid ~80%. As the percentage of stones with calcium phosphate and oxalate make the bulk; serum alkaline phosphatase, serum calcium and phosphate levels need to be checked.

2. This is a suspected case of renal stones. The biochemical investigations of the patient are normal. Therefore to diagnose the patient, the next step of investigation would be an abdominal KUB film which may show a calculus along the line of the ureters. As it is not in the options, the next step i.e. Renal ultrasound becomes the right answer.

3. Gout is a disease characterized by deposition of sodium monourate crystals in joints. After repeated attacks of gout, urate deposits (tophi) can be found in avascular areas e.g. pinna, tendons, joints, eye. As the serum urate levels are mostly (not always) increased in patients with gout, it becomes the investigation of choice in this patient where no joint involvement is mentioned.

4. As explained in the first question.

Theme 23: Investigation of trauma in children

1. This looks like a case of bowel perforation along with haemorrhage in the peritoneal cavity causing peritonitis and shock. Such cases require urgent transfer to the OT and laparotomy. In the given options, CT scan of the abdomen is the best investigation in the case scenario.

2. This looks like a case of splenic rupture as the child has presented with left hypochondrial pain, pallor, hypotension and tachycardia. These signs of shock are commonly seen in splenic rupture. Again the best investigation for this child would be a CT scan of the abdomen.

Theme 24: Investigation in diabetes

1. Diabetes mellitus is due to lack or diminished effectiveness of endogenous insulin and is characterized by hyperglycaemia. For diagnosis of DM, fasting venous plasma glucose level should be ≥ 7 mmol/L. If in doubt an oral glucose tolerance test should be performed and a value above 11.1 mmol/L is diagnostic of DM. In case the patient comes without any preparation and wishes to know whether he is a diabetic, a random blood glucose level can be checked in which a value ≥ 11.1 mmol/L would be diagnostic of DM.

2. This patient has polyuria and is suspected to have diabetes mellitus. Although urine test for glycosuria is an unreliable test and fasting glucose levels or OGTT should be performed; screening for glycosuria is performed because it is easy and has 99% specificity. Only ~1% of the population has a low renal threshold for glucose.

3. Fasting hypoglycaemia is most commonly due to insulin or sulfonylurea treatment in a known diabetic. In non-diabetics the causes include 'EXPLAIN'– Exogenous drugs, Pituitary insufficiency, Liver failure, Addison's disease, Islet cell tumours, Non-pancreatic neoplasms. The first step in such patients is to document hypoglycaemia by doing a fasting blood sugar level. Such patients need to be admitted and investigated. Investigations would include blood sugar, C-peptide and insulin levels.

4. As explained in the first question.

Theme 25: Management of ectopic pregnancy

1. Ectopic pregnancy is defined as the fertilized ovum getting implanted outside the uterine cavity. The patient in the question has presented with signs of shock—BP 70/50 and a pulse rate of 140/min. This must be a case of ruptured ectopic pregnancy leading to shock which can be fatal. Immediate laparotomy is necessary as only clamping the bleeding artery would control the shock.

2. Golden rule is always think of an ectopic in a sexually active woman with abdominal pain or bleeding, as in this case. The suspicion is further heightened by the fact that on USG examination the uterus is empty. The only and a very good non-invasive test to further support the diagnosis is a quantitative 24 hours β HCG. If β HCG > 6000 IU/L in the patient, ectopic pregnancy is very likely.

3. In this case there are no substantial or typical presentations to support the diagnosis of ectopic pregnancy. The lady has 5 weeks of amenorrhoea whereas patients generally present with ~8 weeks of amenorrhoea. β HCG in the patient is 5000, whereas a βHCG > 6000 IU/L is more supportive of an ectopic. Therefore to confirm the diagnosis, laparoscopy needs to be done which would not only confirm the diagnosis but would also be used as treatment modality.

Theme 26: Control of hypertension

1. All patients with malignant hypertension or a sustained BP > 160/180 mmHg should be treated. Start with drugs of proven benefit like β blockers or thiazides. ACE inhibitors are more effective in co existing diabetes or ischaemic heart disease. In this patient although reduction of alcohol intake to < 20 U/wk and to stop smoking should be advised, we need to treat his hypertension first. As there are no thiazides in the options, the best drug to control his BP would be a β blocker.

2. Obesity is defined as BMI > 30. In this patient as the BMI is 33, a reduction in weight through exercise is imperative in the proper treatment of her hypertension. Her BP being 160/100, is just on the borderline which defines the indication for drug therapy for the treatment of hypertension. The amount of alcohol intake is also on the borderline. Therefore the only modality of treatment to control her hypertension is through exercise.

3. Diuretics are the 1st choice in the treatment of hypertension. In case if a drug fails to control hypertension, switch over to another drug or combine drugs. Common combinations include thiazide diuretics with ACE inhibitors or β blockers with calcium channel blockers. In this case as diuretics have not been able to control his hypertension an ACE inhibitor can be added to the regime.

4. This is not such a tricky question as it seems to be. The patient in this case does not himself suffer from cardiovascular disorder, he simply has a family history of the same, putting him into the risk group. Therefore he requires a life-style change which would include most importantly diet control and exercise.

Theme 27: Psychiatry: Management

1. Patients who are on antipsychotics need to visit their doctor regularly due to many reasons: (a) the doctor may add or substitute a drug to the present treatment according to the patients response to the drug (b) All antipsychotics have side effects which need to be monitored frequently e.g. haloperidol can cause malignant neurolept syndrome which can be fatal (c) the doctor may advice to taper the dose of an antipsychotic with the help of bringing in other alternative modalities such as cognitive therapy.

2. Once the patient has been well controlled on his anti psychotic drug, the doctor may wish to start lithium carbonate as prophylaxis. The dose of lithium needs to be adjusted to keep the plasma levels between 0.7 to 1.0 mmol/L. Initially lithium levels are checked weekly until the dose remains constant for 4 weeks, then monthly for 6 months and then every 3 months as must be in this case. So the patient now needs to visit his doctor after 3 months.

Theme 28: Diagnosis of cervical pathology

1. Cervical cancer has a pre-invasive phase, the CIN. The history of multiple sexual partners recently which is a risk factor for cervical carcinoma, is suggestive of that the patient is having cervical intraepithelial neoplasia. Early tumour is a friable mass which bleeds to touch, as in this patient. Had the patient given a long history of multiple sexual partners the diagnosis would have been cervical carcinoma.

2. Cervical ectropion also known as erosion is a normal phenomenon. It is seen temporarily due to hormonal influence during puberty, with the use of OCPs (as in this patient) or during pregnancy. As columnar epithelium is soft and glandular, it is prone to bleeding, excess mucus production and to infection. Treatment is with cautery if the condition is very disturbing otherwise no treatment is required.

3. Golden rule: All postmenopausal bleeding must be investigated as the cause may be endo-metrial carcinoma. Postmenopausal bleeding is an early sign of endometrial carcinoma. Further investigations require endometrial smear and uterine USG. Diagnosis is made by uterine sampling or curettage. All parts of the uterine cavity must be sampled. For stage I and II, total hysterectomy with bilateral salpingo-oophorectomy is done. Radiotherapy is given if the patient is unfit for surgery. For stages III and IV radiotherapy and high dose progestogens are used.

4. As in this case the presentation of the patient is with vaginal discharge with unpleasant odour, which in not very specific for any organism, we can safely mark chlamydial infection as the answer. Chlamydia tracho-matis is the most common bacterial STD in industrialized countries. Women under the age of 25 years age have the highest prevalence. In women it causes cervicitis and PID. It is treated with Doxycycline and Erythromycin. In pregnancy, Azithromycin and Ofloxacin may be used.

5. The mention of postmenopausal i.e. old age and post coital bleeding suggests that the lady is suffering from atrophic vaginitis. Vaginal dryness due to fallen oestrogen levels, can lead to vaginal and urinary infections, dyspareunia, traumatic bleeding, stress incontinence and prolapse.

Theme 29: Cause of respiratory pathology

1. Cystic fibrosis is an autosomal recessive condition caused by mutation in cystic fibrosis transmembrane conductance regulator (CFTR) gene on chromosome 7. It leads to defective chloride secretion and increased sodium absorption across the epithelium. The changes in the composition of airway surface liquid predisposes the lung to chronic pulmonary infections and bronchiectasis. At present prenatal diagnosis is offered only to parents who are known carriers, usually because they have an affected child already. Screening can be done using fetal DNA from amniotic fluid cells or from chorionic villous sampling. Clinical features include failure to thrive, meconium ileus in neonates, cough, wheeze, recurrent chest infections, bronchiectasis, haemoptysis, respiratory failure, pancreatic insufficiency (diabetes mellitus, steatorrhoea), distal intestinal obstruction, gallstones, cirrhosis, sinusitis, nasal polyps, male infertility, etc.
   Sweat test is positive in cystic fibrosis; Na > 60 mmol/L and sweat Cl >70 mmol/L on two occasions. Management is symptomatic.

2. Respiratory distress syndrome is due to insufficient surfactant production due to which the lungs are unable to stay expanded. Reinflation between breaths exhausts the baby and respiratory failure ensues. It presents as worsening tachypnoea in the first few hours of birth. CXR shows diffuse granular patterns with air bronchograms. Treatment is by intubation and giving surfactant by ET tube.

3. Patients with alpha-1 antitrypsin deficiency usually present with dyspnoea and weight loss, cor pulmonale and polycythaemia. CXR shows bilateral basal emphysema with paucity of pulmonary vessels. Lung function tests are typical for emphysema. It is associated with an increase in incidence of bronchiectasis, glomerulonephritis and probably inflammatory bowel disease. Treatment depends largely on the avoidance of stimuli especially smoking which causes repeated pulmonary inflammation.

4. The presentation of symptoms with relation to winters is suggestive of asthma. Asthma implies airway obstruction which is reversible. Patient may present with wheeze, dyspnoea or cough. Treatment of asthma in > 5 years old: Occasional β agonists → add inhaled steroid or cromoglycate → add inhaled salmeterol or increased fluticasone → add trial of theophylline or oral long acting β agonist or inhaled ipratropium → oral prednisolone.

Theme 30: Investigation in acid peptic disease

1. This is a patient of gastric ulcer which occurs mainly in the elderly, as in this case and occurs on the lesser curvature of the stomach. Patients generally present with epigastric pain which occurs in the night, after meals, as in this case and is relieved by antacids. Upper GI endoscopy must be performed in all patients presenting with 'alarm' symptoms which includes >45 years of age, weight loss, vomiting, haematemesis, anaemia and dysphagia.

2. Fundoplication is a surgery for gastro oesophageal reflux in which the aim is to re-establish the lower oesophageal sphincter tone. After the surgery, around 1/3rd of the patients develop new symptoms of dysphagia, bloating, increased flatulence or dyspepsia. Therefore in this patient who complains of pain in stomach after the surgery, endoscopy is required to confirm the success of the surgery done.

3. In the question, there is no mention of the treatment received by the patient till now. As the patient has had a positive *H. pylori* status, *H. pylori* serology needs to be done before starting the treatment of the patients for peptic ulcer. *H. pylori* is associated with 80–90% of the cases of peptic ulcer and eradication of *H. pylori* is a must for complete treatment of the peptic ulcer.

4. In this question again, there is no mention of the treatment received for *H. pylori*. Therefore his *H. pylori* status needs to be checked at first, before any treatment is planned for his dyspeptic symptoms. 80–90% of the patients with peptic ulcer have *H. pylori* infection. Patients with peptic ulcer may present with complications such as haematemesis. *H. pylori* eradication in such patients is imperative for definitive treatment. *H. pylori* eradication is done by 'triple therapy'

which includes Lansoprazole 30 mg 12 hourly with Clarithromycin 500 mg 12 hourly with Amoxicillin 1 gm 12 hourly (or Metronidazole 40 mg 12 hourly). All these drugs are given for 1 week.

Theme 31: Treatment for upper GI conditions

1. Gastro oesophageal reflux and dyspeptic symptoms are reported by a large number of women throughout pregnancy. Antacids containing calcium, magnesium or aluminium may be useful and are considered safe. Studies on H_2 blockers and proton pump inhibitors are either inadequate or have shown some adverse effects over animal embryos.

2. Barrett's oesophagus is seen due to chronic reflux oesophagitis in which squamous mucosa shows metaplastic change. The risk of adenocarcinoma increases 40 folds. Therefore regular endoscopy and biopsy are required for early diagnosis of the malignancy. Its treatment requires intensive antireflux measures including long term proton pump inhibitors.

3. Benign oesophageal stricture can be due to gastro oesophageal reflux disease, corrosives, surgery or radiotherapy. It is treated by endoscopic balloon dilatation.

4. The risk factors for carcinoma oesophagus include spicy hot diet, alcohol excess, tobacco, Barrett's oesophagus, plummer–vinson syndrome. Patients may present with dysphagia, weight loss, retrosternal chest pain, hoarseness and cough. Oesophagoscopy with biopsy is diagnostic. Treatment aims at removal of the tumour and restoring continuity. In this case as there is no metastasis, oesophageal excision would suffice.

5. The risk factors for carcinoma oesophagus include spicy hot diet, alcohol excess, tobacco, Barrett's oesophagus, plummer–vinson syndrome. Patients may present with dysphagia, weight loss, retrosternal chest pain, hoarseness and cough. Oesophagoscopy with biopsy is diagnostic. Treatment aims at removal of the tumour and restoring continuity. In this case as there are metastases, surgery itself would be inadequate and the patient will eventually require radiotherapy with or without surgery

Theme 32: Management of injury to upper limb

1. In cases of pulled elbow the child is typically between 1–4 years of age with history of being lifted by the arms. Radial head in such cases slips out of the annular ligament. Elbow rotation i.e. manipulation is all that is required.

2. This is a case of scaphoid fracture which is commonly seen but missed on radiographs as in this case. There is tenderness 2 cm distal to Lister's tubercle of the radius. Special oblique 'scaphoid' view is required. Treatment in such cases require a plaster cast and repeat X-rays after 2 weeks, which may show a fracture.

3. Infantile torticollis generally results from birth damage to sternocleidomastoid muscle. The child presents with a tilted head with the ear nearer the shoulder on the affected side. 97% of such children have a self limiting disease. The rest can benefit from physiotherapy.

4. This is a case of semilunar cartilage or meniscal tear. Medial cartilage tears follow twists to a flexed knee as in this case. Adduction and internal rotation causes lateral cartilage tears. Extension is limited i.e. knee is locked. Mc Murray's test is positive. The child needs to get admitted in this case to get further investigations such as MRI which would show the tear location, morphology, length and its depth. Moreover MRI would help predict tears which require surgical repair.

Theme 33: Management in case of ischaemic limb

1. Atrial fibrillation is a risk factor for embolism which can cause acute ischaemia and present as the six P's—Pale, Pulseless, Painful, Paralysed, Paraesthetic, Perishing with cold, as in this case. This condition is an emergency and requires urgent surgical embolectomy (Fogarty catheter) or local thrombolysis.

2. This is a case of diabetic foot with foot ulceration on one side. Foot ulceration usually presents as painless punched out ulcer in an area of thick callous with pus, oedema, erythema and malodour. As gangrene has already ensued in this patient the only treatment modality remaining is amputation.

3. Compartment syndromes are one of the causes of ischaemia. Tell tale signs of redness, mottling, blisters, swelling and pain on passive muscle stretching must be looked for. A vicious cycle of pressure → hypoxia → necrosis → increased pressure ensues. Prompt fasciotomy breaks the cycle and prevents contracture.

4. This is a patient with occlusive disease of the artery in the foot. Arteriography also shows lack of blood supply. Treatment includes arterial bypass or arteriovenous grafting.

Theme 34: Management of osteoporosis

1. Obesity implies a BMI of more than 30. Obesity shortens life, aggravates diabetes, gout, osteoarthrosis, heartburn, hypertension, hyperlipidaemia, sleep apnoea and DVT. Weight loss in obese diminishes BP and osteoarthrosis. Drugs used in the treatment of obesity include orlistat and sibutramine. Surgery is reserved for morbid obesity e.g. BMI > 40 or in BMI > 35 with associated cardiovascular risk factors.

2. The lady herself does not suffer from osteoporosis; she just has a family history. In such cases only preventive measures need to be considered. Exercise, calcium rich diet, avoiding smoking and excess alcohol are such preventive measures.

3. Osteoporosis implies reduced bone density. Treatment of osteoporosis includes HRT, biphosphonates, vitamin D and calcium supplements. HRT is not indicated in women with past history of DVT or pulmonary embolism or breast cancer or increased risk of breast cancer. Etidronate, a biphosphonate is licensed for treating and preventing osteoporosis. Since it is mentioned in the question itself, this patient should be given calcium supplement for treating osteoporosis.

Theme 35: Head injury: Diagnosis

1. Head injury is graded as mild, moderate or severe on the basis of glasgow coma scale (GCS).
   Mild head injury – GCS 13–15.
   Moderate head injury – GCS 9–12.
   Severe head injury – GCS ≤ 8.
2. Since the child is alert and oriented, it implies a full GCS score. Moreover no abnormality has been revealed on examination. Head injury is graded as mild, moderate or severe on the basis of glasgow coma scale (GCS).
   Mild head injury – GCS 13–15.
   Moderate head injury – GCS 9–12.
   Severe head injury – GCS ≤ 8.
3. Fracture base of skull may involve the anterior or middle cranial fossa. Both may present with haemotympanum. In addition, anterior fossa fractures present with subconjunctival haematoma, anosmia, epistaxis and CSF rhinorrhoea; whereas middle cranial fossa fractures present with CSF otorrhoea or rhinorrhoea, ossicular disruption, VII and VIII cranial nerve palsies and Battle's sign (bruising behind the ear occurring 36 hours after head injury).
4. Following points favour the diagnosis of extradural haematoma: (i) Usually occur due to trauma which may cause fracture temporal or parietal bone which further causes laceration of middle meningeal artery and vein. (ii) the injury initially produces no loss of consciousness, but later is followed by deterioration of consciousness. This 'lucid interval' pattern is typical of extradural bleeds. CT Scan of the head shows a biconvex lens shaped haematoma. Urgent evacuation of the clot through multiple burr holes with ligation of the bleeding vessel later is the management in such patients.
5. As explained in the first question.

Theme 36: Diagnosis of drug abuse

1. Patients of opiate withdrawal syndrome may present with anxiety, restlessness, irritability, insomnia and craving for opiates. Sweating may be profuse. Piloerection leads to the appearance of 'goose-flesh'. Nausea and vomiting may be accompanied by anorexia, abdominal pain and diarrhoea. Pupil dilatation, elevations of blood pressure, body temperature and respiratory rate may be observed. Methadone, a synthetic opiate with an action lasting more than 24 hours, is used in such patients. Most patients after dose adjustment would require a daily stabilization dose of less than 60 mg of methadone.
2. The signs of alcohol withdrawal i.e. delirium tremens, include tachycardia, hypotension, tremors, seizures, visual or tactile hallucinations. The symptoms of nausea, sweating, mood changes, vomiting etc. usually appear within 6 hours of stopping alcohol. The symptoms fluctuate but peak on 3rd to 4th day of withdrawal and subside over a week. Such patients need to be admitted and given generous amounts (e.g. 10 mg 6 hourly) of diazepam in initial 3 days. Thereafter the doses are tapered off.

Theme 37: Analgesia in terminally sick

1. The analgesic 'ladder' consists broadly of three steps. Step I includes non-opioid analgesics like aspirin, paracetamol and NSAIDs. Step II includes weak opioids such as codeine, dihydrocodeine and dextropropoxyphene. Step III includes strong opioids such as morphine, diamorphine and hydromorphine. The presentation in the patient is suggestive of bony metastasis in which even strong opioids are usually ineffective for pain relief. Radiotherapy is the mainstay in such patients for pain relief. 8–30 Gy dosage is delivered in 1, 2, 5 or 10 fractions.

2. One of the guidelines for successful pain control post operatively is to allow the patient to be incharge of pain control. Patient controlled analgesia promotes well being and does not lead to overuse. Patient controlled continuous parenteral morphine delivery systems are useful.

3. The analgesic 'ladder' consists broadly of three steps. Step I includes non-opioid analgesics like aspirin, paracetamol and NSAIDs. Step II includes weak opioids such as codeine, dihydrocodeine and dextropropoxyphene. Step III hydromorphine. Patients who have undergone a major surgery or have a carcinoma in terminal stages, experience severe degrees of pain. Such a pain normally responds only to the highest level of the analgesic 'ladder'. IV opioids need to be given in such patients.

4. As explained above.

Theme 38: Management of cardiac conditions

1. The commonest arrhythmia in pregnancy is supraventricular tachycardia. The occurrence of arrhythmia in pregnancy, requires hospital assessment and management. Prophylactic anti-arrhythmic therapy is given for the same indications as in the non pregnant state. Adenosine is given IV in paroxysmal supraventricular tachycardias when conventional non-pharmacological measures have failed. Since even adenosine has shown no response in this case, verapamil should be tried. Verapamil is a calcium antagonist which has a negative chronotropic action. There have been no reports of teratogenicity.

2. Diuretics are the mainstay in the management of cardiac failure. If symptoms are mild, frusemide is started as 40–80 mg IV slowly. Larger doses are required in renal failure. If the pulmonary oedema is refractory to loop diuretics or if large doses of loop diuretics are being used, thiazide diuretics e.g. metolazone 5–20 mg/day PO should be added.

3. ACE inhibitors such as lisinopril 2.5–20 mg/day PO or enalapril may be the first choice in the management of hypertension in patients with coexisting LVF or in diabetics with micro albuminuria or proteinuria. Side effects of ACE inhibitors include cough, hyperkalaemia, renal failure, first-dose hypotension and angio-oedema. Their use is contraindicated in renal artery stenosis and aortic stenosis.

4. Asymmetric septal hypertrophy causes left ventricular outflow tract obstruction in hypertrophic obstructive cardiomyopathy. It shows an autosomal dominant inheritance pattern. Patients with HOCM may have angina, dyspnoea, palpitations, syncope and even sudden death. Pulse is jerky with double apex beat, harsh ejection systolic murmur and 'a' wave in JVP. β blockers or verapamil are used in symptomatic patients. Dual-chamber pacing is used if symptomatic despite drugs.

Theme 39: Diagnosis of respiratory disorders

1. Weight reduction is the first step in the management of obstructive sleep apnoea syndrome which is characterized by intermittent closure or collapse of the pharyngeal airway which causes apnoeic episodes during sleep. The typical patient is a fat, middle aged man with complaints of snoring, daytime somnolence, morning headache or poor sleep quality.

2. Pneumothorax is collection of air in the pleural space. It often occurs spontaneous by especially in young thin men due to rupture of subpleural bulla. In this question the patient is breathless which means that he may be suffering from asthma, COPD, TB, pneumonia, lung abscess or sarcoidosis which are also causative factors in the occurrence of pneumothorax. The patient will typically complains of sudden onset dyspnoea and pleuritic chest pain. Patient will have reduced chest expansion, hyperresonance to percussion and decreased breath sounds on the affected area. Mild pneumothorax does not require any treatment, but moderate to severe pneumothorax require aspiration.

3. This is a patient with Coarctation of aorta. Headache, epistaxis, cold extremities and claudication with exercise may be seen in such patients. Hypertension in upper limbs and delayed pulsation in the femoral arteries is detected. A CXR may show a dilated left subclavian artery and a dilated descending aorta. Indentation of the aorta at the site of coarctation and pre and post stenotic dilatation (the 'Z' sign) is pathognomic of the entity. Notching of the ribs may also be seen which is due to erosion by dilated collateral vessels.

4. The presentation of this patient with fever, cough, chest pain is suggestive of pneumonia. Other features that may be present in patients with pneumonia are malaise, anorexia, cough, purulent sputum, haemoptysis, pleuritic chest pain, tachypnoea, hypotension and signs of consolidation. Investigations required are CXR, sputum for microscopy and cultures and pleural aspirate (if present) for culture. Treatment involves antibiotics according to sensitivity patterns.

5. Dressler's syndrome develops 2–10 weeks after an MI. The patient may suffer from recurrent fever, chest pain, pleural and pericardial rub, pleural effusions, anaemia and raised ESR. Treatment is with NSAIDs and steroids.

6. Cystic fibrosis is an autosomal recessive condition caused by mutation in cystic fibrosis transmembrane conductance regulator (CFTR) gene on chromosome 7. It leads to defective chloride secretion and increased sodium absorption across the epithelium. The changes in the composition of airway surface liquid predisposes the lung to chronic pulmonary infections and bronchiectasis. At present prenatal diagnosis is offered only to parents who are known carriers, usually because they have an affected child already. Screening can be done using fetal DNA from amniotic fluid cells or from chorionic villous sampling. Clinical features include failure to thrive, meconium ileus in neonates, cough, wheeze, recurrent chest infections, bronchiectasis, haemoptysis, respiratory failure, pancreatic insufficiency (diabetes mellitus, steatorrhoea), distal intestinal obstruction, gallstones, cirrhosis, sinusitis, nasal polyps, male infertility, etc.

Sweat test is positive in cystic fibrosis; Na > 60 mmol/L and sweat Cl >70 mmol/L on two occasions. Management is symptomatic.

Theme 40: Diagnosis of urinary retention

1. Urinary tract infection implies presence of a pure growth of more than 10^5 colony forming units/mL. Infection may occur at the bladder (cystitis), prostate (prostatitis) or kidney (pyelonephritis). Female sex, sexual intercourse, diabetes, immunocompromised status, pregnancy, menopause, urinary tract obstruction and renal stones are some of the risk factors. Patients may present with frequency, dysuria, urgency, haematuria, fever, vomiting, loin pain, ARF, low backache. *E. coli* is the most common organism causing UTI. Treatment is with trimethoprim 200 mg 12 hourly PO for 3 days in patients with cystitis. Cefuroxime is given in cases of pyelonephritis and ciprofloxacin for prostatitis.

2. Urinary tract obstruction may be due to luminal, mural or extramural causes. Luminal causes of obstruction include stones, blood clot, sloughed papillae, renal, ureteric or bladder tumours. Mural causes include congenital or acquired stricture, neuromuscular dysfunction and schistosomiasis. Extramural causes are abdominal or pelvic mass or tumour, retroperitoneal fibrosis. Since the patient has haematuria in this case, clot retention is the most probable cause of urinary retention.

3. Benign prostatic hypertrophy is a common problem. Decrease in urinary flow is associated with increased frequency, urgency and voiding difficulty. Treatment involves mainly surgical (e.g. TURP, TUIP, TULIP, Retropubic prostatectomy) and in some cases medical (e.g. α blockers, 5 α reductase inhibitors) approach.

4. Prostatic carcinoma is the 2nd most common malignancy in men. Incidence increases with age and is associated with increased levels of testosterone and a positive family history. Patients may present with nocturia, hesitancy, poor stream or urinary obstruction. Weight loss and bone pain are suggestive of metastasis. PR examination may reveal hard, irregular prostate gland. Diagnosis is by measuring serum prostate specific antigen levels and doing transrectal USG and biopsy. The presentation of a hugely enlarged prostate with sudden retention of urine is suggestive of spinal cord compression. Radiotherapy is given in patients with prostatic carcinoma who have bone metastasis or spinal cord compression.

5. Multiple sclerosis is a chronic disorder which consists of plaques of demyelination and axon loss at sites throughout the CNS. Patients may present with unilateral optic neuritis–pain on eye movements and rapid deterioration in central vision, nystagmus, fatigue, weakness or spasticity in limbs, constipation, frequency and urgency, impotence, ataxia, dementia, vertigo, even depression. No test is pathognomic and diagnosis is essentially clinical. Symptoms may worsen by heat or exercise. There is no cure but methylprednisolone shortens relapse and β interferon decreases relapse rate.

Theme 41: Pre operative investigations

1. A pre-operative CXR is required in all those patients with known cardiorespiratory disease, pathology or symptoms or if the patient is > 65 years age. Since the patient has already got a normal chest X-ray, the anaesthetist would like to know about her functional lung volumes for which spirometry is required. In obstructive defects such as asthma and COPD, FEV_1 is reduced more than FVC and the FEV_1/FVC ratio is < 80%.

2. Risk factors for deep vein thrombosis include elderly age group, pregnancy, synthetic oestrogen, pelvic or orthopaedic surgery, past DVT, malignancy, obesity, immobility and thrombophilia. Since this patient is on chronic use of OCPs, she must be investigated with an arteriography to rule out DVT. OCPs should be stopped 6 weeks pre-operatively.

3. This a case of stable angina. Angina is due to myocardial ischaemia and presents as central chest heaviness, tightness or pain which is brought on by exertion. It may also be precipitated by emotion, cold weather and heavy meals. Stable angina is induced by exertion and relieved by rest. Unstable i.e. crescendo angina is of increasing frequency or severity and occurs with minimal exertion or even at rest. An exercise ECG is required in this case which would show the ischaemic changes.

Five

January 2003
Question Paper

Theme 1: Causes of shock

Options:

a. Gram negative septicaemic shock
b. Cardiogenic shock
c. Hypovolemic shock
d. Anaphylaxis

For each presentation below, choose the SINGLE most appropriate cause of shock from the above list of options. Each option may be used once, more than once, or not at all.

1. A young boy after eating peanuts suddenly develops difficulty in breathing with red and oedematous lips.
2. A patient had an accident and fracture of pelvis and femur. His BP is 100/70 and pulse rate is 90/minute.
3. A patient had a myocardial infarction. He is presently in shock.
4. A middle aged man haś been operated for a perforated gall bladder. He becomes progressively drowsy with warm peripheries. His BP is 90/60 and pulse rate is 110/minute.

Theme 2: Management of epistaxis

Options:

a. Anterior nasal packing
b. Posterior nasal packing
c. Neomycin cream
d. Pinching the nose
e. Reassurance
f. Vitamin K
g. FFP
h. Ice pack on the nose

For each presentation below, choose the SINGLE most appropriate management from the above list of options. Each option may be used once, more than once, or not at all.

1. A patient on warfarin, comes to you with nose bleeds. His INR is 0.9.
2. A boy has come with slight bleeding from nose 2 days ago. On examination the nose showed redness and crusting.
3. A patient has come with a BP of 230/110 and bleeding from nose. His circulatory system has been stabilised and anterior nasal packing is done. He continues to bleed.
4. A girl has come with slight bleeding from anterior part of nose. By the time she reaches A & E, bleeding has stopped.

Theme 3: Fractures of wrist joint

Options:

a. X-ray of the wrist: scaphoid view
b. Refer to orthopaedician immediately
c. Bandage and discharge
d. Isotope scan
e. Do nothing

For each presentation below, choose the SINGLE most appropriate management from the above list of options. Each option may be used once, more than once, or not at all.

1. Boy fell from tree now has come with painful wrist. X-rays taken were normal.
2. Patient had a fall. X-ray shows perilunate fracture .
3. Patient had a fall. X-ray of the wrist joint is normal, tenderness is present in the anatomical snuff box.
4. Patient had a fall. X-ray showed displacement of the radial head.

Theme 4: Relation to obesity

Options:

a. Obstructive sleep apnoea
b. Type I DM
c. Type II DM
d. Alcohol
e. Cushing's disease
f. Hypothyroidism
g. Polycystic ovary disease

For each presentation below, choose the SINGLE most appropriate diagnosis from the above list of options. Each option may be used once, more than once, or not at all.

1. Weight loss would help night sleep and this condition and improve family relations.
2. Weight loss would even help to stop the medications.
3. Stop of this would help in weight loss and vitamin deficiency.
4. Surgery in this condition in a female would help in weight loss and improve this condition.

Theme 5: Delayed milestones: Diagnosis

Options:

a. Fragile X syndrome
b. Tay–Sach's disease
c. Bacterial meningitis
d. Hypothyroidism
e. Prematurity
f. Duchenne's muscular dystrophy
g. Fetal alcohol syndrome

For each presentation below, choose the SINGLE most appropriate diagnosis from the above list of options. Each option may be used once, more than once, or not at all.

1. A 4 years old boy can write his name and draw a circle and square. He walks with lordosis and he cannot run.
2. A 3 year old boy has delayed milestones. His uncle and brother also have this condition.
3. Girl can sort out cube 49 and is 97 percentile for her weight, but her head circumference is lower than normal.
4. A six months old child, can smile, but has head lag.
5. Child was normal but then milestones were delayed after a fever.

Theme 6: Psychiatric management

Options:

a. Methadone
b. Propranolol
c. Diazepam
d. Acamprosate
e. Zopiclone
f. Risperidone
g. Amitriptyline
h. Rebreathe in air bag

For each presentation below, choose the SINGLE most appropriate management from the above list of options. Each option may be used once, more than once, or not at all.

1. A girl has developed oral numbness and limb paraesthesias after an argument with her friend.
2. A patient who is a heroin addict is now in ward. He is in withdrawal and wants you to help him.
3. An alcoholic patient who has been detoxified feels that he wants to remain off it, but is scared that he may relapse.
4. A female with complaints of pain in the chest, tightness, feeling like dying and sinking feeling, wants some medication for her condition.
5. Patient has to go for an interview, has sweaty palms and palpitations asks for your help.
6. Patient having restlessness, pacing up and down after death of her husband, presents with difficulty in falling asleep.

Theme 7: Diagnosis of psychiatric disorders

Options:

a. Post-traumatic stress disorder
b. Postnatal psychosis
c. Thought broadcasting
d. Insertion
e. Echo
f. Hallucination
g. Illusion
h. Paranoid delusion
i. Judgement
j. Insight
k. Low mood
l. Flight of ideas

For each presentation below, choose the SINGLE most appropriate diagnosis from the above list of options. Each option may be used once, more than once, or not at all.

1. Patient keeps on talking to you non stop and jumps from one topic to another.
2. Patient after the birth of her child feels sad and does not want to feed the baby.
3. Patient has the belief that his neighbour is planning an attack.
4. An old woman has been admitted and feels that the staff of the hospital knows what she is thinking all the time.
5. Patient who lost her husband is sad now and avoids eye contact.
6. A man has psychiatric problem and he knows that he needs a treatment.

Theme 8: Diagnosis of vomiting in pregnancy

Options:

a. Hyperemesis gravidarum
b. Hydatiform mole
c. Cholecystitis
d. Ectopic pregnancy
e. Brain tumour
f. Pre eclampsia
g. Migraine

For each presentation below, choose the SINGLE most appropriate diagnosis from the above list of options. Each option may be used once, more than once, or not at all.

1. A 12 weeks pregnant woman has been continuously vomiting. She comes with a furred tongue, signs of dehydration and uraemia.
2. A 14 weeks pregnant woman comes to you with severe vomiting. USG of the uterus shows absence of fetal heart motion. The uterus is 18 weeks to date.
3. Patient comes to your with severe vomiting, dizziness and photophobia. She is in the 34th week of her pregnancy. She tells you that she has had these symptoms since 14 weeks and on examination her pulse rate is 60 /minute.
4. A pregnant woman had nausea and vomiting since week 18 and these symptoms have got worse since two weeks. She is anorexic, is vomiting and has slight jaundice.

Theme 9: Nerve injury

Options:

a. Axillary nerve
b. Musculocutaneous nerve
c. Radial nerve
d. Ulnar nerve
e. Common peroneal nerve
f. Sciatic nerve
g. Median nerve
h. Femoral nerve
i. Facial nerve
j. Glossopharyngeal nerve

For each presentation below, choose the SINGLE most appropriate affected nerve from the above list of options. Each option may be used once, more than once, or not at all.

1. Patient has history of fracture shoulder. Now he has decreased sensation on the lateral aspect of the deltoid muscle.
2. Patient had fracture of fibula and now has lost his ability to dorsiflex. He has sensation loss on the lateral side of his lower leg.
3. Patient had fracture of medial epicondyle and now come with decreased sensation of 5th and 4th finger.
4. Patient has some fracture of humerus and comes with signs and symptoms of wrist drop.
5. Old man had a fall and fracture or dislocation of hip. He now has weakness in his hamstrings.

Theme 10: Pain relief

Options:

a. Allopurinol
b. Radiotherapy
c. TENS
d. IM diamorphine
e. Oral NSAIDs
f. Paracetamol
g. Prednisolone
h. Physiotherapy
i. Home exercise
j. IM steroids in joint

For each presentation below, choose the SINGLE most appropriate analgesia from the above list of options. Each option may be used once, more than once, or not at all.

1. Patient with carcinoma prostate and now has secondaries to the back presents with severe pain. No NSAIDs or morphine have helped. He wishes to continue his work.
2. Patient with carcinoma lung with secondaries now has come with an unilateral swollen arm, all other medications have failed.
3. A 50 year old woman has come with painful shoulder joint and hip joint.
4. A 30 year old busy executive has got pain on lateral aspect of thigh. He shows no improvement with NSAIDs. X-ray taken was normal.
5. A man is on frusemide and got pain in his joint.

Theme 11: Mechanism of abortion

Options:

a. Immunological
b. Genetic
c. Anatomical
d. Endocrine
e. Drug-induced

For each presentation below, choose the SINGLE most appropriate mechanism of abortion from the above list of options. Each option may be used once, more than once, or not at all.

1. Patient having 6 abortions in mid trimester.
2. Patient having some problem with the deformed child. She married her cousin.
3. Patient has recurrent abortions. She is obese and has hirsutism.

Theme 12: Investigation of leg ulcers

Options:

a. Pyoderma gangrenosum
b. Bowen's disease
c. Venous stasis
d. Arteriography
e. Melanoma biopsy

For each presentation below, choose the SINGLE most appropriate investigation/ diagnosis from the above list of options. Each option may be used once, more than once, or not at all.

1. Patient having pain on walking. His leg and foot are pale and with the 4th and 5th digit blackened.
2. Patient with diarrhoea and abdominal pain had a small round ulcer with central necrotic tissue.
3. Female fat obese and having oedema of leg now has a small ulcer on medial aspect of her ankle.
4. A 60 years old man with a pigmented skin lesion on his shin.

Theme 13: Head pathology: Diagnosis

Options:

a. Intracerebral haematoma
b. Brainstem injury
c. Extradural haematoma
d. Subdural haematoma
e. Acute SDH
f. Vertibrobasilar ischaemia
g. Migraine
h. Depressed fracture of skull
i. Subarachnoid haemorrhage

For each presentation below, choose the SINGLE most appropriate diagnosis from the above list of options. Each option may be used once, more than once, or not at all.

1. Motorcyclist with accident is brought to casualty with head injury. GCS is 3 and his blood pressure is 180/100 and heart rate of 56/minute. His pupil is dilated and sluggish to light. No neurological sign except his plantars are going up.
2. A 27 year old young male, after a heavy bout of alcohol fell down on the road and then got up and walked home. His wife found him on the floor and cannot rouse him. He has fluctuating consciousness.
3. A 67 years old man had recent falls, became agitated and confused.
4. An old lady has dizziness and vertigo and walking reeling to one side.
5. Female has come to A & E with vomiting and severe pain in the back of the head.
6. Patient hit on the head with a hammer, now comes with vomiting.
7. A young man fell over and there is injury on his temple scalp.

Theme 14: Diagnostic tests: loss of vision

Options:

a. MRI temporal lobe
b. MRI pituitary
c. MRI occipital lobe
d. Doppler carotid artery
e. ESR
f. MRI parietal lobe

For each presentation below, choose the SINGLE most appropriate investigation from the above list of options. Each option may be used once, more than once, or not at all.

1. A patient comes with repeated history of loss of vision in one eye and it improves after a few hours.
2. A patient with bitemporal hemianopia and complaints of increase in shoe size.
3. A patient has come with vomiting and upper quadrantopia.
4. Patient having pain while brushing her hair and now comes with loss of vision in one eye.

Theme 15: Management of injuries

Options:

a. Laparotomy
b. Refer to surgeon
c. Admit and observe
d. Give IV fluids: 1 litre in 30 min
e. IV fluids: 2 litres in 30 min
f. Reassurance and send home

For each presentation below, choose the SINGLE most appropriate management from the above list of options. Each option may be used once, more than once, or not at all.

1. A boy has come with injury by fall on handle of cycle and had got pain and tenderness in left upper side of abdomen. USG of spleen shows a small sized haematoma or infarct in the splenic capsule.
2. A patient who was hit by a ball, comes with severe pain in the epigastrium.
3. A patient was stabbed in a fight and now comes with his hanging omentum. His blood pressure is 110/70 and heart rate 80/minute.
4. A patient with history of fall has come with tenderness in left side of abdomen and fracture of two right sided ribs. Patient is in shock.
5. A patient had some sort of injury to his abdomen. After 2 litres of fluid IV, his BP is low and pulse rate is high.

Theme 16: Management/Investigation of seizures

Options:

a. Start anticonvulsants
b. Reassurance
c. Anxiolytic treatment
d. Valvular surgery
e. EEG
f. ECG
g. IV glucose

For each presentation below, choose the SINGLE most appropriate management/ investigation from the above list of options. Each option may be used once, more than once, or not at all.

1. A 50 years old man had haemoptysis and cough for some time and now come with a first fit.
2. An 8 year old girl falls down in the assembly. She is pale and losses consciousness for one minute. She often falls in dentist visit.
3. A boy has recurrent periods of breathholding spells where he becomes blue and loses consciousness. This happens when he is separating from his parents while going to the school.
4. A 30 year old female has 2-3 episodes of falling down, she also has got a loud murmur on inspiration.
5. A 50 year old woman has episodes of seizures starting in the left thumb and then going to whole body. She loses consciousness.
6. A 10 years old boy behaves strangely and his teacher says that he is not concentrating at the moment.
7. A young man has some kind of seizure and his heart rate drops down to 50/minute.
8. A young boy has seizure, he is a diabetic. His blood glucose is 2mmol/L.

Theme 17: Haematemesis: Diagnosis

Options:

a. Mallory–Weiss tear
b. Alcoholic cirrhosis
c. Gastric erosion
d. Peptic ulcer
e. Duodenal ulcer
f. Diverticulosis
g. Benign gastric ulcer

For each presentation below, choose the SINGLE most appropriate diagnosis from the above list of options. Each option may be used once, more than once, or not at all.

1. A 55 year old patient has been drinking 15 units of alcohol per day. He now comes with massive haematemesis.
2. Patient comes with massive haematemesis after eating a lot and a bout of alcohol.
3. Patient suffering from rheumatoid arthritis, comes with vomiting which contains streaks of blood.
4. A 50 years old manager had epigastric discomfort for some time and his stool are tarry. He is otherwise normal.

Theme 18: Investigation in drug side effects

Options:

a. Drug serum levels
b. Thyroid function tests
c. Liver function tests
d. Serum prolactin levels
e. Urea and electrolytes
f. Increase/decrease levels of insulin
g. ECG
h. CXR
i. USG abdomen

For each presentation below, choose the SINGLE most appropriate investigation from the above list of options. Each option may be used once, more than once, or not at all.

1. A patient on lithium now comes to you with tremors of hand.
2. A patient on lithium now comes with weight gain and constipation.
3. A patient on phenytoin for epilepsy now comes with dizziness, blurred vision and ataxia.
4. A male patient on phenothiazines now comes with painful and lactating breasts.
5. A man took an overdose of his Aspirin. He is conscious since then.

Theme 19: Hearing problem

Options:

a. Ototoxicity
b. Presbyacusis
c. Salicylate levels
d. Fracture petrous temporal bone
e. Wax in ears
f. Acoustic neuroma
g. Blast injury
h. Syringing

For each presentation below, choose the SINGLE most appropriate diagnosis from the above list of options. Each option may be used once, more than once, or not at all.

1. A patient who has been on gentamycin comes with ringing of ears.
2. A patient took some treatment for his headache. He now comes with tinnitus.
3. A boy was hit and fell down. He was hit somewhere behind his ear and now comes with difficulty in hearing and tinnitus.
4. Vagrant comes to A&E with diminished hearing particularly after a shower.
5. A patient who is anaesthetic to his cornea reflex has a diminished hearing. CT showed a widened ear canal.

Theme 20: How would you help this lady

Options:

a. Home redecoration
b. Advice on posture
c. Neck collar
d. Review the dose of anti hypertensive
e. Review the dose of anti diabetic
f. Rearrange home
g. Vision testing

For each presentation below, choose the SINGLE most appropriate management from the above list of options. Each option may be used once, more than once, or not at all.

1. A lady is on aspirin, endofloridazole 7.5 mg comes to you with repeated falls while trying to get out of bed.
2. A lady is on various medications. One of them which is glibenclamide. She comes to you with sweating and altered consciousness.
3. A lady 85 year old, lives alone. She fell down while trying to put up her curtains. Her neighbours tell that she has been seen walking into objects.

Theme 21: Diagnosis of anal condition

Options:

a. Anal haematoma
b. Ischaemic colitis
c. Proctalgia fugax
d. Ca rectum
e. Squamous cell carcinoma of anus
f. Crohn's disease
g. Ulcerative colitis
h. Anal fissure
i. Haemorrhoids

For each presentation below, choose the SINGLE most appropriate diagnosis from the above list of options. Each option may be used once, more than once, or not at all.

1. A patient comes to you with intermittent sensations of electric pain in the rectum.
2. A young girl with history of constipation cannot pass stools. PR is impossible because of the pain.
3. A young woman has constipation and painless fresh blood after defecation
4. A woman of 29 years of age has diarrhoea and colic abdominal pain. She has tags in her anal examination.
5. A patient with weight loss presents with change in bowel habits. Rigid sigmoidoscopy shows an ulcer.

Theme 22: Diagnosis of rectal condition

Options:

a. Rectal haematoma
b. Carcinoma of rectum
c. Ischaemia colitis
d. Ulcerative colitis
e. Crohn's disease

For each presentation below, choose the SINGLE most appropriate diagnosis from the above list of options. Each option may be used once, more than once, or not at all.

1. A 50 year old patient with diarrhoea and pain in the abdomen.
2. On proctosigmoidoscopy an ulcer is found 10 cm from the rectum.
3. An elderly man with history of myocardial infarction presents with chronic, intermittent bleeding per rectum. PR examination was found to be normal.
4. A patient comes with history of fever and diarrhoea. On biopsy granuloma found.

Theme 23: Method of contraception

Options:

a. Abstinence
b. Mirena coil
c. Norethisterone
d. OCPs
e. Progesterone only pills
f. IUCD
g. Depot preparations
h. Tubal ligation
i. Vasectomy
j. Rhythm method
k. Withdrawal
l. Ovulation testing
m. Condom
n. Diaphragm

For each presentation below, choose the SINGLE most appropriate method of contraception from the above list of options. Each option may be used once, more than once, or not at all.

1. A 47 year old woman with 9 month history of amenorrhoea now comes wanting to have contraception. She says that her husband is not reliable with condoms.
2. A 26 year old lady with irregular periods of 24 to 40 day variations. She does not want children for the next two years. She comes to you saying that she wants a natural method of contraception.
3. A 37 year old lady with 2 children and a hectic life-style comes to you for contraception. She wants reliable method since she was pregnant when she was on the oral combined contraceptives last time.
4. A lady who is 26 years old has 2 kids, the youngest 6 months. Says she wants to be sterilized. She has separated from her husband and she does not want to put on weight since the oral combined contraception did before.

Theme 24: Investigation in fever

Options:

a. Thick and thin blood films
b. USG abdomen
c. Lumbar puncture
d. Lyme serology
e. Brucellosis
f. CXR
g. ECG
h. ABG

For each presentation below, choose the SINGLE most appropriate investigation from the above list of options. Each option may be used once, more than once, or not at all.

1. A patient returned from Zambia, now has fever with rigors and seizures.
2. A young girl presents with fever, rash and neck stiffness.
3. An 18 year old boy has come back from Mexico after working in a farm there and now has fever with splenomegaly.
4. A girl went out in the forest for a walk. She had a tick bite and has fever at the moment.

Theme 25: Management in post-operative condition

Options:

a. Catecholamine
b. Dopamine
c. Laparotomy
d. Antibiotics
e. Wide excision of affected tissue
f. Percutaneous drainage
g. Insert stent
h. Excision of the dead tissue
i. Flucloxacillin
j. Ventilatory support

For each presentation below, choose the SINGLE most appropriate management from the above list of options. Each option may be used once, more than once, or not at all.

1. A middle aged woman had operation on the perforated. She has been unwell since the operation. She has difficulties in breathing. Despite of the full support from the high independent unit, her PaO_2 is 6.
2. Patient post acute pancreatic attack has on CT scan non-enhancement behind the tail of pancreas.
3. A girl, post chicken pox gets blue discoloration of skin after scratching, it is spreading at the moment .

Theme 26: Nature of anaemia

Options:

a. Folate deficiency
b. B_{12} deficiency
c. Iron deficiency anaemia
d. Sickle cell anaemia
e. Beta-thalassaemia trait
f. G6PD deficiency
g. Hereditary spherocytosis

For each presentation below, choose the SINGLE most appropriate diagnosis from the above list of options. Each option may be used once, more than once, or not at all.

1. A boy has haemoglobin of 8 gm/dL, unconjugated bilirubin as 120. Mother says that anaemia is hereditary in the family.
2. A Greek boy brought by mother says that he looks pale inspite of being normal.
3. A patient presents with severe menorrhagia and tiredness.
4. A four year old boy has been having a funny dietary pattern. He likes cheese and drinks 2 litres of milk a day. He looks pale but is otherwise normal.

Theme 27: Dysphagia: Diagnosis

Options:

a. Achalasia
b. Pill Stricture
c. Barrett's oesophagus
d. Ca oesophagus
e. Post cricoid cancer
f. Pharyngeal pouch
g. GORD
h. Systemic sclerosis
i. Pseudobulbar palsy
j. Myasthenia gravis

For each presentation below, choose the SINGLE most appropriate diagnosis from the above list of options. Each option may be used once, more than once, or not at all.

1. A 34 year old plump woman has difficulty in swallowing food, particularly after drinking alcohol and in the night.
2. A young lady complains of slurring of speech when speaking. At times food begins to fall from her mouth.
3. A 45 year old man has difficulties in swallowing the food to start with, but the rest of the swallow is normal. He does not have regurgitation and has lost weight in the past 4 months.
4. A 55 year old man has difficult in swallowing, and there is lump in his throat while swallowing.
5. A patient is having difficulty in swallowing. He presents with weight loss and substernal cramps.

Theme 28: Investigation in cervical pathology

Options:

a. Cervical smear
b. Cervical biopsy
c. Colposcopy
d. Do nothing

For each presentation below, choose the SINGLE most appropriate investigation from the above list of options. Each option may be used once, more than once, or not at all.

1. A young patient gets post coital bleeding. Speculum examination shows cervical ectropion.
2. A patient attends clinic because of CIN 1.
3. A patient attends clinic because of CIN2.

Theme 29: Respiratory disease: Diagnosis

Options:

a. Pneumonia
b. Pulmonary embolism
c. Pulmonary oedema
d. Rupture of oesophagus
e. MI
f. Pneumothorax

For each presentation below, choose the SINGLE most appropriate diagnosis from the above list of options. Each option may be used once, more than once, or not at all.

1. A patient presents with fever, basal consolidation. The ECG was found to be normal.
2. A patient presents with surgical emphysema .
3. A patient with breathlessness and absent markings on chest X-ray.
4. A patient presents with severe pain in the chest. ECG shows Q waves in lead V3.
5. A patient presents with severe pain in the chest. ECG shows Q waves in V1 to V3.

Theme 30: Diagnosis of chest pain

Options:

a. Occupational asthma
b. Pneumothorax
c. Aortic dissection
d. Interstitial oedema
e. Pulmonary embolism
f. Herpes zoster
g. GORD
h. Carcinoma lung
i. MI

For each presentation below, choose the SINGLE most appropriate diagnosis from the above list of options. Each option may be used once, more than once, or not at all.

1. A carpenter has chronic breathlessness. He does not smoke. He becomes normal when he goes away for holidays.
2. A woman has cough. On examination she has crepts on her lung base.
3. A 50 year old patient comes with severe pain in chest. He now has breathlessness. ECG shows gallop rhythm. CXR shows absent vascular markings in right apical region.
4. A 50 year old man had severe chest pain under the sternum. He later had hemiparesis.

Theme 31: Investigation of asthma in children

Options:

a. Peak flow diary
b. Spirometry
c. Exercise test
d. No investigation needed
e. CXR
f. FBC
g. Patch test

For each presentation below, choose the SINGLE most appropriate investigation from the above list of options. Each option may be used once, more than once, or not at all.

1. A young girl has 2 episodes of breathlessness so far and she is on short acting bronchodilator therapy. Now she is fine. Mother had eczema.
2. A boy comes with sudden breathlessness and has trachea deviated to the left.
3. A girl in the A&E. She is too breathless to have her peak flow checked.
4. A boy has asthma and he is given some short acting dilator inhaler. His parents don't know when he should use it.

Theme 32: Anatomy of renal failure

Options:

a. Bladder
b. Prostate
c. Papilla
d. Medullary
e. Interstitium
f. Ureter
g. Renal artery
h. Cortex

For each presentation below, choose the SINGLE most appropriate aetiology from the above list of options. Each option may be used once, more than once, or not at all.

1. A woman has not passed her urine for many hours now. On examination there is a mass palpable suprapubically.
2. An old man has difficulty in passing urine and dripping for long time.
3. A woman with sickle cell disease has not passed urine for many hours.
4. A woman has proteinuria and oedema.
5. A patient presents with hypertension and a small kidney on one side.

Theme 33: Investigation of haematuria

Options:

a. Ultrasound
b. Microscopy and sedimentation
c. ASO titre
d. Creatinine
e. IVU
f. Urine osmolarity

For each presentation below, choose the SINGLE most appropriate investigation from the above list of options. Each option may be used once, more than once, or not at all.

1. A man came with haematuria. He says this runs in the family.
2. A boy has fever, oliguria and oedema.
3. A 56 year old woman had operation on her uterine cancer years ago. She now comes with haematuria.
4. A man has been unwell for long time. He now comes with hypertension and haematuria.

Theme 34: Diagnosis of haematuria

Options:

a. Bladder cancer
b. HSP
c. SLE
d. Polycystic kidney

For each presentation below, choose the SINGLE most appropriate diagnosis from the above list of options. Each option may be used once, more than once, or not at all.

1. A chronic smoker presents with painless haematuria.
2. A 40 year old woman has haematuria. She has got non-blanching purpura on her legs and back.
3. A man with haematuria. His father also had haematuria.

Theme 35: Management of cardiac patients

Options:

a. Nitrates
b. Beta blockers
c. ACE inhibitors
d. Surgical intervention
e. Valve replacement

For each presentation below, choose the SINGLE most appropriate management from the above list of options. Each option may be used once, more than once, or not at all.

1. A patient has angina and he is on nitrates. He is having pains once a week although he has been taking his medication.
2. An old woman has pains in her chest. Angiography shows 3 severe atherosclerotic lesions.
3. A 65 year old woman has ejection systolic murmur and heaving undisplaced apex beat. She complains of breathlessness.

Theme 36: Diagnostic test for breast lump

Options:

a. FNAC
•b. Ultrasound
c. Mammography
d. CT scan of the spine
e. X-ray of the spine
f. Ductography
g. Excision biopsy
h. CXR
i. FBC
j. CA 13.5

For each presentation below, choose the SINGLE most appropriate investigation from the above list of options. Each option may be used once, more than once, or not at all.

1. A young, 24 year old woman presents with a breast lump. She has other lumps in the outer quarter of her breast.
2. A young woman presents with a breast lump that varies in size according to her menses.
3. A 56 year old woman has blood stained nipple discharge. The discharge is from a solitary duct. Ultrasound and mammography are normal.
4. A 48 year old woman presents has a breast lump in the upper outer quarter of her breast. Mammography showed a solid lump.
5. An old woman had breast cancer which was operated a few years ago. Now she has numbness on her chest.

Theme 37: Diagnosis of gastroenterology findings

Options:

a. Campylobacter diarrhoea
b. Gastroenteritis
c. UTI
d. Carcinoma colon
e. Acute appendicitis
f. Salmonella infection

For each presentation below, choose the SINGLE most appropriate diagnosis from the above list of options. Each option may be used once, more than once, or not at all.

1. A young boy has fever, nausea and vomiting for 24 hours.
2. A pregnant teacher has diarrhoea and vomiting. All her children have had same symptoms.
3. A young boy has bloody diarrhoea and vomiting for one day.

Theme 38: Pre-operative investigations

Options:

a. ECG
b. CXR
c. FBC
d. Blood glucose
e. Angiography
f. CT
g. LFTs
h. U&E
i. 24 hour ambulatory BP measurements

For each presentation below, choose the SINGLE most appropriate pre-operative investigation from the above list of options. Each option may be used once, more than once, or not at all.

1. An old patient is due for his prostatectomy. He complains of palpitations.
2. A woman due for her operation. She is menorrhagic and tired.

Theme 39: Investigation after bites and stings

Options:

a. Thick and thin blood films
b. Lymes disease serology
c. Leptospirosis serology
d. Hepatitis A serology
e. Hepatitis B serology
f. Skin swab test
g. Skin prick test

For each presentation below, choose the SINGLE most appropriate investigation from the above list of options. Each option may be used once, more than once, or not at all.

1. A 28 year old policeman is brought to A&E after being bitten by a drug addict while catching a thief. There is a deep wound at his right hand.

2. A 16 year old girl after forest walking, had to remove an insect form her leg. She now presents with a red raised ulcer.

3. A 52 year old businessman presents with fever and rigors after coming back from 10 days' long meeting at Zambia.

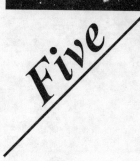

Five

January 2003 Answers

Theme 1: Causes of shock

1. **(d)** Anaphylaxis
2. **(c)** Hypovolaemic shock
3. **(b)** Cardiogenic shock
4. **(a)** Gram negative septicaemic shock

Theme 2: Management of epistaxis

1. **(f)** Vitamin K
2. **(d)** Pinching the nose
3. **(b)** Posterior nasal packing
4. **(e)** Reassurance

Theme 3: Fractures of wrist joint

1. **(d)** Isotope scan
2. **(b)** Refer to orthopaedician immediately
3. **(a)** X-ray of the wrist: Scaphoid view
4. **(b)** Refer to orthopaedician immediately

Theme 4: Relation to obesity

1. **(a)** Obstructive sleep apnoea
2. **(c)** Type II DM
3. **(d)** Alcohol
4. **(e)** Cushing's disease

Theme 5: Delayed milestones: Diagnosis

1. **(f)** Duchenne's muscular dystrophy
2. **(a)** Fragile X syndrome
3. **(d)** Hypothyroidism
4. **(e)** Prematurity
5. **(c)** Bacterial meningitis

Theme 6: Psychiatric management

1. **(h)** Rebreathe in air bag
2. **(a)** Methadone
3. **(d)** Acamprosate
4. **(b)** Propranolol
5. **(b)** Propranolol
6. **(c)** Diazepam

Theme 7: Diagnosis of psychiatric disorders

1. **(l)** Flight of ideas
2. **(b)** Postnatal psychosis
3. **(h)** Paranoid delusion
4. **(c)** Thought broadcasting
5. **(a)** Post-traumatic stress disorder
6. **(j)** Insight

Theme 8: Diagnosis of vomiting in pregnancy

1. **(a)** Hyperemesis gravidarum
2. **(b)** Hydatiform mole
3. **(g)** Migraine
4. **(c)** Cholecystitis

Theme 9: Nerve injury

1. **(a)** Axillary nerve
2. **(e)** Common peroneal nerve
3. **(d)** Ulnar nerve
4. **(c)** Radial nerve
5. **(f)** Sciatic nerve

Theme 10: Pain relief

Options:

1. **(b)** Radiotherapy
2. **(h)** Physiotherapy
3. **(e)** Oral NSAIDs
4. **(d)** IM diamorphine
5. **(e)** Oral NSAIDs

Theme 11: Mechanism of abortion

1. **(a)** Immunological
2. **(b)** Genetic
3. **(d)** Endocrine

Theme 12: Investigation of leg ulcers

1. **(d)** Arteriography
2. **(a)** Pyoderma gangrenosum
3. **(c)** Venous stasis
4. **(e)** Melanoma biopsy

Theme 13: Head pathology: Diagnosis

1. **(b)** Brainstem injury
2. **(e)** Acute SDH
3'. **(d)** Subdural haematoma
4. **(f)** Vertebrobasilar ischaemia

5. **(i)** Subarachnoid haemorrhage
6. **(h)** Depressed fracture of skull
7. **(c)** Extradural haematoma

Theme 14: Diagnostic tests: Loss of vision

1. **(d)** Doppler carotid artery
2. **(b)** MRI pituitary
3. **(a)** MRI temporal lobe
4. **(e)** ESR

Theme 15: Management of injuries

1. **(b)** Refer to surgeon
2. **(c)** Admit and observe
3. **(b)** Refer to surgeon
4. **(e)** IV fluids: 2 litres in 30 min
5. **(a)** Laparotomy

Theme 16: Management/Investigation of seizures

1. **(e)** EEG
2. **(f)** ECG
3. **(b)** Reassurance
4. **(f)** ECG
5. **(e)** EEG
6. **(e)** EEG
7. **(f)** ECG
8. **(g)** IV glucose

Theme 17: Haematemesis: Diagnosis

1. **(a)** Mallory–Weiss tear
2. **(a)** Mallory–Weiss tear
3. **(c)** Gastric erosion
4. **(d)** Peptic ulcer

Theme 18: Investigation in drug side effects

1. **(a)** Drug serum levels
2. **(b)** Thyroid function tests
3. **(a)** Drug serum levels

4. **(d)** Serum prolactin levels

5. **(e)** Urea and electrolytes

Theme 19: Hearing problem

1. **(a)** Ototoxicity
2. **(c)** Salicylate levels
3. **(d)** Fracture petrous temporal bone
4. **(e)** Wax in ears
5. **(f)** Acoustic neuroma

Theme 20: How would you help this lady

1. **(d)** Review the dose of anti hypertensive
2. **(e)** Review the dose of anti diabetic
3. **(c)** Vision testing

Theme 21: Diagnosis of anal conditions

1. **(c)** Proctalgia fugax
2. **(h)** Anal fissure
3. **(i)** Haemorrhoids
4. **(f)** Crohn's disease
5. **(d)** Carcinoma of rectum

Theme 22: Diagnosis of rectal condition

1. **(e)** Crohn's disease
2. **(b)** Carcinoma of rectum
3. **(a)** Angiodysplasia
4. **(e)** Crohn's disease

Theme 23: Method of contraception

1. **(b)** Mirena coil
2. **(k)** Withdrawal
3. **(f)** IUCD
4. **(h)** Tubal ligation

Theme 24: Investigation in fever

1. **(a)** Thick and thin blood films
2. **(c)** Lumbar puncture

3. **(e)** Brucellosis

4. **(d)** Lyme serology

Theme 25: Management in post-operative condition

1. **(j)** Ventilatory support
2. **(h)** Excision of the dead tissue
3. **(i)** Flucloxacillin

Theme 26: Nature of anaemia

1. **(g)** Hereditary spherocytosis
2. **(d)** Sickle cell anaemia
3. **(c)** Iron deficiency anaemia
4. **(c)** Iron deficiency anaemia

Theme 27: Dysphagia: Diagnosis

1. **(g)** GORD
2. **(j)** Myasthenia gravis
3. **(e)** Post cricoid cancer
4. **(f)** Pharyngeal pouch
5. **(a)** Achalasia

Theme 28: Investigation in cervical pathology

1. **(d)** Do nothing
2. **(b)** Cervical biopsy
3. **(c)** Colposcopy

Theme 29: Respiratory disease: Diagnosis

1. **(a)** Pneumonia
2. **(d)** Rupture of oesophagus
3. **(f)** Pneumothorax
4. **(e)** MI
5. **(e)** MI

Theme 30: Diagnosis of chest pain

1. **(a)** Occupational asthma
2. **(d)** Interstitial oedema
3. **(e)** Pulmonary embolism

4. **(c)** Aortic dissection

Theme 31: Investigation of asthma in children

1. **(a)** Peak flow diary
2. **(d)** No investigation needed
3. **(d)** No investigation needed
4. **(c)** Exercise test

Theme 32: Anatomy of renal failure

1. **(a)** Bladder
2. **(b)** Prostate
3. **(c)** Papilla
4. **(e)** Interstitium
4. **(g)** Renal artery

Theme 33: Investigation of haematuria

1. **(a)** Ultrasound
2. **(c)** ASO titre
3. **(e)** IVU
4. **(a)** Ultrasound

Theme 34: Diagnosis of haematuria

1. **(a)** Bladder cancer
2. **(b)** HSP
3. **(d)** Polycystic kidney

Theme 35: Management of cardiac patients

1. **(d)** Surgical intervention
2. **(d)** Surgical intervention
3. **(e)** Valve replacement

Theme 36: Diagnostic test for breast lump

1. **(c)** Mammography
2. **(b)** Ultrasound
3. **(f)** Ductography
4. **(a)** FNAC
4. **(d)** CT scan of the spine

Theme 37: Diagnosis of gastroenterology findings

1. **(c)** UTI
2. **(b)** Gastroenteritis
3. **(a)** Campylobacter diarrhoea

Theme 38: Pre-operative investigations

1. **(a)** ECG
2. **(c)** FBC

Theme 39: Investigation after bites and stings

1. **(f)** Skin swab test
2. **(b)** Lyme disease serology
3. **(a)** Thick and thin blood films

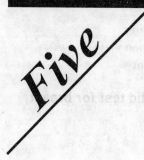

Theme 1: Causes of shock

1. Anaphylactic shock is an IgE mediated hypersensitivity reaction. Release of histamine and other agents causes cyanosis, urticaria, capillary leak, wheeze and oedema of larynx, lids, tongue and lips as in this case. Treatment, after securing the airway, is by giving IM adrenaline 0.5 mg i.e. 0.5 ml of 1:1000.

2. Hypovolaemic shock can be due to bleeding, fluid loss or heat exhaustion. In this case bleeding is the cause of shock as there is a fracture of pelvis and femur. There may not be any obvious bleeding in a simple fracture of femur but bleeding into the thigh of > 1 litre in adults is invariable.

3. Cardiogenic shock is primarily due to failure of the heart to maintain circulation. MI is one of the causes of cardiogenic shock. Other causes include arrhythmias, cardiac tamponade, tension pneumothorax, myocarditis, valve destruction, pulmonary embolism and aortic dissection.

4. Septicaemia commonly relates to colonisation and translocation in the GIT. It is often seen after anastomotic breakdown. Gram negative bacilli are mainly responsible but staphylococcus aureus and fungi may be involved.

Theme 2: Management of epistaxis

1. Warfarin inhibits the reductase enzyme responsible for regenerating the active form of vitamin K, thus producing a state analogous to vitamin K deficiency. In this case as the INR is 0.9 which is infact on the lower side of the normal range (0.9–1.2), giving only vitamin K in this case would suffice.

2. First aid in case of epistaxis is to sit up, head tilted downwards to prevent blood trickling backwards and firm pressure on the cartilagenous part of the nose (not the bridge) for 10–15 min. Then assess the patient for shock and treat the cause.

3. The fact that his circulatory system has been stabilized implies that his blood pressure has been brought under control. Now because, he continues to bleed despite an anterior nasal packing, suggests complicated epistaxis i.e., posterior epistaxis. The gold standard in such patients is to visualise the bleeding point with endoscopy and then directly treat with bipolar cautery. In case a bleeding site cannot be found, posterior nasal packing should be done.

4. As the bleeding has stopped in this patient, nothing needs to be done; simply reassurance will do. But before the girl is discharged, one should rule out all avoidable causes of epistaxis and advise accordingly.

Theme 3: Fractures of wrist joint

1. The presentation of trauma and site of pain are very suggestive of a fracture. The X-rays taken are normal. We can easily presume that the scaphoid view has also been taken therefore the only certain way to reach the diagnosis now is isotope scan.

2. A fall on the palm of the outstreched and dorsiflexed hand may dislocate the whole carpus backwards in relation to the radius and lunate. This is a perilunate dislocation of the wrist. Clinically the patient will have stiff wrist and finger with swollen and tender wrist. If the lunate has dislocated it may compress the median nerve. Isolated dislocation of the lunate can usually be treated by closed reduction. If this fails, open reduction is mandatory. Avascular necrosis of the lunate (Kienbock's disease) may occur after this injury. Trans-scaphoid perilunate dislocation should be treated by open reduction and internal fixation.

3. The language of the question suggests that although an X-ray has been taken, scaphoid view radiograph has not yet been taken. As the site of tenderness is in the anatomical snuff box it is very suggestive of scaphoid fracture. Therefore a scaphoid view radiograph is required here.

4. In fractures of the radial head, the elbow is tender and swollen. Undisplaced fractures can be treated in a collar and cuff sling but if the fracture is displaced, internal fixation or excision of the radial head may be needed. Radial nerve palsy, though is a rarity but a serious complication in such cases. The patient needs to be referred to an orthopaedician.

Theme 4: Relation to obesity

1. Weight reduction is the first step in the management of obstructive sleep apnoea syndrome which is characterized by intermittent closure or collapse of the pharyngeal airway which causes apnoeic episodes during sleep. The typical patient is a fat, middle aged man with complaints of snoring, daytime somnolence, morning headache or poor sleep quality.

2. Type II DM or NIDDM is seen in older age group patients especially who are obese. Obesity probably causes insulin resistance by the associated increased rate of release of non esterified fatty acids causing post receptor defects in insulin's action. The first step in the management of NIDDM is weight loss and exercise.

3. Weight loss and vitamin B deficiency are well known facts which occur due to alcoholism. Alcoholism can cause fatty liver, hepatitis, cirrhosis, Korsakoff's psychosis $\pm$ Wernicke's encephalopathy. Alcohol withdrawal with the help of benzodiazepines and multiple high potency vitamins given IM may reverse the effects caused due to alcoholism.

4. Cushing's disease is treated by selective removal of pituitary adenoma via a trans-sphenoidal or very rarely transfrontal approach. Cushing's disease is due to adrenal hyperplasia due to excess ACTH from pituitary tumour. 90% of pituitary causes are microadenomas. Cushing's disease is commoner in women with a peak age incidence at 30–50 years.

Theme 5: Delayed milestones: Diagnosis

1. Duchenne's muscular dystrophy presents in boys of 1–6 years of age with waddling gait. Selective wasting causes calf pseudohypertrophy. Scoliosis and chest infections occur later. Creative kinase is increased. IQ levels are not affected. Aim is to keep the boy walking with knee–ankle–foot orthoses. Spinal fixation with Luque operation or bracing helps in scoliosis.

2. Fragile X syndrome is also known as Martin-Bell syndrome. This is the most common form of inherited cognitive impairment. Patient may present with large testes, high forehead, a big jaw, facial asymmetry, long ears and a short temper.

3. Hypothyroidism in paediatric age group can be:
   i. Congenital-thyroid dysgenesis, dyshormonogenesis, maternal antithyroid drugs.
   ii. Acquired–Prematurity, Hashimoto's thyroiditis, Down syndrome, hypopituitarism. Patient may present with neonatal jaundice, widely opened posterior fontanelle, dry skin, inactivity, excessive sleeping, little crying, constipation, delayed growth and mental retardation, protuding tongue, hypotonia and short stature.

4. A neonate whole calculated gestational age from the last menstrual period is less than 37 weeks is considered to be premature or preterm. Smoking, tobacco, poverty, malnutrition, history of prematurity, genitourinary infections, pre eclampsia, multiple pregnancy, polyhydramnios, placenta praevia, abruption, uterine malformations, all are risk factors for prematurity. Such neonates are usually small in size with a relatively large head, large fontanelle, small face, abundant lanugo, absent breast nodule, testes not yet descended into the scrotal sac. Neonatal reflexes such as Moro, sucking and swallowing are sluggish. There is hypotonia and head lag persisting for longer age limits. Such infants are also susceptible to various infections.

5. The presentation of delayed milestones after a fever is suggestive of an acquired cause. Out of the options given above, bacterial meningitis is the only suitable answer. Complications due to meningitis in children include disseminated sepsis, subdural effusion, hydrocephalus, ataxia, paralysis, deafness, mental retardation, epilepsy and brain abscess.

Theme 6: Psychiatric management

1. This is a case of hypocalcaemia due to hyperventilation. Such patient will present with perioral paraesthesiae, carpopedal spasm (especially if brachial artery is occluded), neuromuscular excitability, depression or tetany. As the aetiology in this case is hyperventilation, rebreathing in an airbag would relieve the symptoms and normalize the calcium levels.

2. Patient on narcotic withdrawal will present with 'cold turkey'– dilated pupils, diarrhoea, vomiting, tachycardia, sweating, cramps and piloerection. Opiate withdrawal can be eased with methadone given as 20–70 mg/12 hourly PO reducing by 20% every 2 days. Methadone is a long acting opioid that possesses almost all physiological properties of Heroin.

3. Acamprosate is used in the treatment of alcohol withdrawal. It decreases craving in alcoholics and can treble abstinence rates. It is contraindicated in pregnancy and liver failure. It can cause diarrhoea, vomiting and libido dysfunction.

4. Panic attack or disorder is a type of anxiety. Patient will complaint of tension, feelings of impending doom, trembling, sense of collapse, insomnia, poor concentration, goose flesh, hyperventilation, sweating, headaches, palpitations and poor appetite. Treatment is with cognitive behavioural therapy and with anxiolytics e.g. propranolol, benzodiazepines.

5. As explained above.

6. This is a case of acute stress reaction. It is the immediate normal emotional response to a major stress. The symptoms are anxiety, depression, irritability, poor sleep, difficulty in concentration, restlessness, palpitations and tremors. Usually they resolve spontaneously within a few days. If the reaction is severe, as in this case, an anxiolytic or hypnotic drug could be prescribed for 2–3 days.

Theme 7: Diagnosis of psychiatric disorders

1. Flight of ideas is seen in patients with mania. Other features that may be present in patients with mania are grandiose delusions, increased need for sleep, increased sexual desire, spending sprees, euphoria, hyperactivity, increased appetite and disinhibition. Less severe states are termed hypomania. Sedation with chlorpromazine may be needed. Lithium carbonate has a prophylactic effect in prevention of recurrent mania.

2. The risk of developing postnatal depression or psychosis is three times increased in those with no recent pregnancy. If mild, they are termed postnatal 'blues'. Most postnatal depression resolves within 6 months. Treatment options include fluoxetine, cognitive–behavioural counselling, adding lithium, ECT and even transdermal oestrogen patches.

3. This is a case of paranoid delusion. Delusions are beliefs that are held unshakably, irrespective of counter argument and which are unexpected, considering the patients' cultural background. Delusions are often secondary. Primary delusions arrive fully formed and with no antecedent events or experiences to account for it.

4. Thought broadcasting, as in this case, is a 1st rank symptom in schizophrenia. Other 1st rank symptoms in schizophrenia include thought insertion, thought withdrawal, passivity, hearing voices commenting on actions, primary delusions and somatic hallucinations.

5. Post traumatic stress disorder is an intense, prolonged and sometimes delayed reaction to a stressful event. Patient may present with anxiety, depression, obsessive recall, alcohol abuse, irritability, bed wetting, detachment, diminished interest and inability to feel normal emotions.

6. The fact that the patient knows that he is suffering from a psychiatric problem and that he needs treatment for it implies that the person has insight.

Theme 8: Diagnosis of vomiting in pregnancy

1. Hyperemesis gravidarum is seen mostly in young patients, non smokers, primiparas, with molar or multiple pregnancies, with patients working outside home. Patient may present with weight loss, dehydration, hypovolaemia, electrolyte disturbance, polyneuritis, liver and renal failure. Patient should be admitted and given antiemetics. Patient may require enteral feeding, IV thiamine and parenteral nutrition.

2. Hydatiform mole is a gestational disease in which the fertilized ovum forms abnormal trophoblast tissue but not fetus. The tumour consists of proliferative chorionic villi which have swollen up and degenerated. It produces HCG in large quantities which gives rise to exaggerated pregnancy symptoms e.g. hyperemesis or first trimester pre-eclampsia. Uterus is large for dates and feels doughy with no fetal heart sounds. USG shows 'snow-storm' in the uterus and no fetus.

3. Migraine classically presents with visual or other aura lasting around 15 min followed within an hour by unilateral, throbbing headache. Some patients may have nausea, vomiting and sometimes photophobia or phonophobia but no aura ('common migraine'). Around 20% of pregnant women will experience migraine. Obstetric complications are not increased in migraine sufferers. Pregnant women having migraine attacks should be treated with analgesics, anti-emetics and where possible by avoiding triggering factors.

4. Pregnancy exacerbates gall stone formation due to biliary stasis and increased cholesterol in bile. Symptoms of subcostal pain, nausea and vomiting are similar to the non-pregnant state. USG confirms the diagnosis. 90% of the cases resolve conservatively. Laparoscopic cholecystectomy may be required in some patients.

Theme 9: Nerve injury

1. Injury to the shoulder and a region of anaesthesia over the lower part of shoulder or deltoid area is suggestive of an anterior shoulder dislocation with injury to the axillary nerve. (Cutaneous branch of the axillary nerve supplies the upper lateral part of the arm).

2. Lateral popliteal nerve is also known as common peroneal nerve (L4–S2). A lesion or injury to the nerve causes equinovarus with inability to dorsiflex the foot and toes–'foot drop'. Sensory loss is seen over the dorsum of the foot.

3. Ulnar nerve can be damaged in association with a medial epicondyle fracture. Ulnar nerve (C8–T1) is the nerve of finger abduction and adduction. There is sensory loss over the little finger and variable area of ring finger.

4. Fracture of the shaft of the humerus is often caused by a fall on an outstreched hand. Radial nerve is the nerve of extension of the elbow, wrist and fingers. Its injury can cause wrist drop.

5. Sciatic nerve (L4–S2) supplies the hamstring muscles, hip abductors and all muscles below the knee. Injury to the nerve may cause severe lower leg and hamstring weakness, flail foot and severe disability and loss of sensation below the knee laterally.

Theme 10: Pain relief

1. The symptomatic treatment for carcinoma prostate includes analgesia and treating associated hypercalcaemia. Radiotherapy is given for bone metastases or spinal cord compression which would otherwise cause severe pain to the patient.

2. Although the initial medication for pain due to swollen arm in a patient with lung carcinoma would be palliation with NSAIDs; opioid analgesia will be required if NSAIDs fail. If the drug therapy fails then physiotherapy is the next step in protocol.

3. The condition of the patient is suggestive of rheumatoid arthritis involving the larger joints. The treatment at such an advanced stage would require oral drugs for pain relief. NSAIDs are the drugs of 1st choice in this condition.

4. Pain not relieved by NSAIDs needs to be treated with opiates. As in the options the opiate mentioned is IM diamorphine, it becomes the obvious answer.

5. The patient is on frusemide which suggests gout as the diagnosis for this patient. The drug of choice in pain alleviation for such patient is NSAIDs.

Theme 11: Mechanism of abortion

1. There are multiple causes of miscarriages. These include chromosomal abnormalities, endocrine disorders, abnormalities of the uterus, infections, chemical agents, psychological disorders and immunological disorders. Antiphospholipid syndrome is an immunological disorder with antiphospholipid antibodies (Lupus anticoagulant, anticardiolipin antibodies) with past arterial thrombosis, venous thrombosis or recurrent pregnancy loss.

2. This is a case of consanguinity. It is one of the indications for genetic counselling. In autosomal recessive diseases such as infantile polycystic kidney disease, Huntington's chorea, etc. both parents must be carriers for the offspring to be affected. In such cases consanguinity (marrying relatives) increases the risk.

3. There are multiple causes of miscarriages. These include chromosomal abnormalities, endocrine disorders, abnormalities of the uterus, infections, chemical agents, psychological disorders, immunological disorders. Various endocrine disorders which may cause miscarriages include diabetes, hypothyroidism, luteal phase deficiency and polycystic ovarian syndrome. This case looks like a case of polycystic ovarian syndrome which is characterized by hyperandrogenism, oligo-ovulation and polycystic ovaries. Acne, male pattern baldness and hirsutism can be seen in such patients.

Theme 12: Investigation of leg ulcers

1. The condition of the patient suggests chronic ischaemia causing punched out painful ulcers. Investigation required for this patient would be ABPI and then arteriography, DSA or colour duplex imaging to assess the extent and location of stenosis and quality of distal vessels ('run off').

2. Pyoderma gangrenosum implies recurring nodulopustular ulcers around 10 cm wide, with tender red/blue overhanging edges. They are seen in patients with Crohn's disease. These ulcers heal with cribriform scars and are seen on legs, abdomen and face. Saline cleansing with high dose oral or intralesional steroids are required.

3. The site i.e. medial aspect of the ankle is a favourite place for gravitational ulcers which are mostly related to superficial venous disease. Minimal trauma to the legs can lead to ulceration which then takes months to heal.

4. The age and the presentation of the lesion requires biopsy to rule out melanoma in this patient. Malignant melanomas are caused due to excessive UV exposure. For diagnosis, the 'Glasgow 7' signs include (i) change in size (ii) change in shape (iii) change in colour (iv) diameter > 7 mm (v) inflammation (vi) oozing or bleeding from the lesion (vii) itching or odd sensation in the lesion. Excision biopsy with a margin of normal skin should be done. 1 cm of normal skin around the melanoma should be excised for every millimeter of depth of the lesion, upto a maximum of 3 cms.

Theme 13: Head Pathology: Diagnosis

1. This is a clear cut case of Brainstem injury/ herniation. The points in favour are the GCS score of 3 (suggesting coma), a raised BP of 180/100 with a fallen PR of 56/minute i.e. Cushing's response, dilated pupils and positive Babinski sign.

2. Although subdural haematomas are generally found in the elderly, this young patient is an alcoholic and we can very well presume that he has had many falls in the past. The most important point that moves the diagnosis in the favour of subdural haematoma is his fluctuating consciousness which is typically seen in this condition.

3. Again in this patient the old age factor and number of recent falls points towards the diagnosis of subdural haematoma. It is due to bleeding from bridging veins between cortex and venous sinuses. The elderly are more vulnerable due to brain shrinkage which makes bridging veins more susceptible to rupture.

4. The old lady here complains of dizziness and vertigo which would have a DD of diseases such as Ménière's disease, motion sickness, vestibular schwannoma, acute labyrinthitis, ototoxicity. The sign that clinches the diagnosis is the ipsilateral ataxia i.e. walks reeling to one side which is seen in vertebrobasilar ischaemia.

5. The condition of the patient with which she present to A & E would include a DD of migraine and SAH. But because the lady gives no history of similar attacks, no history of aura and complains of pain in the occipital region which is a very common site of pain in patients with SAH; the diagnosis becomes that of SAH which can occur spontaneously.

6. The condition of the patient in this case makes a DD of depressed fracture and extradural haematoma. As there is no mention of lucid interval the diagnosis becomes that of depressed fracture skull.

7. Although in this patient one would again like to diagnose the patient as depressed fracture skull, the GMC has given a pointer in the form of site of injury i.e. the temporal region which is the commonest site involved in extradural haemorrhage.

Theme 14: Diagnostic tests: Loss of vision

1. Causes of sudden painless loss of vision include ischaemic optic neuropathy, central retinal artery occlusion, vitreous haemorrhage, optic neuritis and central retinal vein occlusion. Carotid artery doppler helps in the diagnosis to rule out carotid artery stenosis causing such recurrent loss of vision.

2. Acromegaly presents between 30–50 years. Patients have coarse oily skin, large tongue, prominent supraorbital ridge, prognathism, increase in shoe size, thick spade like hands, deep voice, arthralgia, proximal muscle weakness, parastheisae due to carpal tunnel syndrome, progressive heart failure, goitre and sleep apnoea in some. Investigations required are oral GTT, serum IGF–1 and MRI pituitary fossa. Trans-sphenoidal surgery is the treatment of choice. Dopamine agonists can be used as adjuncts.

3. Visual loss according to the site involved in the visual pathway
   i. Ipsilateral complete loss of vision– Optic nerve atrophy.
   ii. Bitemporal hemianopia– central chiasma– Pituitary tumour.
   iii. Binasal hemianopia– Lateral chiasma.
   iv. Contralateral superior quadrantanopia– Temporal lobe.
   v. Contralateral inferior quadrantanopia– Parietal lobe.
   vi. Homonymous hemianopia–Optic tract or radiation, visual cortex or anterior occipital lobe involvement.

4. Giant cell arteritis, also known as temporal arteritis can present with malaise, jaw claudication with tender scalp or temporal arteries in which pulses may be absent. The unaffected eye is also at risk if prompt treatment is not started. ESR more than 40 is very suggestive of the diseases. Oral prednisolone 80 mg/day is started promptly.

Theme 15: Management of injuries

1. In this patient the diagnosis is very clear— Trauma to the spleen. The vitals of the boy remain stable and moreover there is a haematoma and that too a small one. Therefore it becomes a surgeons' prerogative to decide whether there is a need for laparotomy or not. Therefore refer the patient to a surgeon.

2. In this patient we do not know about the extent of intra-abdominal injury. So the patient needs to be admitted, observed and needs to undergo investigations to rule out any rupture of GI tract, spleen or pancreatic trauma.

3. The patient in this condition would have required a laparotomy but his stable vitals are a clue given by the GMC to refer the patient to a surgeon who can then do an elective laparotomy.

4. The presentation of the patient with pain in left side of abdomen, 2 right sided fractured ribs and patient in shock after trauma, suggests splenic rupture. Before laparotomy is undertaken, the shock needs to be rectified and hence, IV fluids become the management of choice.

5. The condition of the patient here suggests an internal haemorrhage in the abdomen with shock. Despite all efforts the shock has not been controlled as his BP is still low, the patient require urgent laparotomy for definitive treatment.

Theme 16: Management/Investigation of seizures

1. For a patient who presents with 1st seizure, a protocol needs to be followed for diagnosis and proper treatment. History, basic investigations such as U & E, LFT, Blood sugar, Electrolytes and Imaging (CT/MRI Brain) are required in that order before an EEG is undertaken.

2. The presentation of the girl looks like a vasovagal syncope. Therefore an ECG should be done in this case.

3. Breathholding spells generally occur between the ages 6 months and 5 years. They occur mostly during crying when the breath is held in expiration and the child becomes cyanosed and limp. The only measures required, are, to avoid the precipitating factors resulting in breathholding spells. An attack can also be aborted by a strong physical stimulus like a pinch applied at the onset of the spell.

4. A loud murmur on inspiration suggests a right heart murmur (left heart murmurs are accentuated in expiration). Though the most appropriate investigation would have been an Echocardiogram, it is not in the options. Therefore ECG becomes the next most appropriate option.

5. The presentation sounds like that of a partial secondary generalized seizure with evidence of focal origin starting from the thumb and then moving to the whole body. Therefore an EEG would be the most appropriate investigation.

6. GMC has given a lot of clues in the question to diagnose this as an absence or petitmal seizure. The patient, suddenly stops talking in mid sentence and then carries on where left off. It is seen in childhood. The investigation required is an EEG.

7. As the nature of the attack is not clear, one cannot be very sure but his bradycardia does warrant an ECG to look for any cardiovascular cause for the seizure.

8. Seizure can be due to various reasons and hypoglycaemia and hyperglycaemia are two important causes. As the boy is a diabetic with hypoglycaemia (his blood glucose is 2 mmol/L), he would require IV glucose to treat the condition.

Theme 17: Haematemesis: Diagnosis

1. The mention of severe vomiting pushes the diagnosis towards Mallory—Weiss tear. In such cases vomiting causes haematemesis via an oesophageal tear.
2. As explained above.
3. The treatment of rheumatoid arthritis includes NSAIDs which on prolonged use can cause gastric erosion and vomiting. The presentation here of vomiting with streaks of blood is sufficient enough to clinch the diagnosis.
4. The age, the job and the site of pain all support the diagnosis of an Acid Peptic disease. The mention of tarry stools provides the clue that the blood is coming in contact with hydrochloric acid and therefore the diagnosis is peptic ulcer.

Theme 18: Investigation in drug side effects

1. Features of hyperthyroidism are seen in case of lithium toxicity. Therefore, in this case one needs to check the serum drug levels.
2. As compared to the above case scenario, the patient in this case is showing features suggestive of hypothyroidism. It is seen if the patient is on long term lithium medication. Hence, in this condition we need to do the thyroid function tests which should be checked every 6 months after starting treatment with Lithium.
3. Plasma level of phenytoin needs to be monitored carefully in each patient as there is marked variation in dose requirements between individuals and the saturation kinetics of the drug which gives rise to an exponential dose-blood level relationship. The common side effects of phenytoin toxicity include ataxia, nystagmus, tremors, dystonia, gum hypertrophy and hirsutism.
4. Phenothiazines are antipsychotic drugs which are used to treat schizophrenia and mania. Their mechanism of action is by blocking the central dopamine receptors. Their side effects include impotence, extrapyramidal effects, gynaecomastia and galactorrhoea (due to increased S. prolactin levels). Therefore his S. prolactin levels need to be measured.
5. Salicylate or aspirin overdose leads to tinnitus, vertigo, vomiting, dehydration and hyperventilation. Treatment includes gastric lavage, activated charcoal, alkaline diuresis and haemodialysis in severe poisoning (plasma levels > 700 mgs/dL). Therefore, to treat the patient properly one needs the serum salicylate levels in hand along with the values of blood pH, urea and electrolytes.

Theme 19: Hearing problem

1. Gentamycin is an aminoglycoside antibiotic which is both ototoxic and nephrotoxic. Ringing of the ears in this case is suggestive of ototoxicity due to gentamycin use.

2. Tinnitus is a well known feature of toxicity of salicylate. The patient must have overdosed himself to get rid of the headache and hence he now complains of tinnitus. For proper evaluation of the patient, salicylate levels need to be checked.

3. Tinnitus can be due to hearing loss, presbyacusis, noise induced, head injury, otosclerosis, Ménière's disease, anaemia, hypertension, aspirin, loop diuretics, aminoglycosides quinine. In this patient the history clearly guides use to the cause of tinnitus as head injury (fracture petrous temporal bone).

4. The presentation of diminished hearing after a shower is almost diagnostic of wax impaction. Wax impaction is commonly seen in people with unhygienic lifestyles. Its treatment would include softening the wax with oil drops daily for a week and then syringing the ear or suction with the help of a microscope.

5. Acoustic neuromas are slow growing, benign lesions that behave as a SOL. Also known as Vestibular Schwannoma. They cause: ipsilateral tinnitus and sensorineural deafness by compressing the cochlear nerve Giddiness is common. Trigeminal nerve compression may cause facial numbness. Nearby cranial nerves may be affected especially V, VII, IX and X with ipsilateral cerebellar signs. MRI is the best investigation but CT can also clinch the diagnosis. Enlargement or erosion of the internal auditory meatus can be visualized. Surgical treatment is difficult.

Theme 20: How would you help this lady

1. Postural hypotension is a common cause of poor mobility and falls. The causes are autonomic neuropathy, drugs such as diuretics (as in this case), nitrates antidepressants. The patient typically falls after meals, on exercise or on getting off the bed (as in this case). Treatment would include stopping or reviewing the dose of the drug which is causing postural hypotension.

2. Hypoglycaemia by definition is plasma glucose < 2.5 mmol/L. It typically present as sweating, hunger, tremors, drowsiness, personality change, fits and rarely with focal symptoms. Causes of hypoglycaemia include drugs— insulin or oral hypoglycaemics (as in this patient), pituitary insufficiency, liver failure, Addison's disease, insulinoma, non-pancreatic neoplasms. In this patient one would need to review the dose of oral hypoglycaemics to prevent further such episodes.

3. Causes of falls include poor visual acuity, postural hypotension, arrhythmias, carotid bruits, parkinsonism, proximal myopathy, instability in knees. Patients with recurrent falls should get themselves investigated for these causes. The mention of 'walking into objects' is suggestive of a poor visual acuity. Hence the lady should get her vision tested.

Theme 21: Diagnosis of anal conditions

1. Proctalgia fugax is a disease characterized by attacks of severe idiopathic pain arising in the rectum. The pain is described as stabbing cramp-like. It often occurs when the patient is in bed at night. It seems to occur commonly in patients suffering from anxiety or undue stress and is also said to afflict young doctors! It is probably due to segmental cramp in the pubococcygeus muscle. It is unpleasant, incurable but fortunately harmless.

2. Anal fissure or Fissure-in-ano, is a midline longitudinal split in squamous lining of the lower anus often present with a mucosal tag at the external aspect–'the sentinel pile'. Mostly it is due to hard faeces or constipation. Defecation or PR examination is very painful, as in this patient.

3. The patient in this case is suffering from haemorrhoids. Constipation with prolonged straining is the key causative factor. As there are no sensory fibres above the dentate line, piles are not painful. Moreover because the bleeding is from the capillaries, it is bright red in colour.

4. Crohn's disease is an inflammatory GI condition characterized by transmural granulomatous inflammation. Mostly seen in the terminal ileum and proximal colon with skin lesions in between. Smoking increases the risk 3–4 folds. Patients present with abdominal pain, weight loss, diarrhoea, aphthous ulcers, abdominal tenderness, RIF mass and perianal abscesses or tags. Small intestinal obstruction or toxic dilatation can occur as complications. One must investigate by sigmoidoscopy, rectal biopsy and barium enema which may show cobble stoning, 'rose thorn' ulcers. Prednisolone is used for mild attacks. For severe attacks, patient needs to be admitted and given IV hydrocortisone $\pm$ metronidazole $\pm$ rectal hydrocortisone.

5. Rectal carcinoma is the 4th most common malignancy in women. Local spread occurs circumferentially and within 2 years complete encirclement would have taken place. Spread via the venous system occurs late. Patients present with bleeding which is the earliest and most common symptom along with a sense of incomplete defecation (tenesmus). Alteration in the bowel habit, weight loss and pain abdomen at a later stage are also seen. 90% of all neoplasms can be felt digitally. Proctosigmoidoscopy will always show the carcinoma. A histological examination will not only confirm the diagnosis but also stage it. A sphincters' saving operation (anterior resection) is usually done for tumours of upper 2/3rd of the rectum. For tumours involving the lower 1/3rd of the rectum, a permanent colostomy (abdominoperineal excision) is often required.

Theme 22: Diagnosis of rectal condition

1. Crohn's disease is an inflammatory GI condition characterized by transmural granulomatous inflammation. Mostly seen in the terminal ileum and proximal colon with skin lesions in between. Smoking increases the risk 3–4 folds. Patients present with abdominal pain, weight loss, diarrhoea, aphthous ulcers, abdominal tenderness, RIF mass and perianal abscesses or tags. Small intestinal obstruction or toxic dilatation can occur as complications. One must investigate by sigmoidoscopy, rectal biopsy and barium enema which may show cobble stoning, 'rose thorn' ulcers. Prednisolone is used for mild attacks. For severe attacks, patient needs to be admitted and given IV hydrocortisone $\pm$ metronidazole $\pm$ rectal hydrocortisone.

2. Rectal carcinoma is the 4th most common malignancy in women. Local spread occurs circumferentially and within 2 years complete encirclement would have taken place. Spread via the venous system occurs late. Patients present with bleeding which is the earliest and most common symptom alongwith a sense of incomplete defecation (tenesmus). Alteration in the bowel habit, weight loss and pain abdomen at a later stage are also seen. 90% of all neoplasms can be felt digitally. Proctosigmoidoscopy will always show the carcinoma. A histological examination will not only confirm the diagnosis but also stage it. A sphincter saving operation (anterior resection) is usually done for tumours of upper 2/3rd of the rectum. For tumours involving the lower 1/3rd of the rectum, a permanent colostomy (abdominoperineal excision) is often required.

3. Angiodysplasia is a vascular malformation which is associated with ageing. Angiodysplasias occur particularly in the ascending colon and caecum of elderly patients over 60 years of age. The malformations consist of dilated tortuous submucosal veins. Inspection of the mucosa is unremarkable. Bleeding is usually chronic and intermittent. There is an association with aortic stenosis (which can present as angina, dyspnoea, heaving apex beat). Colonoscopy may show the characteristic lesion in the caecum or ascending colon. Superior and inferior mesenteric angiography shows the site and extent of the lesion. To localize and confirm the source of haemorrhage, ^{99m}Tc labelled red cells are used.

4. As explained in first question.

Theme 23: Method of contraception

1. Mirena coil is an IUCD carrying levonorgestrel. It inhibits implantation and makes periods lighter. It lasts around 5 years. The risk of ectopic pregnancy is less. The risk of an STD also decreases. One–fifth of the patients may experience reversible amenorrhoea on its use.

2. Out of the given options, rhythm method and withdrawal are two natural methods of contraception. As in this case the lady has irregular periods, rhythm method cannot be applied therefore withdrawal is the only alternative.

3. It has been clearly mentioned in the question that the lady has a hectic life style which implies that she cannot take daily OCPs. Moreover it has been further specified that she had got pregnant the last time, she was on OCPs. That also suggests that she must have forgotten to take the pill due to her hectic lifestyle. Therefore an IUCD implantation being the next best alternative is the choice.

4. The most common method of sterilization in UK is with Filshie clips. The tubes may be ringed, clipped or diathermied or else the tubes may be divided and ligated through a mini-laparotomy incision. An IUCD should be left in place till the next period just in case an already fertilized ovum is present.

Theme 24: Investigation in fever

1. The history of travel to Africa (an endemic area for malaria) along with the presenting features of rigors and fever suggests the diagnosis of malaria. The mention of fits in the question points towards cerebral malaria which is a complication seen in plasmodium falciparum infection. Diagnosis requires serial thin and thick blood films taken at the time of fever. Thick films help in rapid detection of malarial parasites, while thin films help in identification of the plasmodium subtype. Treatment is with Quinine + Tetracycline/Doxycycline/Clindamycin.

2. The presentation of neck stiffness and fever suggests the diagnosis of meningitis. The presence of rash along with other features is suggestive of meningococcal meningitis. Lumbar puncture is critical to diagnosis. Treatment of Meningococcal meningitis is with Benzylpenicillin.

3. Brucellosis is a Zoonosis common in Middle-east and typically affects the farmers or vets. It may present as fever, sweats, malaise, anorexia, vomiting, weight loss, hepatospleno-megaly, diarrhoea, backache, rash, orchitis or myalgia. Diagnosis is by blood culture and serology. Treatment is by Doxycycline and streptomycin.

4. Lyme disease is a tick borne infection caused by Borrelia burgdorferi. The patient will invariably give a history of travel to the forest. It presents as erythema chronicum migrans, arthralgia, malaise, myocarditis, heart block, meningitis, ataxia, amnesia and neuropathy. Diagnosis is by clinical signs, symptoms and serology. Treatment is by Doxycycline. To avoid getting the disease, the limbs should be properly covered and insect repellants used.

Theme 25: Management in post-operative condition

1. Indications for ventilation include a GCS of $\leq$ 8, $PaO_2 < 9$ kPa in air, $PaCO_2 > 6$ kPa, spontaneous hyperventilation and respiratory irregularity.
2. Secondary infection of the necrotic tissue in the pancreatic bed produces an abscess 1 or 2 weeks after the initial attack in 3% of cases. Operative debridement of the area and excision of the dead pancreatic tissue offers the best chance of recovery.
3. Toxic epidermal necrolysis (Lyle's syndrome, scalded skin syndrome) is usually acute in onset and may be preceded by toxic erythema or blistering. Pressure and shearing stress on the skin tend to encourage the extension of blisters. It can be due to staphylococcal infection or due to a drug reaction. Treatment includes administration of antistaphylococcal agents, fluid and electrolyte management and local care to the denuded skin.

Theme 26: Nature of anaemia

1. Hereditary spherocytosis is an autosomal dominant disease with RBC membrane defect which makes them osmotically fragile. Patients present with splenomegaly and increased risk of gallstones. Diagnosis is by the Hb levels which are between 8–12 gm/dL and by osmotic fragility tests. Treatment is with folate replacements and in some cases with splenectomy.
2. Sickle cell anaemia results due to substitution of glutamate with valine at position 6 of beta chain of haemoglobin, leading to formation of HbS. HbS polymerizes when deoxygenated, causing RBCs to sickle. Sickle cells are fragile and haemolyse, thus leading to anaemia and jaundice. Splenomegaly may be seen in children. (After 10 years, spleen shrinks due to infarction). Other features include, painful swelling of hands and feet (hand and foot syndrome), later leg ulcers, osteomyelitis, renal failure may occur. Patients may also be simply anaemic without any other features.
Serum electrophoresis detects HbS.
Treatment includes Hydroxyurea if frequent crises (causes increased production of fetal haemoglobin) or simply blood transfusions to keep HbS level < 30%.
3. The patient here is suffering from chronic blood loss which is causing an iron deficiency anaemia. It is seen in upto 14% of menstruating women. Treatment would require treating menorrhagia and oral iron supplements in the form of ferrous sulphate. Hb should rise by 1 gm/dL/week.
4. This is another case of iron deficiency anaemia though the reason in this case is rarely seen. The child is on a dietary pattern of large amounts of milk with affects iron absorption from the GIT. Moreover milk and its products such as cheese (in this case) are poor sources of iron, adding further to the severity of iron deficiency.

Theme 27: Dysphagia: Diagnosis

1. Gastro oesophageal reflux diseases is due to dysfunction of the lower oesophageal sphincter. It is associated with smoking, alcohol, hiatus hernia, pregnancy, obesity, big meals, systemic sclerosis. Patient generally presents with heartburn, acid brash, water brash, odynophagia and nocturnal asthma. Barium swallow does not show any strictures.

2. Myasthenia gravis is an antibody mediated autoimmune disease causing muscle weakness. Antiacetyl choline receptor antibodies are seen in 90% of patients. Patients are generally young increased with—muscle fatigability which progresses to permanent weakness. Voice weakens on counting aloud till 50. Male: Female ratio is 1:2. Tensilon test is positive if edrophonium injection improves muscle power within minutes. Treatment options include pyridostigmine, prednisolone, thymectomy and plasmapheresis.

3. Out of the given options, the presentation and age of the patient are suggestive of a post cricoid cancer. It is usually associated with plummer–vinson syndrome. It is frequently circumferential with metastasis to both sides of the neck. Patients typically complain of increasing dysphagia. Diagnosis can be confirmed by laryngopharyngoscopy and biopsy. Treatment requires surgery followed by radiotherapy.

4. Pharyngeal pouch is a protusion through Killian's dehiscence. Patients suffering from this condition are usually elderly. It is twice as common in men as in women. Initially symptoms are identical with those of a foreign body in the throat. Later regurgitation of undigested food at unpredictable times is the chief complaint. Still later patient can complaint of gurgling noises in the neck especially on swallowing. Such pouches can sometimes be seen to enlarge when the patient drinks.

Patients have progressive loss of weight due to semistarvation.

5. Achalasia is failure of oesophageal peristalsis and failure of relaxation of the lower oesophageal sphincter. This causes dysphagia, regurgitation, substernal cramps and weight loss. Barium swallow shows dilated tapering oesophagus (typical 'rats tail' appearance). Treatment is with endoscopic balloon dilatation or Heller's cardiomyotomy.

Theme 28: Investigation in cervical pathology

1. Cervical ectropion also known as erosion is a normal phenomenon. It is seen temporarily due to hormonal influence during puberty, with the use of OCPs (as in this patient) or during pregnancy. As columnar epithelium is soft and glandular, it is prone to bleeding, excess mucus production and to infection. Treatment is with cautery if the condition is very disturbing otherwise no treatment is required.
2. Cervical cancer has a pre invasive phase—CIN i.e. Cervical Intraepithelial Neoplasia. Papanicolaou smears identify women who need cervical biopsy. Papanicolaou smears can show dyskaryosis which reflects CIN. The main cause of cervical cancer is Human Papilloma virus (HPV 16, 18 and 33). Prolonged usage of OCPs has been implicated as an important co-factor. Patients with smears suggestive of CIN II or III will undergo colposcopy while those with minor changes as mild atypia or inflammation will have a repeat smear.
3. As explained above.

Theme 29: Respiratory disease: Diagnosis

1. The presentation of the patient with fever and basal consolidation on CXR is almost diagnostic of pneumonia. Other features that may be present in patients with pneumonia are malaise, anorexia, cough, purulent sputum, haemoptysis, pleuritic chest pain, tachypnoea, hypotension and signs of consolidation. Investigations required are CXR, sputum for microscopy and cultures and pleural aspirate (if present) for culture. Treatment involves antibiotics according to sensitivity patterns.
2. Perforation of oesophagus can result from inexpert use of an oesophagoscope. The most frequent cause of perforation is a sharp foreign body plus instrumentation to remove it. Patient would complain of general distress, dysphagia and dyspnoea. A chest radiography (as in this case) would reveal presence of air in the mediastinum, pleural cavity or in the neck which may be palpable (surgical emphysema). Urgent surgery under antibiotic cover should be performed and repair done.
3. Pneumothorax is collection of air in the pleural space. It often occurs spontaneous by especially in young thin men due to rupture of subpleural bulla. In this question the patient is breathless which means that he may be suffering from asthma, COPD, TB, pneumonia, lung abscess or sarcoidosis which are also causative factors in the occurrence of pneumothorax. The patient will typically complains of sudden onset dyspnoea and pleuritic chest pain. Patient will have reduced chest expansion, hyperresonance to percussion and decreased breath sounds on the affected area. Mild pneumothorax does not require any treatment, but moderate to severe pneumothorax require aspiration.
4. Myocardial infarction is usually due to occlusion of a coronary artery resulting from

rupture of an atheromatous plaque. Patient usually present with acute chest pain lasting > 20 minute. MI is associated with nausea, sweatiness, dyspnoea and palpitations. In elderly or diabetics, MI may also present without chest pain (silent MI). On examination there may be pallor, distress, sweatiness and 4th heart sound. ECG changes—Q waves (as in this case) signify transmural infarction. Hyperacute T waves and ST elevation are also seen. Non Q wave infarct means a subendocardial infarct. Other investigations required are cardiac enzymes CK, AST, LDH which are elevated. Troponin T is also elevated. Treatment involves aspirin stat, analgesia with morphine, O_2, thrombolysis with streptokinase or t-PA.

5. As explained above.

Theme 30: Diagnosis of chest pain

1. The presentation of the patient with breathlessness which disappears when he goes away for holidays i.e. is off from his work, is suggestive of occupational asthma due to dust from the wood.

2. This is a case of pulmonary oedema. Pulmonary oedema can be due to cardiogenic (e.g. LVF, MS, arrhythmias) causes or non-cardiogenic causes (e.g. ARDS, fluid overload, head injury). Patients present with dyspnoea, orthopnoea, pink frothy sputum, pallor, tachycardia, pulsus alternans, increased JVP, fine lung crepts and wheeze (cardiac asthma). CXR shows bilateral shadowing, Kerley B lines as linear opacities.

3. Pulmonary embolism usually arises from a venous thrombus in the pelvis or legs. Risk factors include history of DVT, OCPs, immobility and hypercoagulability. Patients may present with breathlessness, pleuritic chest pain, fever, haemoptysis, tachycardia, gallop rhythm, hypotension, raised JVP and pleural rub. ECG may be normal. CXR may show oligaemia of the affected segment, dilated pulmonary artery. The investigation of choice is CT pulmonary angiography. If unavailable V/Q scan should be done. Low molecular weight heparin is used to anticoagulate.

4. Dissection of the thoracic aorta can present as tearing chest pain radiating to the back. It can lead to hemiplegia (if carotids are occluded), unequal arm pulses and BP, paraplegia (if anterior spinal artery is occluded) and anuria (if renal arteries are occluded). Aortic incompetence and inferior MI may develop. CT, MRI or transoesophageal echo-cardiography are required for the diagnosis.

Theme 31: Investigation of asthma in children

1. Although the child at present has no breathlessness, peak flow diary needs to be maintained. It gives a fair idea about the effectivity of the drugs being taken and can also give an idea about the improvement or deterioration in the condition of the patient.

2. This is a case of tension pneumothorax. It can be spontaneous especially in young thin men or can be due to asthma, COPD, TB, pneumonia, lung abscess, carcinoma, cystic fibrosis, sarcoidosis, trauma or iatrogenic. Patients may present with sudden onset dyspnoea, pleuritic chest pain, reduced expansion, hyperresonance to percussion and diminished breath sounds on the affected side. Trachea is deviated away from the affected side in tension pneumothorax. A CXR should not be performed if a tension pneumothorax is suspected as it will delay the necessary treatment. Treatment is with needle aspiration and chest drain if aspiration fails.

3. Signs of severe asthma include
   i. Too breathless to speak or feed
   ii. Respiratory rate ≥ 50 breaths/minute.
   iii. Pulse rate ≥ 140/minute
   iv. Peak flow $\leq 50\%$ of predicted value.
   Such patients require urgent treatment without wasting any time in investigations.

4. Since the child does not have any symptoms of asthma at the moment, exercise induced symptoms can be generated. Once the symptoms are perceivable, the inhaler can be used and the change be noted both by the parents and the child.

Theme 32: Anatomy of renal failure

1. A pelvic mass can be due to full bladder, bladder carcinoma, fibroid, fetus, ovarian cyst, ovarian cancer, uterine cancer. The presentation of not passing her urine for many hours is suggestive of urinary obstruction causing a full bladder which is palpable as a suprapubic mass.

2. The presentation in this case could be either due to a BPH or prostatic carcinoma. As there is no specific pointer in the question which suggests a carcinoma, BPH becomes the only option. BPH is a common problem. Decrease in urinary flow is associated with increased frequency, urgency and voiding difficulty. Treatment involves mainly surgical, but in some cases medical approach.

3. Sickle cell disease causes renal complications that arise mainly as a result of sickling of RBCs in the microvasculature. This causes local infarction and hence papillary necrosis. Functional tubule defects in patients with sickle cell disease are likely due to injury to renal tubules.

4. Combination of proteinuria of > 3 gm/day, hypoalbuminaemia (albumin < 30 gm/L) and oedema comprises nephrotic syndrome. Hypoalbuminaemia results in increased intravascular oncotic pressure, leading to leakage of extracellular fluid from blood to the interstitium. The neuronal and hormonal responses promote renal salt and water retention hence triggering further leakage of fluid to the interstitium.

5. Renovascular disease is one of the causes of hypertension. Atherosclerosis is seen in around three-fourth of all patients with renovascular disease. Patients may have abdominal bruit, carotid or femoral bruits and absent leg pulses. Renal angiography is the gold standard investigation. Percutaneous transluminal renal angioplasty or surgery is required in such cases.

Theme 33: Investigation of haematuria

1. Adult polycystic kidney disease is an autosomal dominant condition with genes on chromosomes 16 & 4. Patients present with renal enlargement with cysts, abdominal pain, haematuria, UTI, renal calculi, hypertension or renal failure. An abdominal USG is sufficient to diagnose.

2. Acute nephritis presents with haematuria and oliguria. β haemolytic streptococcus is usually the cause. A sore throat around 2 weeks before is very suggestive of the aetiology. Patients may also have fever, hypertension. oedema or loin pain. Antistreptolysin 'O' titres are helpful in the diagnosis. Treatment includes restriction of protein if oliguric, penicillin for streptococcal infection and nitroprusside for encephalopathy.

3. The history of uterine cancer in the patient presenting with haematuria is suggestive of renal metastasis. Intravenous urogram or pyelogram is done for defining renal anatomy. IVU in this patient will be able to show a filling defect in the kidney.

4. Renal causes of haematuria with hypertension include diabetic nephropathy, CGN, chronic interstitial nephritis, PKD and renovascular disease. Ultrasound is the usual initial imaging method in renal medicine. It can show a small kidney in CRF and large kidney in renal masses, cysts or hypertrophy. It can also show hydronephrosis (due to renal obstruction or reflux), perinephric collections (due to trauma) and bladder residual volume.

Theme 34: Diagnosis of haematuria

1. Transitional cell carcinomas may arise in the bladder, ureter or renal pelvis. They usually present after 40 years of age. Male: Female ratio is 4:1. Smoking, cyclophosphamide, phenacetin, azodyes, β naphthalene, schistosomiasis are known risk factors. Patients present with painless haematuria, frequency, urgency, dysuria or obstruction. Cystoscopy with biopsy is diagnostic.

2. Henoch–Schönlein (anaphylactoid) purpura generally presents with purple spots or nodules which do not disappear on pressure i.e. intradermal bleeding. They are generally seen over buttocks and extensor surfaces. It may follow a respiratory infection. It may present with nephritis, joint involvement, abdominal pain and intussusception.

3. Adult polycystic kidney disease is an autosomal dominant condition with genes on chromosomes 16 & 4. Patients present with renal enlargement with cysts, abdominal pain, haematuria, UTI, renal calculi, hypertension or renal failure. An abdominal USG is sufficient to diagnose.

Theme 35: Management of cardiac patients.

1. One of the indications for referral of a patient with angina, is angina uncontrolled by drugs. Overall risk of death is around 15% for refractory angina despite medical therapy. Indications for consideration of invasive intervention in patients with angina include poor prognosis such as with pulmonary oedema, refractory symptoms, positive exercise tolerance test and a non-Q wave infarct.

Percutaneous transluminal coronary angioplasty (PTCA) involves balloon dilatation of the stenotic vessel. Poor response or intolerance to medical therapy and refractory angina in patients not suitable for CABG, are indications for PTCA. Indications for coronary artery bypass grafting (CABG) include left main stem disease, multivessel disease, multiple severe stenoses, distal vessel disease, patient unsuitable for angioplasty, failed angioplasty, refractory angina, MI and pre-operatively in valvular or vascular surgery.

2. Indications for coronary artery bypass grafting (CABG) include left main stem disease, multivessel disease, multiple severe stenoses, distal vessel disease, patient unsuitable for angioplasty, failed angioplasty, refractory angina, MI and pre-operatively in valvular or vascular surgery.

3. The presentation of the patient is suggestive of aortic stenosis. Senile calcification is the most common cause of aortic stenosis. Prompt valve replacement is recommended in both symptomatic and asymptomatic patients. Valves can be mechanical, xenografts or homografts. Xenograft valves are made of porcine or pericardium. Homografts are cadaveric grafts.

Theme 36: Diagnostic test for breast lump.

1. Breast carcinoma usually does not present in such young age groups. But breast carcinoma commences most frequently in the upper, outer quadrant, as in this case. Breast carcinoma should be investigated for in this patient. The most significant features of carcinoma seen on mammography are:
   i. a solid lesion with ill defined edges or stellate configuration
   ii. asymmetry of density, vascularity or stromal architecture
   iii. true microcalcification
   iv. distortion of the skin or outline of the breast
   v. increased skin thickness
   vi. a single, dilated duct
   vii. large lesion of nodular outline
   viii. changes on serial mammography.

2. This is a clear cut case of fibrocystic breast disease as the symptom (feeling of lumpiness) is related with the timing of menses. It is one of the benign breast disorders. Only reassurance is needed. But because a mass due to fibrocystic disease is frequently indistinguishable from carcinoma, suspicious lesions should be investigated further. Mammography may be helpful but the breast tissue in young women is usually too radiodense to permit a worthwhile study. Therefore ultrasonography is required to differentiate a cystic from a solid mass.

3. Since ultrasound and mammography which have already been done show normal study ductography should be performed in this case. A blood stained discharge may be due to duct ectasia or duct papilloma or carcinoma. Ductography demonstrates duct anatomy and pathology by injection of radio-opaque contrast medium into a major lacteal duct and taking a radiograph.

4. Golden rule: All solid breast lumps need histological or cytological assessment. Since mammography shows a solid lump, FNAC should be done. Fine-needle aspiration cytology is the least invasive technique for obtaining a cell diagnosis. The aspirate is smeared onto a slide which is air dried and visualized.

5. Bones are the most common site of secondary deposits in breast carcinoma. It occur through blood stream in the lumbar vertebrae, femurs, thoracic vertebrae, ribs and skull. The presentation of the patient in this case is suggestive of spinal metastasis, most likely thoracic metastasis. A CT scan of the spine is required to rule out secondary deposits.

Theme 37: Diagnosis of gastroenterology findings

1. Urinary tract infection implies presence of a pure growth of more than 10^5 colony forming units/mL. Infection may occur at the bladder (cystitis), prostate (prostatitis) or kidney (pyelonephritis). Female sex, sexual intercourse, diabetes, immunocompromised status, pregnancy, menopause, urinary tract obstruction and renal stones are some of the risk factors. Patients may present with frequency, dysuria, urgency, haematuria, fever, vomiting, loin pain, ARF, low backache. *E. coli* is the most common organism causing UTI. Treatment is with trimethoprim 200 mg 12 hourly PO for 3 days in patients with cystitis. Cefuroxime is given in cases of pyelonephritis and ciprofloxacin for prostatitis.

2. Ingestion of certain bacteria, viruses and toxins (bacterial and chemical) is a common cause of gastroenteritis. Contaminated food and water are common sources. The history should include details of food and water taken, process of cooking, time until onset of symptoms and whether fellow-diners were affected. As the children are also affected in this case, gastroenteritis is very likely. Stool microscopy and culture are required for diagnosis. Oral fluid intake should be maintained. Antiemetics and antidiarrhoeals are given for severe symptoms. Antibiotics are indicated in patients who are systemically unwell.

3. Campylobacter infection is one of the causes of bloody diarrhoea with vomiting. Campylobacter enteritis is a zoonosis like salmonellosis. The infection is usually transmitted indirectly via contaminated meat, milk or water. After an incubation period of 2–5 days, the illness starts either with abdominal pain and diarrhoea or with a prodrome of fever, headache and influenza-like symptoms. Diagnosis depends on the isolation of

campylobacters from faeces. Antibiotics are effective only if given early in the disease when patient is acutely ill. Erythromycin is the drug of choice given 500 mg twice daily for 5 days.

Theme 38: Pre-operative investigations

1. ECG is indicated pre-operatively in all patients who are above 65 years of age (since patients have a high incidence of 'silent ischaemia'), have poor exercise tolerance, have history of myocardial infarction, hypertension, rheumatic fever, Kawasaki's disease or any other heart disease.

2. The mention of menorrhagia and tiredness are suggestive of anaemia. Menorrhagia is increased menstrual blood loss (defined as > 80 ml/cycle) which can lead to iron deficiency anaemia. Such patients may present with tiredness, dyspnoea, palpitations, headache, tinnitus, anorexia, dyspepsia and bowel disturbance. Such patients must have a full blood count pre-operatively. If the haemoglobin level is less than 10 gm/dL, anaesthetist should be informed. Patients should be further investigated and treated appropriately.

Theme 39: Investigations after bites and stings

1. Human bites are said to be the most dangerous and can result in serious infection. Common human organism includes Eikenella corridens. Staphylococci are also common. Skin swab culture taken from the wound is thus necessary (also to determine sensitivity to antibiotics).

2. Lyme disease is a tick-borne infection caused by Borrelia burgdorferi. It presents with erythema chronicum migrans which is a small papule developing into a large erythematous ring with central fading. It lasts 48 hours–3 months. Other features include malaise, lymphadenopathy, arthralgia, myocarditis, meningitis, ataxia, etc. Diagnosis is by clinical signs and symptoms and serology.
Treatment for skin rash is by doxycycline 100 mg/12 hours for 10–21 days.
For later complications, high dose IV Benzyl penicillin/cefotaxime/ceftriaxone can be given.

3. Malaria is one of the most common causes of fever and illness in the tropics. Travellers going to malaria-endemic areas can acquire the infection. Hence, chemoprophylaxis with chloroquine is advised. Chemoprophylaxis should begin a week before arrival in the malarious area and continued for at least 4 weeks or preferably 6 weeks after leaving the malarious area.
Serial thick and thin blood films are taken at the time of fever. Thick films help in rapid detection of malarial parasites, while thin film helps in identification of the plasmodium subtype.

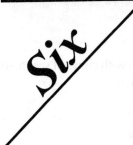

September 2002 Question Paper

Theme 1: Management of diarrhoea in children

Options:

a. 5% dextrose
b. 0.9 %saline
c. 5% dextrose and 0.45% saline
d. 50 ml per kg ORT over 4 hours
e. 150 ml per kg ORT over 4 hours
f. 150 ml per kg ORT over 24 hours
g. Ciprofloxacin
h. Trimethoprim-Sulphamethoxazole
i. Anti-diarrhoeals
j. Anti-emetics
k. Lactose free diet

For each presentation below, choose the SINGLE most appropriate management from the above list of options. Each option may be used once, more than once, or not at all.

1. An 8 month old child with history of diarrhoea 8 episodes in the last 24 hours.
2. A child presenting with diarrhoea and vomiting for past 3 days.
3. A child presenting with Shigella dysentery.
4. A bottle fed baby presenting with diarrhoea and urine reducing substance positive.

Theme 2: Diagnosis of injury in children

Options:

a. Fracture
b. Non accidental injury
c. Accidental injury
d. Normal finding
e. Henoch-Schönlein purpura
f. ITP
g. Leukaemia
h. Sickle cell anaemia
i. Osteogenesis imperfecta

For each presentation below, choose the SINGLE most appropriate diagnosis from the above list of options. Each option may be used once, more than once, or not at all.

1. A 10 year old boy with history of fall from cycle. On examination lower leg swelling and deformation.
2. An 8 month old child with large blue patch on the bottom. Father is Caucasian and mother is African.
3. A 10 year old girl brought to the A&E by her stepfather. On examination girl has petechial lesions around her waist and ankles.

4. A 5 year old girl develops sore foot after playing football at her school. GP is concerned about patches of different colours on her lower legs. Otherwise the girl's examination is normal.

5. An 11 month old infant with spiral fracture of the humerus. X-ray done shows absence of callus formation.

Theme 3: Investigation of wrist fractures

Options:

a. Isotope scan
b. X-ray wrist AP , lateral with views of scaphoid
c. Refer to Orthopaedician
d. X-ray thumb
e. Plaster cast of wrist
f. Discharge with advice
g. Physiotherapy

For each presentation below, choose the SINGLE most appropriate investigation from the above list of options. Each option may be used once, more than once, or not at all.

1. A 10 year old boy comes with history of fall on his hand. X-ray of the thumb reveals no fracture.

2. A 12 year old boy comes with history of fall on his hand.

3. An 18 year old comes with history of fall on his hand. X-ray wrist reveals impacted fracture lower hand on the left.

4. An 8 year old boy comes with history of fall on his hand and complains of pain in the wrist joint. X-rays of the area reveal no fracture.

Theme 4: Investigation of dyspepsia

Options:

a. 24 hour ambulatory oesophageal pH monitoring
b. Oesophageal manometry
c. Endoscopy
d. Fecal occult blood
e. No investigation needed at present
f. Helicobacter pylori serology
g. Barium meal

For each presentation below, choose the SINGLE most appropriate investigation from the above list of options. Each option may be used once, more than once, or not at all.

1. A 50 year old obese woman with history of pain in the epigastrium which comes on at night and wakes her up. She also complains of cough and water brash.
2. A woman with history of pain in the stomach after a fundoplication operation.
3. A woman with long history of peptic ulcer disease with positive *H.pylori*. She has not had an examination for the past 4 years, now presents for a check up.
4. A 36 year old man who has been treating himself for dyspeptic symptoms for several years.
5. A 47 year old man who has a stressful job presents with history of epigastric pain for past 2 years. He smokes about 20 cigarettes per day.

Theme 5: Diagnosis of antepartum haemorrhage

Options:

a. Abruptio placenta
b. Placenta praevia
c. Vasa praevia
d. Velamentous insertion
e. Show
f. Carcinoma cervix
g. Trauma

For each presentation below, choose the SINGLE most appropriate diagnosis from the above list of options. Each option may be used once, more than once, or not at all.

1. A 21 year old primi with history of hypertension presents with acute abdominal pain. On examination uterus is tender to palpation and BP is 90/40.
2. A 20 year old primi with history of painless, bright red vaginal bleed over past 3 hours. On examination the fetus is in transverse lie.
3. A 26 year old in labour with blood and mucus per vaginum.
4. A 38 year old woman, 4th gravida with history of blood and mucus per vaginum. On examination vagina red and ulcerated.
5. A 27 year old primi with history of post coital bleed.

Theme 6: Diagnosis of head injury

Options:

a. Extradural haematoma
b. Subdural haematoma
c. Mild head injury
d. Moderate head injury
e. Severe head injury
f. Fracture base of skull
g. Subarachnoid haemorrhage
h. Coma

For each presentation below, choose the SINGLE most appropriate diagnosis from the above list of options. Each option may be used once, more than once, or not at all.

1. A 45 year old alcoholic with history of recurrent falls was brought to A&E by his wife in a confused state.
2. A 23 year old footballer brought to the A&E. Was talking to the paramedics well after injury but subsequently lost consciousness.
3. A 7 year old boy with history of fall from cycle. Lost consciousness initially but alert, oriented now. Examination reveals no abnormality.
4. A 38 year old man presents with a history of fall. On examination haemotympanum present.
5. A 42 year old man fell down. On examination GCS-13.

Theme 7: Investigation in vaginal bleed

Options:

a. Endometrial sampling
b. 21 day progesterone
c. Full blood count
d. Colposcopy
e. D&C
f. Vaginal ultrasound
g. Laparotomy
h. Abdominal USG
i. Urine examination

For each presentation below, choose the SINGLE most appropriate investigation from the above list of options. Each option may be used once, more than once, or not at all.

1. A 45 year old woman who attained menopause 2 years back, presents with an episode of vaginal bleed. She gives no recent history of sexual intercourse.
2. A 14 year old girl, menarche at 12 years has been having regular periods so far. Past 4 cycles, she has been having heavy bleed and appears exsanguinated now.
3. A 33 year old West Indian woman with history of menorrhagia and dysmenorrhoea.
4. A 23 year old woman on OCPs presents with vaginal bleed.

Theme 8: Management of burns

Options:

a. Escharotomy
b. Intravenous fluids
c. Intubation
d. Aspiration of blisters
e. Deroof blisters
f. Estimation of COHb level
g. Fasciotomy
h. Debridement
i. Cold irrigation

For each presentation below, choose the SINGLE most appropriate management from the above list of options. Each option may be used once, more than once, or not at all.

1. A man presents with full and partial thickness burns from his elbows to hands.
2. A man rescued from burning house with singed nostrils asking for his other family members.
3. A man presents with burns over his chest and anterior aspect of his thigh.
4. A patient presented with scalds with large tense blisters.

Theme 9: Mechanism of action of contraceptives

Options:

a. Inhibition of tubal motility
b. Inhibition of ovulation
c. Production of hostile cervical mucus
d. Inhibition of implantation
e. Spermicidal
f. Causes miscarriage
g. Inhibition of ovulation and thickening of cervical mucus

For each contraceptive below, choose the SINGLE most appropriate mechanism of action from the above list of options. Each option may be used once, more than once, or not at all.

1. COCPs.
2. IUCD.
3. Mirena coil.
4. POP.
5. Vaginal sponge.
6. Depot Progesterone.

Theme 10: Management of visual loss

Options:

a. Eye operation
b. Laser treatment
c. Intraocular steroids
d. Oral steroids
e. Intravenous steroids
f. β-blocker drops
g. No treatment effective
h. Systemic antibiotics

For each presentation below, choose the SINGLE most appropriate management from the above list of options. Each option may be used once, more than once, or not at all.

1. A 68 year old male with 3 month history of pain and diminished vision in left eye. Pain increases towards evening. Peripheral vision constricted. On examination glaucomatous cupping seen.

2. A 58 year old male with right sided headache and pain right eye.

3. A 45 year old diabetic with proliferative retinopathy of right eye. Left eye shows retinal haemorrhage on fundoscopy.

4. A 78 year old female with decreased visual acuity. On retinoscopy the macula shows pigmentation bilaterally.

5. A 44 year old woman with history of SLE has diminished vision .

Theme 11: Management of post menopausal conditions

Options:

a. Vaginal oestrogens
b. Cyclical OCPs
c. Continuous OCPs
d. Ring pessary
e. Transdermal oestrogen patch
f. POP
g. Biphosphonates
h. Prevent infection measures

For each presentation below, choose the SINGLE most appropriate management from the above list of options. Each option may be used once, more than once, or not at all.

1. A 78 year old woman sexually active complains of dyspareunia and vaginal dryness.

2. A 45 year old woman who has attained menopause 2 years back complains of weight gain and depression.

3. A 54 year old woman who has had irregular period for last 3 months complains of flushing, mood swings and weight gain.

4. An 84 year old woman with 14 issues complains of feeling of something coming down per vaginum.

5. A 32 years old woman with menopausal symptoms, underwent hysterectomy for some pathology. She cannot take oral preparations.

6. A 53 year old woman who has attained menopause complains of constipation, excess thirst. X-ray shows bone rarefaction.

7. A post menopausal diabetic woman presents with frequent vaginal and vulval pruritus.

Theme 12: Investigation of acute abdomen

Options:

a. Chest X-ray
b. Serum amylase
c. Abdominal USG
d. Laparotomy
e. Laparoscopy
f. TOE
g. CT
h. Observation only
i. ECG

For each presentation below, choose the SINGLE most appropriate investigation from the above list of options. Each option may be used once, more than once, or not at all.

1. A male with history of APD (acid peptic disease) presents with 24 hour history of acute abdominal pain. On examination board like rigidity in the abdomen and no bowel sounds.
2. A man with history of intermittent claudication and IHD presents with tearing pain in the abdomen radiating to back. On examination BP is 90/ 40.
3. A female presents with history of pain that started in the loin. Pain is radiating to the groin now.
4. A 14 year old boy with history of abdominal pain periumbilically. Pain had spread to the right iliac fossa. Now he complains of no pain. On examination a mass is palpable in right iliac fossa.
5. A man with history of injury to upper abdomen. On examination a mass is palpable in the epigastrium.

Theme 13: Diagnosis of deafness

Options:

a. Acoustic neuroma
b. Noise induced deafness
c. Temporary shift of threshold of hearing
d. AOM with effusion
e. Ménière's disease
f. Otosclerosis
g. Adenoids
h. Trauma
i. Ototoxicity

For each presentation below, choose the SINGLE most appropriate diagnosis from the above list of options. Each option may be used once, more than once, or not at all.

1. An 18 year old presents with deafness of 1 day duration after a night out at the local dance club.
2. An 8 year old girl found to be deaf at a school hearing test. After 1 week mother notices that the girl is fine and can hear well.
3. A 40 year old man with history of vomiting, vertigo and tinnitus. On examination low sensorineural deafness of left ear.
4. A 23 year old lactating mother presents with hearing loss. After 9 months post partum, she can hear well again.
5. A 40 year old man with family history of deafness. Examination reveals conductive deafness in the left ear.

14. Theme: Investigation of epilepsy

Options:

a. CT scan
b. Blood glucose
c. EEG
d. ECG
e. MRI
f. Blood levels of anticonvulsant

For each presentation below, choose the SINGLE most appropriate investigation from the above list of options. Each option may be used once, more than once, or not at all.

1. A 14 year old girl with well controlled epilepsy so far presents with recurring seizures. Dose of valproate on which the girl is, has been increased several times. Still she has convulsions.

2. An 8 year old boy with history of 2 episodes of seizures in his sleep. The seizures start as twitching of mouth followed by generalized convulsions lasting for about 3 mins. He is all right in the morning.

3. A 12 year old boy with generalized tonic clonic convulsions lasting for about 5 min.

4. A 23 year old man with history of diplopia, headache and seizures.

Theme 15: Investigation of stroke

Options:

a. Blood cultures
b. Echocardiography
c. Doppler ultrasound of neck
d. CT scan
e. ECG

For each presentation below, choose the SINGLE most appropriate investigation from the above list of options. Each option may be used once, more than once, or not at all.

1. A 32 year old woman one week after cholecystectomy presents with left sided weakness. On examination she has a murmur precordially and is febrile, temperature being 37.7 deg C.

2. A 42 year old woman presents with hemiparesis. Examination reveals a bruit in the neck.

3. A 23 year old woman presents with neck stiffness. No complains of vomiting. She is noted to be drowsy.

4. A 70 year old women presents with 12 days history of weakness which has somewhat resolved. Her pulse is irregularly irregular. Rest of the CVS examination is normal.

Theme 16: Diagnosis of dementia

Options:

a. Huntington's chorea
b. Alzheimer's dementia
c. Pseudodementia
d. Multi infarct dementia
e. AIDS dementia

For each presentation below, choose the SINGLE most appropriate diagnosis from the above list of options. Each option may be used once, more than once, or not at all.

1. Commonest dementia in UK.
2. Dementia characterized by senile plaques and neurofibrillary tangles.
3. Dementia responsive to antidepressants.
4. Family history of dementia and characterized by early death.
5. Dementia common in hypertensives.

Theme 17: Investigation of thyroid conditions

Options:

a. THRH
b. TSH
c. T_3 levels
d. No investigation required at present
e. USG
f. FNAC

For each presentation below, choose the SINGLE most appropriate investigation from the above list of options. Each option may be used once, more than once, or not at all.

1. A woman is presently taking thyroxine for hypothyroidism. Has come for assessment of thyroid function.
2. A 13 year old girl with diffuse swelling of thyroid. No symptoms of dysthyroid function.
3. A woman presents with thyroid swelling, sweating and tremors of hands.
4. A 32 year old man presents with swelling on one side of thyroid gland.
5. A man presented with unilateral swelling of thyroid. USG shows nodular lesion which is not cystic.

Theme 18: Diagnosis of nerve injury

Options:

a. Musculocutaneous nerve
b. Common peroneal nerve
c. Sciatic nerve
d. Axillary nerve
e. Median nerve
f. Femoral nerve
g. Radial nerve
h. Facial nerve
i. Glossopharyngeal nerve
j. Ulnar nerve

For each presentation below, choose the SINGLE most appropriate affected nerve from the above list of options. Each option may be used once, more than once, or not at all.

1. A man with history of fall. Injury to shoulder. On examination region of anaesthesia over the lower part of shoulder is noted.
2. A child with history of fall. He has injured his arm. X-rays reveal a fracture mid-shaft of humerus. He now presents with wrist drop.
3. A man presents with history of injury to lower leg. On examination there is restriction of dorsiflexion of left foot and region of anaesthesia over the foot.
4. A man presents with injury to medial epicondyle of humerus. There is region of anaesthesia on the dorsum of hand.
5. A man presents with injury to back of his upper thigh. Weakness of hamstrings are noted on examination.
6. A man presents with loss of taste sensation in the anterior two thirds of tongue.
7. A woman presents with loss of voluntary movements in the lower part of face. Sensation and movements are preserved in the upper part of face.

Theme 19: Diagnosis of chest pain

Options:

a. Pericarditis
b. Musculoskeletal pain
c. Pneumonia
d. Stable angina
e. Unstable angina
f. Myocardial infarction
g. Herpes
h. Gastritis
i. Aortic aneurysm

For each presentation below, choose the SINGLE most appropriate diagnosis from the above list of options. Each option may be used once, more than once, or not at all.

1. A patient who is post MI presents with chest pain related to movement.
2. A man presents with cough, fever, chest pain, which is more on inspiration.
3. A woman who used to have chest pain on walking some distance now presents with chest pain even at rest.
4. A 45 year old diabetic presents with 2 hour history of central, crushing chest pain.
5. A man presents with chest pain on climbing up the stairs.

Theme 20: Investigations of chest pain/dyspnoea

Options:

a. V/Q scan
b. ECG
c. Echocardiogram
d. Spiral CT
e. Chest X-ray
f. USG abdomen
g. Stress ECG
h. Lung function tests

For each presentation below, choose the SINGLE most appropriate investigation from the above list of options. Each option may be used once, more than once, or not at all.

1. A 25 year old woman with 3 day history of cough, sputum, fever and chest pain.
2. A 30 year old woman on OCPs with history of deep vein thrombosis presents with dyspnoea.
3. A 45 year old man presents with history of crushing chest pain.
4. A 25 year old woman who has been on OCPs for the last 6 months presents with palpitations. Further examination reveals a murmur.

Theme 21: Diagnosis of pneumonia

Options:

a. Streptococcus pneumoniae
b. Legionella
c. Mycoplasma
d. Pneumocystis carinii
e. Mycobacterium tuberculosis
f. Haemophilus influenzae

For each presentation below, choose the SINGLE most appropriate etiology from the above list of options. Each option may be used once, more than once, or not at all.

1. A woman presents with 3 day history of cough and purulent sputum. On examination she is found to be febrile.
2. An 18 year old boy returns home after stay in some country. He presents with fever, cough and diarrhoeal episodes.
3. A woman presents with fever and cough. Blood investigation shows cold agglutinins.
4. An IV drug abuser presents with fever, rigor and chills. CXR shows fine, perihilar mottling.

Theme 22: Terminal Care

Options:

a. Benzodiazepines
b. Hyoscine
c. Haloperidol
d. NSAIDs
e. Palliative X-ray therapy
f. Lactulose
g. Biphosphonates

For each presentation below, choose the SINGLE most appropriate management from the above list of options. Each option may be used once, more than once, or not at all.

1. A patient with carcinoma bronchus presents with intractable hiccups.
2. A man with excessive salivary and bronchial secretions presents with rattly breathing due to excess secretions. Relatives are concerned.
3. A woman with terminal hepatocellular carcinoma presents with ascites and hepatic encephalopathy.
4. A man with carcinoma prostate presents with intractable backache.
5. A woman with multiple myeloma presents with thirst and constipation.

Theme 23: Metabolic parameters in renal conditions

Options:

a. Haemolytic uraemic syndrome
b. CRF
c. Renal tubular acidosis
d. Nephrotic syndrome
e. Acute glomerulonephritis
f. SLE
g. Diabetic nephropathy

For each presentation below, choose the SINGLE most appropriate diagnosis from the above list of options. Each option may be used once, more than once, or not at all.

1. Increased urea, increased creatinine, anaemia, fragmented RBCs, hypertension.
2. Increased urea, increased creatinine, hyperkalaemia.
3. Proteinuria, hypoalbuminaemia.
4. Hypertension, haematuria.
5. Hypertension, glomerular crescents on microscopy.

Theme 24: Diagnosis of chronic abdominal conditions

Options:

a. Ulcerative colitis
b. Irritable bowel syndrome with diarrhoea
c. Irritable bowel syndrome with constipation
d. Sigmoid colon carcinoma
e. Appendicular mass
f. Diverticular disease
g. Crohn's disease
h. Acid peptic disease

For each presentation below, choose the SINGLE most appropriate diagnosis from the above list of options. Each option may be used once, more than once, or not at all.

1. A 72 year old man presenting with confusion. On examination faeces filled in colon. History of weight loss and tiredness present.
2. A 22 year old woman presents with diarrhoea for the past 7 months. She has abdominal pain which is relieved by passing motion.
3. A 14 year old boy with history of pain in the right iliac fossa. Now there is a mass present on examination.
4. A man presents with history of bloody diarrhoea and mucus for the past 6 months. Colonoscopy shows granular mucosa.

Theme 25: Management of backache

Options:

a. Bed rest
b. Traction
c. Surgery
d. Admit in hospital
e. Skeletal metastasis
f. Neurological problem

For each presentation below, choose the SINGLE most appropriate management from the above list of options. Each option may be used once, more than once, or not at all.

1. A man who has moved a cupboard in his house some time back presents with history of backache ever since.
2. A man with history of sudden onset lower backache. He now presents with loss of sensation in his perineum and inability to pass urine.
3. A man presents with history of fall yesterday. He has backache and urinary retention ever since. CXR shows suspicious lesions–one in the apex of the lung and the other at base.

Theme 26: Epistaxis

Options:

a. Maxillary sinusitis
b. Carcinoma maxillary antrum
c. Sepsis
d. Fracture ethmoid
e. Fracture nasal bone
f. Allergic rhinitis
g. Vasomotor rhinitis
h. Rhinitis medicamentosa

For each presentation below, choose the SINGLE most appropriate diagnosis from the above list of options. Each option may be used once, more than once, or not at all.

1. A woman with 3 month history of headache, pain over maxillary antrum and epistaxis. X-ray of sinus reveals clouding.
2. A woman presenting with headache, nasal discharge and blocked nose since one week. Tenderness over maxillary sinus is present.
3. An 11 year old boy with history of fall. He had epistaxis initially but now only clear fluid dripping from his nostrils.
4. A man who had a nasal polyp surgery a week back, now presents to the A&E with epistaxis.

Theme 27: Side effects of drugs

Options: ·

a. Aplastic anaemia
b. Check blood levels
c. TFTs
d. LFTs
e. Steven's Johnson syndrome
f. Blue tinted vision
g. Optic neuritis
h. Hypotension

For each presentation below, choose the SINGLE most appropriate side effect/ investigation from the above list of options. Each option may be used once, more than once, or not at all.

1. Chloramphenicol causes this.
2. A woman with history of manic depressive illness on lithium treatment, presents with tremors of hand.
3. A woman who is on lithium treatment, presents with depression, weight gain, cold intolerance and lethargy.
4. A woman with carcinoma breast with cerebral metastasis, on carbamazepine treatment for convulsions, presents with confusion.

Theme 28: Diagnosis in haematology

Options:

a. CLL
b. CML
c. ALL
d. Autoimmune haemolytic anaemia
e. Myeloproliferative disorder
f. Sickle cell anaemia
g. ITP
h. Haemophilia

For each presentation below, choose the SINGLE most appropriate diagnosis from the above list of options. Each option may be used once, more than once, or not at all.

1. An elderly person presenting with massive lymphadenopathy and splenomegaly.
2. An elderly man presents with splenomegaly and is philadelphia chromosome positive.
3. A woman presents with antibodies in blood.

Theme 29: Diagnosis of urinary obstruction

Options:

a. BPH
b. Carcinoma prostate
c. Clot retention
d. Bladder stone
e. Urethral stricture

For each presentation below, choose the SINGLE most appropriate diagnosis from the above list of options. Each option may be used once, more than once, or not at all.

1. A 65 year old man who has been drinking large pints of beer since afternoon now presents to A&E with inability to pass urine.
2. A man with history of painless haematuria and weight loss now presents with acute inability to pass urine.
3. A man with history of weight loss and backache now has progressive difficulty in passing urine.

Theme 30: Investigation in malignancies

Options:

a. PSA
b. PLAP
c. Skeletal survey
d. Thallium scan
e. Technitium scan
f. Abdominal USG
g. CA 125
h. CEA
i. α fetoprotein

For each presentation below, choose the SINGLE most appropriate investigation from the above list of options. Each option may be used once, more than once, or not at all.

1. A man with prostatic carcinoma on GnRH analogues now comes for follow up.
2. A man diagnosed as carcinoma prostate now presents with severe backache.
3. A man with carcinoma prostate which has spread beyond the capsule now presents with renal failure.

Theme 31: Diagnosis of Acid-Base disturbances

Options:

a. Metabolic acidosis
b. Metabolic alkalosis
c. Respiratory acidosis
d. Respiratory alkalosis
e. Hypokalaemia
f. Renal failure

For each presentation below, choose the SINGLE most appropriate diagnosis from the above list of options. Each option may be used once, more than once, or not at all.

1. A man having projectile vomiting due to pyloric stenosis presents with hypokalaemia and base excess.
2. A man with villous adenoma of rectum presents with diarrhoea.
3. A 45 year old man with pulmonary embolism presents with tachycardia, hypotension and breathlessness.
4. A man presenting with pallor, dry skin and anuria.

Theme 32: Management of asthma

Options:

a. Intravenous steroids
b. Short acting inhaled β-agonist
c. Short acting β-agonist (nebulizer)
d. Long acting β-agonist
e. Sodium cromoglycate
f. Leukotriene receptor antagonist
g. Inhaled steroids
h. Theophylline
i. IV Aminophylline
j. Avoid smoking
k. Avoid allergen

For each presentation below, choose the SINGLE most appropriate management from the above list of options. Each option may be used once, more than once, or not at all.

1. A boy presenting with acute severe asthma to A & E.
2. A boy has been diagnosed for the first time with asthma. He now comes to you for medication.
3. A man who has nocturnal wheeze inspite of being on twice daily β-agonists.
4. A 6 year old girl who presents with wheeze when brother plays with his friend's cat.
5. A 3 year old girl whose parents are smokers coughs everytime they smoke.

Theme 33: Management of cancer pain

Options:

a. TENS
b. NSAIDs
c. Palliative X-ray
d. Opiates
e. Calcium supplements
f. Pamidronate
g. HRT

For each presentation below, choose the SINGLE most appropriate management from the above list of options. Each option may be used once, more than once, or not at all.

1. A man with carcinoma prostate complains of backache which prevents him from sleeping. He is already on opiates.
2. A woman with multiple myeloma presents with features of hypercalcaemia. X-ray shows bony rarefaction and this is causing her great pain.
3. A woman with carcinoma breast has pain in her elbow.

Theme 34: Management of shingles

Options:

a. IV Aciclovir
b. Oral Aciclovir
c. Amitriptyline
d. SSRIs
e. Paracetamol

For each presentation below, choose the SINGLE most appropriate management from the above list of options. Each option may be used once, more than once, or not at all.

1. A woman presenting with ophthalmic herpes.
2. A boy with lymphoma has developed herpes.
3. A woman presenting with Herpetic neuralgia.
4. A man presents with pain along the distribution of intercostal nerves but no lesion over the region.

Theme 35: Management of meningitis

Options:

a. Parenteral Penicillin
b. Plasma expansion
c. CT scan
d. Lumbar puncture
e. Sputum for AFB

For each presentation below, choose the SINGLE most appropriate management from the above list of options. Each option may be used once, more than once, or not at all.

1. An 8 year old child presents with fever and rash over his whole body. GP is waiting for paediatricians advice.
2. A child with meningitis has been started on antibiotics. He is still febrile and drowsiness has increased.
3. A woman returned from Pakistan to meet her family at UK. She now presents with meningitis.
4. An IV drug abuser has high fever, headache and vomiting.

Theme 36: Resuscitation-immediate management post trauma

Options:

a. Splint fracture
b. Gain IV access and intravenous fluids
c. Gain IV access and blood transfusion
d. Intubation and ventilation
e. Open airway
f. CT scan
g. Cervical spine immobilization
h. ECG

For each presentation below, choose the SINGLE most appropriate management from the above list of options. Each option may be used once, more than once, or not at all.

1. A 12 year old girl involved in RTA. Vitals stable, breathing is rattly. Respiratory rate is 30 per minute.

2. A man involved in RTA. He has pallor and tachycardia. Pulse rate is 120 per minute, BP is 90/40. Thigh is deformed and ecchymoses are present over it.

3. A woman involved in RTA. Left side upper abdomen shows injury. She has cold peripheries. BP is 90/40.

4. A man involved in an RTA is brought to A&E. His GCS score is 3.

5. A man involved in RTA is brought to A&E with head injury. Pulse rate is 50 per minute and BP is 140/96.

Theme 37: Complications of myocardial infarction

Options:

a. Atrial fibrillation
b. Ventricular tachycardia
c. Chordae tendinae rupture of mitral valve leaflet
d. Ventricular rupture
e. Pericarditis
f. Pulmonary embolism
g. Acute pulmonary oedema
h. Heart block

For each presentation below, choose the SINGLE most appropriate complication from the above list of options. Each option may be used once, more than once, or not at all.

1. A man post MI presents with syncope. Heart rate is 40 per minute.

2. A man post MI presents with palpitations and breathlessness. On examination his pulse is irregular and rate is 120 per minute.

3. A man post MI presents with chest pain. Positional variation of pain is present. ECG shows saddle like ST elevation in anterior leads.

4. A woman post MI presents with syncope. On examination systolic and diastolic murmur audible at the apex.

5. A man one week post cholecystectomy presents with an MI. Four days after MI he presents with dyspnoea, tachycardia and frothy sputum.

Theme 38: Psychiatry: Diagnosis

Options:

a. Delirium
b. Late onset schizophrenia
c. Alzheimer's dementia
d. Huntington's chorea
e. Korsakoff's psychosis
f. Psychotic depression

For each presentation below, choose the SINGLE most appropriate diagnosis from the above list of options. Each option may be used once, more than once, or not at all.

1. A woman who stays alone, looked after by neighbours presents at a shop at 6 O' clock in the morning. Neighbours say she has had for the past 2 years slow forgetfulness.

2. A man who has been admitted in the medical ward, on the third day screams at staff and nurses saying that they are going to kill him.

3. A man who has had surgery shouts and screams as he regains consciousness.

4. A woman brings her husband to the casualty saying that he has been behaving strangely for the past 3 days. He is a chronic drinker.

5. A man hears voices commanding him to risk his life.

Theme 39: Prevention of bleeding

Options:

a. Apply pressure to site of bleeding
b. Gain IV access and transfuse fluids
c. Gain IV access and immediately transfuse blood

For each presentation below, choose the SINGLE most appropriate management from the above list of options. Each option may be used once, more than once, or not at all.

1. A 5 year old child fell on broken glass. Wrist has been slashed by the glass and profuse bleeding from the wound site. Nurses are trying to get an IV access.

2. A 20 year old woman who had attempted suicide by slashing her wrists claims that she wants to live no more. She is pale.

3. A male with suspected splenic injury involved in a RTA presents with pallor, tachycardia and hypotension.

Theme 40: Pre-operative investigation

Options:

a. Spirometry
b. CXR
c. Angiogram
d. ECG-24 hour monitoring
e. Blood sugar
f. Echocardiogram

For each presentation below, choose the SINGLE most appropriate pre-operative investigation from the above list of options. Each option may be used once, more than once, or not at all.

1. A woman with history of COPD needs to undergo hysterectomy. CXR reveals no abnormality.
2. A woman with diabetes needs a laparotomy to be done.
3. A man who has been posted for a cholecystectomy is a known IHD patient. He now has syncope. ECG taken pre-operatively shows a LBBB.
4. A man with rheumatic heart disease has a mid systolic murmur and click on auscultation. He has been posted for surgery under GA tomorrow.
5. A woman with cough and fever one week back has been posted for a sterilization operation tomorrow.

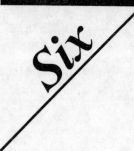

September 2002 Answers

Theme 1: Management of diarrhoea in children

1. **(f)** 150 ml per kg ORT over 24 hours
2. **(c)** 5% dextrose and 0.45% saline
3. **(g)** Ciprofloxacin
4. **(k)** Lactose free diet

Theme 2: Diagnosis of injury in children

1. **(a)** Fracture
2. **(d)** Normal finding
3. **(b)** Non accidental injury
4. **(f)** ITP
5. **(i)** Osteogenesis imperfecta

Theme 3: Investigation of wrist fractures

1. **(b)** X-ray wrist AP , lateral with views of scaphoid
2. **(b)** X-ray wrist AP, lateral with views of scaphoid
3. **(c)** Refer to Orthopaedician
4. **(f)** Discharge with advice

Theme 4: Investigation of dyspepsia

1. **(c)** Endoscopy
2. **(c)** Endoscopy
3. **(f)** Helicobacter pylori serology
4. **(f)** Helicobacter pylori serology
5. **(c)** Endoscopy

Theme 5: Diagnosis of antepartum haemorrhage

1. **(a)** Abruptio placenta
2. **(b)** Placenta praevia
3. **(e)** Show
4. **(f)** Carcinoma cervix
5. **(g)** Trauma

Theme 6: Diagnosis of head injury

1. **(b)** Subdural haematoma
2. **(a)** Extradural haematoma
3. **(d)** Moderate head injury
4. **(f)** Fracture base of skull
5. **(c)** Mild head injury

Theme 7: Investigation in vaginal bleed

1. **(a)** Endometrial sampling
2. **(c)** Full blood count

3. **(f)** Vaginal ultrasound
4. **(d)** Colposcopy

Theme 8: Management of burns

1. **(a)** Escharotomy
2. **(c)** Intubation
3. **(a)** Escharotomy
4. **(b)** Intravenous fluids

Theme 9: Mechanism of action of contraceptives

1. **(b)** Inhibition of ovulation
2. **(d)** Inhibition of implantation
3. **(d)** Inhibition of implantation
4. **(c)** Production of hostile cervical mucus
5. **(e)** Spermicidal
6. **(g)** Inhibition of ovulation and thickening of cervical mucus

Theme 10: Management of visual loss

1. **(f)** β-blocker drops
2. **(d)** Oral steroids
3. **(b)** Laser treatment
4. **(g)** No treatment effective
5. **(a)** Eye operation

Theme 11: Management of post menopausal conditions

1. **(a)** Vaginal oestrogens
2. **(b)** Cyclical OCPs
3. **(b)** Cyclical OCPs
4. **(d)** Ring pessary
5. **(e)** Transdermal oestrogen patch
6. **(g)** Biphosphonates
7. **(h)** Prevent infection measures

Theme 12: Investigation of acute abdomen

1. **(a)** Chest X-ray
2. **(d)** Laparotomy

3. **(c)** Abdominal USG
4. **(h)** Observation only
5. **(c)** Abdominal USG

Theme 13: Diagnosis of deafness

1. **(b)** Noise induced deafness
2. **(c)** Temporary shift of threshold of hearing
3. **(e)** Ménière's disease
4. **(c)** Temporary shift of threshold of hearing
5. **(f)** Otosclerosis

Theme 14: Investigation of epilepsy

1. **(f)** Blood levels of anticonvulsant
2. **(c)** EEG
3. **(c)** EEG
4. **(a)** CT scan

Theme 15: Investigation of stroke

1. **(a)** Blood cultures
2. **(c)** Doppler ultrasound of neck
3. **(a)** Blood cultures
4. **(d)** CT scan

Theme 16: Diagnosis of dementia

1. **(b)** Alzheimer's dementia
2. **(b)** Alzheimer's dementia
3. **(c)** Pseudodementia
4. **(a)** Huntington's chorea.
5. **(d)** Multi infarct dementia

Theme 17: Investigation of thyroid conditions

1. **(b)** TSH
2. **(d)** No investigation required at present
3. **(b)** TSH
4. **(e)** USG
5. **(f)** FNAC

Theme 18: Diagnosis of nerve injury

1. **(d)** Axillary nerve
2. **(g)** Radial nerve

3. **(b)** Common peroneal nerve
4. **(j)** Ulnar nerve
5. **(c)** Sciatic nerve
6. **(h)** Facial nerve
7. **(h)** Facial nerve

Theme 19: Diagnosis of chest pain

1. **(a)** Pericarditis
2. **(c)** Pneumonia
3. **(e)** Unstable angina
4. **(f)** Myocardial infarction
5. **(d)** Stable angina

Theme 20: Investigations of chest pain/ dyspnoea

1. **(e)** Chest X-ray
2. **(a)** V/Q scan
3. **(b)** ECG
4. **(c)** Echocardiogram

Theme 21: Diagnosis of pneumonia

1. **(a)** Streptococcus pneumoniae
2. **(b)** Legionella
3. **(c)** Mycoplasma
4. **(d)** Pneumocystis carinii

Theme 22: Terminal care

1. **(c)** Haloperidol
2. **(b)** Hyoscine
3. **(f)** Lactulose
4. **(e)** Palliative X-ray therapy
5. **(g)** Biphosphonates

Theme 23: Metabolic parameters in renal conditions

1. **(a)** Haemolytic uraemic syndrome
2. **(b)** CRF
3. **(d)** Nephrotic syndrome
4. **(e)** Acute glomerulonephritis
5. **(e)** Acute glomerulonephritis

Theme 24: Diagnosis of chronic abdominal conditions

1. **(d)** Sigmoid colon carcinoma
2. **(b)** Irritable bowel syndrome with diarrhoea
3. **(e)** Appendicular mass
4. **(a)** Ulcerative colitis

Theme 25: Management of backache

1. **(a)** Bed rest
2. **(f)** Neurological problem
3. **(e)** Skeletal metastasis

Theme 26: Epistaxis

1. **(b)** Carcinoma maxillary antrum
2. **(a)** Maxillary sinusitis
3. **(d)** Fracture ethmoid
4. **(c)** Sepsis

Theme 27: Side effects of drugs

1. **(a)** Aplastic anaemia
2. **(c)** TFTs
3. **(c)** TFTs
4. **(d)** LFTs

Theme 28: Diagnosis in haematology

1. **(a)** CLL
2. **(b)** CML
3. **(d)** Autoimmune haemolytic anaemia

Theme 29: Diagnosis of urinary obstruction

1. **(a)** BPH
2. **(c)** Clot retention
3. **(b)** Carcinoma prostate

Theme 30: Investigation in malignancies

1. **(a)** PSA
2. **(e)** Technitium scan
3. **(f)** Abdominal USG

Theme 31: Diagnosis of Acid Base disturbances

1. **(b)** Metabolic alkalosis
2. **(e)** Hypokalaemia
3. **(c)** Respiratory acidosis
4. **(f)** Renal failure

Theme 32: Management of asthma

1. **(c)** Short acting β-agonist (nebulizer)
2. **(b)** Short acting inhaled β-agonist
3. **(d)** Long acting β-agonist
4. **(k)** Avoid allergen
5. **(j)** Avoid smoking

Theme 33: Management of cancer pain

1. **(c)** Palliative X-ray
2. **(f)** Pamidronate
3. **(d)** Opiates

Theme 34: Management of shingles

1. **(b)** Oral Aciclovir
2. **(a)** IV Aciclovir
3. **(c)** Amitriptyline
4. **(c)** Amitriptyline

Theme 35: Management of meningitis

1. **(a)** Parenteral Penicillin
2. **(d)** Lumbar puncture
3. **(d)** Lumbar puncture
4. **(c)** CT scan

Theme 36: Resuscitation-immediate management post trauma

1. **(e)** Open airway
2. **(c)** Gain IV access and blood transfusion
3. **(c)** Gain IV access and blood transfusion
4. **(d)** Intubation and ventilation
5. **(f)** CT scan

Theme 37: Complications of myocardial infarction

1. **(h)** Heart block
2. **(b)** Ventricular tachycardia
3. **(e)** Pericarditis
4. **(c)** Chordae tendinae rupture of mitral valve leaflet
5. **(g)** Acute pulmonary oedema

Theme 38: Psychiatry: Diagnosis

1. **(c)** Alzheimer's dementia
2. **(a)** Delirium
3. **(a)** Delirium
4. **(e)** Korsakoff's psychosis
5. **(b)** Late onset schizophrenia

Theme 39: Prevention of bleeding

1. **(a)** Apply pressure to site of bleeding
2. **(c)** Gain IV access and immediately transfuse blood.
3. **(c)** Gain IV access and immediately transfuse blood.

Theme 40: Pre-operative investigation

1. **(a)** Spirometry
2. **(e)** Blood sugar
3. **(c)** Angiogram
4. **(f)** Echocardiogram
5. **(b)** CXR

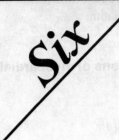

September 2002 Explanations

Theme 1: Management of diarrhoea in children

1. In cases of mild dehydration which is usually evident as decreased urinary output, the child is put on maintenance fluids.

Age (in years)	Weight (in kg)	Water (ml/kg/day)	Na+	K+
< 0.5	< 5	150	3	3
0.5–1	5–10	120	2.5	2.5
1–3	10–15	100	2.5	2.5
3–5	15–20	80	2	2
75	>20	45–75	1.5–2	1.5–2

2. As the child in this case has vomiting along with diarrhoea, energy requirements also need to be fulfilled intravenously. Thus 5% dextrose is given along with saline.

3. Dysentery is the passage of bloody diarrhoea. It may present as abdominal pain, bloody diarrhoea, fever and occasionally neck stiffness. Stool culture is the preferred investigation. Treatment is with fluids PO. As the patient is having dysentery due to shigella, ciprofloxacin BD PO is given for 5 days.

4. A bottle fed baby with diarrhoea and reducing substances in urine indicates lactose intolerance. Treatment is with lactose free diet.

Theme 2: Diagnosis of injury in children

1. History of fall implies that the injury is evidently traumatic or accidental. Lower leg swelling and deformity in this case specifically indicates a fracture. Such patients may also present with pain, swelling, crepitus and limitation of movement. X-rays of the affected site are required. Treatment depends upon the bone involved and the type of fracture.

2. Mongolian spots are bluish, well demarcated spots on the buttocks and trunk. The name is a misnomer as these are not related to Down's syndrome. They usually disappear by 1st birthday.

3. Bruises over the wrist and ankle are suggestive that the child has been tied at the wrists and ankle joints. Moreover, as the child has been brought by her step father, the suspicion of NAI is raised further.

4. In immune thrombocytopenic purpura, antiplatelet autoantibodies lead to phagocytic destruction of platelets. Acute ITP usually occurs in children and presents with sudden self limiting purpura, usually 2 weeks after infection. Antiplatelet IgG autoantibodies are positive on blood investigation and bone marrow shows

many megakaryocytes. If patient is symptomatic or has platelet count $< 20 \times 10^9$/L, prednisolone is given. Splenectomy may be considered. If these fail immunosuppressant e.g. azathioprine, ciclosporin, cyclophosphamide are given.

Note: Henoch schönlein purpura usually presents in association with nephritis i.e. an IgA nephropathy, joint involvement and abdominal pain.

5. Osteogenesis imperfecta (Adair–Dighton syndrome) is a genetic disorder characterized by tendency for frequent fractures in newborns due to weak and brittle bones. It results from defective collagen synthesis and hence absence of callus formation. Associated features are blue sclerae, joint laxity, otosclerosis in adulthood. Fractures unite normally but deformities secondary to malunion may occur. Radiographs may show fractures, osteoporotic bones with thinned out cortex and bowing deformity of long bones. Preventing injury is the best treatment. Intramedullary rods are sometimes used in long bones.

Theme 3: Investigation of wrist fractures

1. Fall on the outstretched hand may produce a fracture of the carpal bones, most commonly the scaphoid bone. This presents with tenderness in the anatomical snuff box (scaphoid fossa). A force transmitted along the 2nd metacarpal may produce pain in the region of the scaphoid bone. It is usually visualized in the oblique view radiograph of the wrist, which is thus necessary in addition to AP and lateral views. Immobilization is done in glass holding position i.e. wrist maintained in little dorsiflexion and radial deviation.

2. As explained above.

3. Compression forces cause impacted fracture. The risk of complications in such fractures are more and there is no mention of the same in the question. Therefore to rule out and treat complications if any, the case should be referred to an orthopaedician.

4. As no fracture is evident at the time of injury, the boy probably has soft tissue injury and should be discharged after being given analgesics and advice to give rest to the affected joint. However a repeat radiograph may be performed after 2 weeks, as a small fracture of the scaphoid may not be visible initially.

Theme 4: Investigation of dyspepsia

1. This is a patient of gastric ulcer which occurs mainly in the elderly and occurs on the lesser curvature of the stomach. Patients generally present with epigastric pain which occurs in the night, after meals and is relieved by antacids. Upper GI endoscopy must be performed in all patients presenting with 'alarm' symptoms which includes >45 years of age, weight loss, vomiting, haematemesis, anaemia and dysphagia.

2. Fundoplication is a surgery for gastro oesophageal reflux in which the aim is to re-establish the lower oesophageal sphincter tone. After the surgery, around 1/3rd of the patients develop new symptoms of dysphagia, bloating, increased flatulence or dyspepsia. Therefore in this patient who complains of pain in stomach after the surgery, endoscopy is required to confirm the success of the surgery done.

3. In the question, there is no mention of the treatment received by the patient till now. As the patient has had a positive *H. pylori* status, *H. pylori* serology needs to be done before starting the treatment of the patients for peptic ulcer. *H. pylori* is associated with 80–90% of the cases of peptic ulcer and eradication of *H. pylori* is a must for complete treatment of the peptic ulcer.

4. In this question the patient is a chronic case of dyspepsia. *H. pylori* is suspected in this case also. Therefore *H. pylori* serology needs to be done.

5. This patient is most probably suffering from a gastric ulcer. Smoking and stress are risk factors predisposing more to a gastric ulcer than a duodenal ulcer. Investigation of choice would be an upper GI endoscopy to rule out malignancy and take multiple biopsies from the rim and base of ulcer for histology and *H. pylori*. Moreover endoscopy is advised in all patients with 'alarm' symptoms e.g. > 45 years of age, weight loss, vomiting, haematemesis, anaemia and dysphagia.

Theme 5: Diagnosis of antepartum haemorrhage

1. Following points favour the diagnosis of abruptio placentae (i) history of hypertension. Pre-eclampsia is a risk factor associated with abruptio placentae. (ii) It presents with acute abdominal pain. Vaginal bleeding may or may not be present (concealed abruptio placentae) (iii) Uterus is tense, tender and rigid on palpation (iv) Anaemia and general condition is out of proportion to visible blood loss.

2. Following points favour the diagnosis of placenta praevia (i) presents with painless, apparently causeless (i.e. with no history of trauma etc) and recurrent bleeding (ii) commonly associated with malpresentation due to low lying placenta. Head is usually floating or is in transverse lie.

3. With the onset of labour, there is profuse cervical secretion. Simultaneously, there is slight oozing of blood from rupture of capillary vessels of the cervix and from decidual surface due to separation of membranes. This expulsion of cervical mucus, mixed with blood is called "show". This is a normal phenomenon in labour.

4. The main cause of cervical carcinoma is HPV 16, 18 and 33. Prolonged pill usage, high parity, many sexual partners, early first coitus, HIV, other STD's and smoking are risk factors. Non menstrual bleeding is a classical symptom. Early tumour is firm which grows as a friable mass and bleeds on touch. Stage I and II of cervical carcinoma are treated with Wertheims's hysterectomy or radiotherapy. Stage III needs both radiotherapy and chemotherapy. For Stage IV only palliative treatment is given.

5. Post coital bleed in 27 years old is most likely due to trauma. Cervical ectropion would have been the most appropriate answer. Cervical ectropion/erosion is noted during puberty, with the OCP use and during pregnancy. Ectropion is prone to bleeding, infection and to mucus production.

Theme 6: Diagnosis of head injury

1. Following points favour the diagnosis of subdural haematoma : (i) more common in elderly as brain shrinkage makes bridging veins more vulnerable (ii) mostly results due to trauma which may have been mild e.g. recurrent falls (iii) presents with fluctuating level of consciousness. CT. Scan of the head shows a concave or crescent shaped hyper-dense clot with or without midline shift. Treatment is with evacuation via burr holes.

2. Following points favour the diagnosis of extradural haematoma: (i) Usually occur due to trauma which may cause fracture temporal or parietal bone which further causes laceration of middle meningeal artery and vein. (ii) the injury initially produces no loss of consciousness, but later is followed by deterioration of consciousness. This 'lucid interval' pattern is typical of extradural bleeds. CT Scan of the head shows a biconvex lens shaped haematoma. Urgent evacuation of the clot through multiple burr holes with ligation of the bleeding vessel later is the management in such patients.

3. Head injury is graded as mild, moderate or severe on the basis of glasgow coma scale (GCS).

    Mild head injury – GCS 13–15.
    Moderate head injury – GCS 9–12.
    Severe head injury – GCS ≤ 8.

4. Fracture base of skull may involve the anterior or middle cranial fossa. Both may present with haemotympanum. In addition, anterior fossa fractures present with subconjunctival haema-toma, anosmia, epistaxis and CSF rhinorrhoea; whereas middle cranial fossa fractures present with CSF otorrhoea or rhinorrhoea, ossicular disruption, VII and VIII cranial nerve palsies and Battle's sign (bruising behind the ear occurring 36 hours after head injury).

5. As explained in the third question.

Theme 7: Investigation in vaginal bleed

1. Golden rule: All postmenopausal bleeding must be investigated as the cause may be endo-metrial carcinoma. Postmenopausal bleeding is an early sign of endometrial carcinoma. Further investigations require endometrial smear and uterine USG. Diagnosis is made by uterine sampling or curettage. All parts of the uterine cavity must be sampled. For stage I and II, total hysterectomy with bilateral salpingo-oophorectomy is done. Radiotherapy is given if the patient is unfit for surgery. For stages III and IV Radiotherapy and high dose progestogens are used.

2. This is probably a case of dysfunctional uterine bleeding which implies heavy and/or irregular bleeding in the absence of a recognizable pelvic pathology. It is associated with anovulatory cycles and therefore is common at the extre-mes of reproductive life. Teenage menorrhagia generally settles without any interference/ treatment as the cycles later become ovula-tory. As the patient in this condition appears exsanguinated, a full blood count is necessary to check her haemoglobin level.

3. Menorrhagia in this patient may be due to IUCD, fibroids, endometriosis, adenomyosis, pelvic infection or polyps. Vaginal ultrasound is indicated if pelvic pathology or uterine pathology is suspected.

4. Cervical ectropion also known as erosion is a normal phenomenon. It is seen temporarily due to hormonal influence during puberty, with the use of OCPs (as in this patient) or during pregnancy. As columnar epithelium is soft and glandular, it is prone to bleeding, excess mucus production and to infection. Treatment is with cautery if the condition is very disturbing otherwise no treatment is required.

Theme 8: Management of burns

1. As the patient in this case suffers from full and partial thickness burns, the swelling and tissue tension due to burns may lead to venous obstruction. There is also a possibility of muscle compartment syndrome therefore escharotomy needs to be done to avoid such complications.

2. Singed nostrils in this case are suggestive of inhalation of hot gases which may cause upper airway obstruction with passage of time. Such patients must be considered for early intubation or surgical airway.

3. Trunk escharotomy needs to be done in this case because of the risk of impairment of chest excursion.

4. Presentation of the patient with scalds and large tense blisters is suggestive of impending fluid loss and dehydration. Immediate replacement with IV fluid is imperative.

Theme 9: Mechanism of action of contraceptives

1. Chief mechanism of action of combined OCPs is inhibition of ovulation. Both oestrogen and progesterone act synergistically on the hypo-thalamo-pituitary axis and prevent the release of GnRH from the hypothalamus through a negative feedback mechanism. Thus, there is no peak release of FSH and LH from the anterior pituitary. So, follicular growth is either not initiated or if initiated, ovulation does not occur.

2. IUCDs (Intra Uterine Contraceptive Devices) induce histological and biochemical changes in the endometrium by causing a non-specific inflammatory reaction. They also increase tubal motility, which results in quick migration of the fertilized ovum into the uterine cavity before the endometrium is receptive. Both these processes result in failure of implantation.

3. Mirena coil is an IUCD which carries levonorgestrel. IUCDs (Intra Uterine Contraceptive Devices) induce histological and biochemical changes in the endometrium by causing a non-specific inflammatory reaction. They also increase tubal motility, which results in quick migration of the fertilized ovum into the uterine cavity before the endometrium is receptive. Both these processes result in failure of implantation.

4. Progesterone only pill (minipill) works mainly by making cervical mucus thick and viscous thus preventing sperm penetration. It has to be taken daily from the first day of the cycle. Chief advantage of POP is that it has no adverse effect on lactation. Also, the side effects due to oestrogen in the combined pills are totally avoided.

5. Vaginal sponge is made of synthetic polyurethane impregnated with non oxynol-9 as spermicide. It acts as a surfactant which either immobilises or kills the sperms. The sponge is inserted immediately before the

coitus into the vagina to cover the cervix. It should not be removed for 6 hours after intercourse. The sponge is for single use only over a 24 hour period.

6. Depot progesterone is given as an injectable contraceptive given intramuscularly. Two preparations are available: Depo-provera (medroxy progesterone acetate) and Noristerat (norethisterone enanthate). It acts by making cervical mucus thick and viscid, thus preventing sperm penetration and also by inhibiting ovulation. However, failure rate is higher than that for combined OCPs and there are chances of irregular bleeding and occasional amenorrhoea.

Theme 10: Management of visual loss

1. This is a case of chronic simple (open angle) glaucoma. Intraocular pressure ≥ 21 mmHg causes optic disc cupping as in this patient. Nerve damage ensues with sausage shaped field defect (scotoma). Nasal and superior fields are lost first and temporal last. High risk group include > 35 years old with positive family history, myopics, diabetic or with thyroid eye disease. Treatment includes beta blocker eye drops, pilocarpine eye drops, carbonic anhydrase inhibitors. If drugs fail surgery is indicated.

2. This is a patient of Giant cell arteritis. The typical patient will present with sudden painless loss of vision, malaise, jaw claudication and with tender scalp on temporal arteries. ESR > 40 is suggestive. Temporal artery biopsy report may be false positive in some cases and therefore is not a reliable investigation. Management includes oral prednisolone promptly as the other eye is at risk.

3. Proliferative Diabetic Retinopathy is caused due to vascular occlusion which leads to proliferation of new vessels in the retina, optic disc and iris. Patient may have cotton wool spots due to occlusion, vascular leakage, hard exudates, flame shaped haemorrhage, blot haemorrhages and is at increased risk of retinal detachment. Treatment requires good control of diabetes and photocoagulation by laser to treat both maculopathy and proliferative retinopathy.

4. This is a patient with age related macular degeneration. It is the most common cause of registrable blindness in UK. There is a loss of visual acuity, visual fields are unaffected. The disc appears normal but there is pigment, fine exudate and bleeding at the macula. Laser photocoagulation can halt the progress but otherwise there is no treatment as yet available for the condition.

5. SLE (systemic lupus erythematosus) is an autoimmune disease in which ANA (anti-nuclear antibodies) are present. Its treatment invariably requires the use of oral steroids which on long term use can cause cataract, as is mentioned in this patient as lens opacities. The only treatment for cataract is surgery.

Theme 11: Management of post menopausal conditions

1. This patient is suffering from senile/atrophic vaginitis. Dyspareunia and senile vaginitis in post menopausal women respond well to local oestrogen cream, which is preferred to oral therapy.

2. Weight gain, 'Premenstrual syndrome' are side effects of hormone replacement therapy. This patient is already complaining of weight gain and depression, therefore continuous HRT is contraindicated, rather cyclical HRT should be given.

3. Non continuous HRT is indicated in this patient as the patient has not yet achieved menopause. She has started having symptoms of flushing with mood swings and weight gain therefore non continuous HRT is indicated.

4. This is a case of vaginal prolapse. Vaginal prolapse in the elderly is preferably treated by Le Fort's repair or colpocleisis. However, if the patient is unfit for surgery, ring pessary may be used to hold the prolapse back. However this form of management is only palliative, not curative.

5. Subcutaneous oestrogen implantation is res-tricted in UK to patients who have undergone hysterectomy with or without oophorectomy. It involves positioning of a pellet of oestradiol in the subcutaneous tissue, usually in the lower abdomen. Such implants are reviewed at 6 monthly intervals and are generally well tolerated. This mode of treatment successfully treats menopausal symptoms and also protects against bone loss.

6. This patient is suffering from osteoporosis. Osteoporosis means decreased bone density. Exercise, calcium rich diet, avoiding smoking and excess alcohol all help in the management of osteoporosis. HRT decreases the risk of fracture if given for 5–10 years post meno-pausally. This patient has already been diag-

nosed with osteoporosis, therefore biphos-phonates are the definitive treatment. It is used both for treating and preventing osteoporosis. It also decreases fracture rate. Alendronate is licensed for osteoporosis treatment in UK.

7. Vaginal pruritus may be due to varied reasons such as psoriasis, lichen planus, infection, infestation (scabies, pubic lice, threadworm), or vulval dystrophy (lichen sclerosis, leukoplakia). As in this case the patient is diabetic, the possibility of the aetiology of the pruritus is likely to be infection. Therefore infection preventive measures should be taken.

Theme 12: Investigation of acute abdomen

1. The presentation of patient in this case with board like rigidity and no bowel sounds is suggestive of peritonitis. Peritonitis may be due to perforation of peptic ulcer, diverticulum, appendix, bowel or gall bladder. History of APD in this case is further suggestive of perforation of peptic ulcer. Erect CXR may show gas under diaphragm. Laparotomy is required in this case.

2. This is a case of ruptured aortic aneurysm. Patients may present with intermittent or continuous abdominal pain radiating to the back, iliac fossae or groins, collapse and an expansile abdominal mass. If in doubt, assume a ruptured aneurysm. Take the patient straight to theatre for a laparotomy and do not waste precious time in X-rays.

3. The presentation of pain starting in the loin and radiating to the groin is suggestive of renal colic. Such patients must have a renal ultra-sound done to rule out nephrolithiasis. Treat-ment is with antispasmodics, IV fluids and analgesics.

4. This is possibly a case of appendicular mass. The presentation of the patient is suggestive of an attack of acute appendicitis. Appendicular mass i.e. inflamed appendix surrounded by omentum, is a complication of acute appendicitis. It can be palpated in the right iliac fossa. Management in such cases is preferably by observation and conservative treatment by Ochsner–Sherran regimen. Patient is kept NPO, a nasogastric tube is passed and IV fluids and antibiotics are started.

5. This can be a case of splenic trauma. As there is no mention of hypotension/shock, urgent laparotomy is not required. Abdominal ultrasound needs to be done to confirm the site and extent of injury.

Theme 13: Diagnosis of deafness

1. Noise induced.
2. Temporary shift of threshold.
3. Ménière's disease is a condition in which there is dilatation of the endolymphatic space of the membranous labyrinth causing vertigo with prostation, nausea, vomiting, tinnitus with or without progressive sensorineural hearing loss. Treatment of acute vertigo requires cyclizine. Surgical decompression of the endolymphatic sac may relieve vertigo, prevent progress of disease and conserve hearing.
4. Temporary shift of threshold.
5. Otosclerosis is an autosomal dominant hereditary disorder with incomplete penetration. Half of the patients have a family history of the disorder, as in this patient. In this condition the vascular spongy bone replaces the normal lamellar bone of otic capsule origin especially around the oral window which fixes the stapes foot plate. Symptoms are usually seen in adulthood and are exacerbated due to pregnancy, menstruation and menopause. Hearing is often better with background noise. Surgical treatment involves stapedectomy or stapedotomy.

Theme 14: Investigation of epilepsy

1. The patient in this case has history of being given increased dosage of the anticonvulsant in the past. The blood levels of the drug need to be checked here for two reasons: (i) to make sure that the drug level in the blood is within the therapeutic range (ii) to avoid reaching toxic levels in the blood.
2. This is a case of secondary generalized seizure, which is a type of partial seizure. EEG being a baseline investigation in epilepsy, needs to be done. CT scan of the head would then be the next investigation. Electroencephalography is useful for distinguishing the various types of seizures. For example, there may be confusion between disturbances of consciousness due to typical absences, and disturbances due to complex partial seizures. The distinction is important not only for the right therapy to be given, but also has prognostic value.
3. This is case of generalized tonic clonic i.e. classical grand mal seizure. Again EEG would be the initial investigation before proceeding to CT Scan of the head. Electroencephalography is useful for distinguishing the various types of seizures. For example, there may be confusion between disturbances of consciousness due to typical absences, and disturbances due to complex partial seizures. The distinction is important not only for the right therapy to be given, but also has prognostic value.
4. This patient is a suspected case of space occupying lesion in the brain which is presenting as headache, diplopia and seizures. To rule out or diagnose an SOL in the brain CT scan of the head needs to be done which will be more diagnostic than an EEG.

Theme 15: Investigation of stroke

1. Golden rule: Fever with a new murmur is endocarditis until proved otherwise. Gall bladder diseases and surgery are risk factors for endocarditis. Infective endocarditis is a well known risk factor for heart emboli which may further be a cause of stroke. The investigation of choice in patients with infective endocarditis is blood culture.

2. Carotid bruits may signify stenosis especially near the origin of the internal carotid artery. The usual cause is an atheroma. The risk of stroke in symptomless patients is very small. As this patient is presenting with hemiparesis, carotid doppler needs to be done to measure the degree of stenosis. Angiography and endarterectomy is justified if stenosis > 80%.

3. Neck stiffness can be seen in subarachnoid haemorrhage, Meningitis and shigella infection. Patient is also drowsy which is suggestive of meningitis. Though lumbar puncture is critical to diagnosis but as there is drowsiness in the patient (a sign of raised ICT), blood culture becomes the first investigation to be done.

4. An irregularly irregular pulse is suggestive of Atrial fibrillation. AF is a risk factor for cardiac emboli which further is a chief cause of stroke. Therefore a CT scan of the head needs to be done to exclude a haemorrhagic stroke before starting aspirin.

Theme 16: Diagnosis of dementia

1. Alzheimer's dementia is the most common form of dementia in UK. Suspect AD in any enduring, acquired deficit of memory and cognition. Onset may be from 40 years though it may be seen earlier in patients suffering from Down's syndrome. On histological examination plaques with neurofibrillary tangles and cortical β-amyloid protein are found. On MRI an increased cortical atrophy in the medial temporal lobe can be seen. In stage I of AD there is falling memory and spatial disorientation. In stage II the personality disintegrates and in stage III the patient is apathetic, wasted and bedridden.

2. As explained above.

3. Pseudodementia is a term applied to patients who are depressed and who apparently are demented. These patients often complain about their memory problems rather them covering then up. Such patients improve dramatically with their improvement in the depressed status.

4. Huntington's chorea is an autosomal dominant condition with onset of the disease in middle age. Initially chorea is noticed which is followed by irritability and then dementia with or without seizures. The life span of these patients is much shorter. The basic pathology in such patient is the reduced number of corpus striatum GABAnergic and cholinergic neurons. There is no treatment as yet available for the disease. Counselling of the patient and the family should be done.

5. This is a case of multi-infarct or vascular dementia in which hypertension is a risk factor. Such patients are characterized by psycho-motor slowing, reduced attention, loss of executive function and personality changes.

Theme 17: Investigation of thyroid conditions

1. In healthy young adults thyroxine is given for the treatment of hypothyroidism. The dose is adjusted clinically so as to normalize the TSH levels which are checked annually. In patients with preexisting heart disease especially the elderly, the dosage needs to be assessed accurately by measuring TSH levels every 4 weekly. If the diagnosis is in question stop thyroxine and recheck TSH in 6 weeks.

2. The normal thyroid gland is impalpable. Goitre implies generalized enlargement of the gland. A simple i.e. euthyroid goitre can be either diffuse hyperplastic or multinodular. Diffuse hyperplastic goitre can be seen at puberty when metabolic demands are high. This is known as puberty goitre. If TSH stimulation ceases, the goitre may regress but can recur later at times of stress e.g. pregnancy. Such goitres are soft, diffuse and do not require any other investigation.

3. This is a case of hyperthyroidism. Patient may present with weight loss, heat intolerance, sweating, diarrhoea, tremors, irritability, emotional lability, psychosis, oligomenorrhoea, tachycardia, AF, lid lag, goitre ± nodules. Investigations include TSH which will be decreased and free T_3 and T_4 which will be increased. Treatment options include carbimazole, propylthiouracil, partial thyroidectomy, radioiodine. Propranolol can be given for symptomatic relief.

4. As the nature of the swelling is not mentioned here, one needs to rule out malignancy. Around 10% of single thyroid lumps are malignant. Other causes of a single thyroid lump include a cyst, adenoma and nodule in a multinodular goitre. Ultrasound of the thyroid needs to be done to see if the swelling is solid, cystic or part of a group of lumps.

5. The possibility of the lesion, being malignant is very high in this case because USG has already shown that the nodular lesion is not cystic. Therefore fine needle aspiration and cytology of the fluid needs to be done to rule out malignancy.

Theme 18: Diagnosis of nerve injury

1. Injury to the shoulder and a region of anaesthesia over the lower part of shoulder or deltoid area is suggestive of an anterior shoulder dislocation with injury to the axillary nerve. (Cutaneous branch of the axillary nerve supplies the upper lateral part of the arm).

2. Fracture of the shaft of the humerus is often caused by a fall on an outstreched hand. Radial nerve is the nerve of extension of the elbow, wrist and fingers. Its injury can cause wrist drop.

3. Lateral popliteal nerve is also known as common peroneal nerve (L4–S2). A lesion or injury to the nerve causes equinovarus with inability to dorsiflex the foot and toes–'foot drop'. Sensory loss is seen over the dorsum of the foot.

4. Ulnar nerve can be damaged in association with a medial epicondyle fracture. Ulnar nerve (C8–T1) is the nerve of finger abduction and adduction. There is sensory loss over the little finger and variable area of ring finger.

5. Sciatic nerve (L4–S2) supplies the hamstring muscles, hip abductors and all muscles below the knee. Injury to the nerve may cause severe lower leg and hamstring weakness, flail foot and severe disability and loss of sensation below the knee laterally.

6. Anterior two thirds of the tongue is supplied by the chorda tympani component of the facial nerve. Loss of taste sensation in this region is due to lesion in the middle ear portion of the facial nerve.

7. The chief function of the VIIth cranial nerve i.e. the facial nerve is the supply of motor fibres to the muscles of facial expression. In Idiopathic (Bell's) palsy, the site of damage to the nerve is probably the labyrinthine portion within the facial canal. Patient can have hyperacusis if nerve to stapedius is involved. LMN lesions, cause loss of frontal wrinkling on ipsilateral side with positive Bell's sign and loss of nasolabial fold. In UMN lesions the function of muscles in upper face are preserved and loss of nasolabial fold is seen in the ipsilateral side with deviation of mouth to the normal side. The chorda tympani fibres are often affected so that taste is impaired on the anterior 2/3rd of the tongue. Treatment requires a short course of dexamethasone and physiotherapy if required.

Theme 19: Diagnosis of chest pain

1. Dressler's syndrome develops 2–10 weeks after an MI. The patient may suffer from recurrent fever, chest pain, pleural and pericardial rub, pleural effusions, anaemia and raised ESR. Treatment is with NSAIDs and steroids.

2. The presentation of this patient with fever, cough, chest pain is suggestive of pneumonia. Other features that may be present in patients with pneumonia are malaise, anorexia, cough, purulent sputum, haemoptysis, pleuritic chest pain, tachypnoea, hypotension and signs of consolidation. Investigations required are CXR, sputum for microscopy and cultures and pleural aspirate (if present) for culture. Treatment involves antibiotics according to sensitivity patterns.

3. Angina is due to myocardial ischaemia and presents as central chest heaviness, tightness or pain which is brought on by exertion. It may also be precipitated by emotion, cold weather and heavy meals. Stable angina is induced by exertion and relieved by rest. Unstable i.e. crescendo angina is of increasing frequency or severity and occurs with minimal exertion or even at rest as in this patient.

4. Myocardial infarction is usually due to occlusion of a coronary artery resulting from rupture of an atheromatous plaque. Patient usually present with acute chest pain lasting > 20 minute. MI is associated with nausea, sweatiness, dyspnoea and palpitations. In elderly or diabetics, MI may also present without chest pain (silent MI). On examination there may be pallor, distress, sweatiness and 4th heart sound. ECG changes—Q waves (as in this case) signify transmural infarction. Hyperacute T waves and ST elevation are also seen. Non Q wave infarct means a subendocardial infarct. Other investigations required are cardiac enzymes CK, AST, LDH which are elevated. Troponin T is also elevated. Treatment involves aspirin stat, analgesia with morphine, O_2, thrombolysis with streptokinase or t-PA.

5. As explained in the third question.

Theme 20: Investigations of chest pain/dyspnoea

1. The presentation of cough with sputum, fever and chest pain is suggestive of pneumonia. The presentation of this patient with fever, cough, chest pain is suggestive of pneumonia. Other features that may be present in patients with pneumonia are malaise, anorexia, cough, purulent sputum, haemoptysis, pleuritic chest pain, tachypnoea, hypotension and signs of consolidation. Investigations required are CXR, sputum for microscopy and cultures and pleural aspirate (if present) for culture. Treatment involves antibiotics according to sensitivity patterns.

2. Pulmonary embolism usually arises from a venous thrombus in the pelvis or legs. Risk factors include history of DVT, OCPs, immobility and hypercoagulability. Patients may present with breathlessness, pleuritic chest pain, fever, haemoptysis, tachycardia, gallop rhythm, hypotension, raised JVP and pleural rub. ECG may be normal. CXR may show oligaemia of the affected segment, dilated pulmonary artery. The investigation of choice is CT pulmonary angiography. If unavailable V/Q scan should be done. Low molecular weight heparin is used to anticoagulate.

3. Myocardial infarction is usually due to occlusion of a coronary artery resulting from rupture of an atheromatous plaque. Patient usually present with acute chest pain lasting > 20 minute. MI is associated with nausea, sweatiness, dyspnoea and palpitations. In elderly or diabetics, MI may also present without chest pain (silent MI). On examination there may be pallor, distress, sweatiness and 4th heart sound. ECG changes—Q waves (as in this case) signify transmural infarction. Hyperacute T waves and ST elevation are also seen. Non Q wave infarct means a subendocardial infarct. Other investigations required are cardiac enzymes CK, AST, LDH which are elevated. Troponin T is also elevated. Treatment involves aspirin stat, analgesia with morphine, O_2, thrombolysis with streptokinase or t-PA.

4. The presence of murmur along with the complaint of palpitations suggests a cardiac aetiology. Therefore an echocardiography needs to be done to assess the site and extent of the pathology.

Theme 21: Diagnosis of pneumonia

1. Pneumonia is an acute lower respiratory tract illness associated with fever, signs and symptoms in the chest and abnormalities on the CXR. Pneumococcal pneumonia is the most common bacterial pneumonia. It is more common in elderly, alcoholics and immuno-suppressed patients. It may present with fever, pleurisy, herpes labialis. CXR may show lobar consolidation. Treatment is with ampicillin or cefuroxime.

2. Legionella colonizes in water tanks kept at < 60°C. Fever, malaise, myalgia precede dry cough and dyspnoea. Patient may have history of travel or stay in a hotel or attending any conference. CXR shows bibasal consolidation. Treatment is with high dose erythromycin.

3. Mycoplasma pneumoniae may present with headache, myalgia, arthralgia followed by dry cough. CXR shows bilateral patchy consolidation. Diagnosis is with mycoplasma serology. Cold agglutinins may cause autoimmune hemolytic anaemia. Treatment is with erythromycin or tetracycline.

4. Pneumocystis carinii pneumonia (PCP) is seen in the immunosuppressed e.g. HIV. It presents as dry cough, exertional dyspnoea, fever and crepts. CXR may show perihilar insterstitial shadowing. Diagnosis is by visualization of the organism. Treatment is with co-trimoxazole IV or pentamidine.

Theme 22: Terminal care

1. Parenteral haloperidol is sometimes used for intractable hiccups.

2. Hyoscine is an anticholinergic drug which is less potent and longer acting than atropine. It is used for oesophageal and gastrointestinal spastic conditions. It decreases secretions from various glands such as sweat, salivary, tracheobronchial and lacrimal glands. Its side effects include dry mouth and blurred vision.

3. Specific treatment of hepatic encephalopathy is aimed at (i) elimination or treatment of precipitating factors (ii) lowering of blood ammonia levels. Lactulose, an osmotic laxative decreases ammonia absorption. Moreover metabolism of lactulose in the gut results in an acidic pH which favours conversion of ammonia to ammonium ion which is poorly absorbed. In addition, lactulose may actually decrease ammonia production.

4. The analgesic 'ladder' consists broadly of three steps. Step I includes non-opioid analgesics like aspirin, paracetamol and NSAIDs. Step II includes weak opioids such as codeine, dihydrocodeine and dextropropoxyphene. Step III includes strong opioids such as morphine, diamorphine and hydromorphine. The presentation in the patient is suggestive of bony metastasis in which even strong opioids are usually ineffective for pain relief. Radiotherapy is the mainstay in such patients for pain relief. 8–30 Gy dosage is delivered in 1, 2, 5 or 10 fractions.

5. This is a patient with hypercalcaemia, due to multiple myeloma. A single dose of pamidronate (biphosphonate) will lower calcium levels over 2–3 days. They inhibit osteoclast activity and so bone resorption.

Theme 23: Metabolic parameters in renal conditions.

1. Haemolytic uraemic syndrome is characterized by microangiopathic haemolytic anaemia, thrombocytopenia and ARF. It is the most common cause of ARF in children. Tests show $\downarrow$ Hb, $\downarrow$ platelets, $\downarrow$ Na^+, $\uparrow$Neutrophils, $\uparrow$ Urea, $\uparrow$ Creatinine, $\uparrow$ Urate, $\uparrow$ bilirubin, $\uparrow$ LDH, $\uparrow$ reticulocytes and fragmented RBCs i.e. schistocytes. Treat hypovolaemia or hypertension.

2. Tests done in CRF may show normocytic, normochromic anaemia, $\uparrow$ urea, $\uparrow$ creatinine, $\uparrow$ phosphate, $\uparrow$ PTH, $\downarrow$ calcium, $\uparrow$ alkaline phosphatase, $\uparrow$ potassium and $\downarrow$ pH.

3. Nephrotic syndrome by definition means combination of proteinuria (> 3 gm/day), hypoalbuminaemia (< 30 gm/L) and oedema.

4. Acute Glomerulonephritis patients can have extracellular fluid volume expansion, oedema, hypertension due to impaired GRF and increased tubular absorption of salt and water. Haematuria is often macroscopic. The classic pathologic correlate of RPGN is crescent formation involving most glomeruli, crescents being half-moon shaped lesions in Bowman's space.

5. As explained above.

Theme 24: Diagnosis of chronic abdominal conditions

1. Sigmoid colon cancer may present as bleeding PR, altered bowel habit, tenesmus, mass PR, abdominal mass, obstruction, perforation, haemorrhage, fistula, weight loss or anaemia. Neoplastic polyps, UC, familial polyposis, previous cancer and low fibre diet are predisposing factors. Sigmoid colectomy is done for tumours of sigmoid colon. Anterior resection can be done for low sigmoid tumours.

2. Irritable bowel syndrome is a group of abdominal symptoms for which no organic cause can be found. Patients are usually 20–40 years old and affects women more than men. Patients may present with central or lower abdominal pain (relieved by defecation), altered bowel habit i.e. constipation alternating with diarrhoea, tenesmus and mucus PR. Generalized abdominal tenderness may be seen. No treatment but symptomatic relief can be provided to the patient.

3. This is possibly a case of appendicular mass. The presentation of the patient is suggestive of an attack of acute appendicitis. Appendicular mass i.e. inflamed appendix surrounded by omentum, is a complication of acute appendicitis. It can be palpated in the right iliac fossa. Management in such cases is preferably by observation and conservative treatment by Ochsner–Sherran regimen. Patient is kept NPO, a nasogastric tube is passed and IV fluids and antibiotics are started.

4. Ulcerative colitis is an inflammatory disorder of the colonic mucosa and it never spreads proximal to the ileocaecal valve. It is more common in non smokers than smokers!. Patients typically present with gradual onset of diarrhoea mixed with blood and mucus. It is also associated with aphthous ulcers, erythema nodosum, pyoderma gangrenosum, conjunctivitis, sacroiliitis and cholangio-

carcinoma. Toxic dilatation of the colon can occur. Sigmoidoscopy shows inflammed, friable mucosa. Barium enema shows loss of haustra and granular mucosa. Treatment is with prednisolone and sulfasalazine.

Theme 25: Management of backache

1. The history of backache in this patient is suggestive of a mechanical cause of backache. Pain is worse on movement and relieved by rest in such patients. Such patients should avoid such precipitants and should learn safe lifting skills with back straight.
2. This is a case of acute cauda equina compression. Such patients present with alternating or bilateral root pain in legs, saddle anaesthesia (bilaterally around anus) and disturbance of bowel and/or bladder function. Surgery is indicated in such patients.
3. The presentation of patient in this case is suggestive of a primary lung carcinoma with bony metastasis which is further leading to acute cord compression. The exact cause and site of the compression can be ascertained by X-rays.

Theme 26: Epistaxis

1. Carcinoma maxillary sinus is more common in men aged 40–60 years. Early features include nasal stuffiness, blood stained nasal discharge, headache, facial paraesthesia and epiphora. Further, spread to the nasal cavity can cause nasal obstruction and epistaxis. Anterior spread causes swelling of the cheek and invasion of facial skin. It may also spread superiorly and inferiorly causing proptosis, diplopia, ocular pain, epiphora, dental pain, loosening of teeth, ulceration of the gingiva etc. X-ray of the sinus may show clouding. Treatment consists of combination of radiotherapy and surgery.

2. Sinusitis is inflammation of the air filled cavities in the bones around the nose. It can be either acute or chronic. Both may present with pain over the affected sinus which increases on bending forwards, discharge from the nose, nasal obstruction or congestion, anosmia, cacosmia and even fever. Treatment is with rest, decongestants, analgesics or function endoscopic sinus surgery (FESS) for chronic cases.

3. Fractures through the roof of the ethmoid labyrinth may cause CSF rhinorrhoea. The nasal discharge would test positive for glucose. Generally such leaks stop spontaneously, if not neurosurgical closure of the dura is indicated.

4. Polypectomy is generally done by endoscopy. One of the post-operative complications is bleeding. Post-operative douches may be given with or without topical steroids.

Theme 27: Side effects of drugs

1. Of all the drugs, chloramphenicol is the most important cause of aplastic anaemia, agranulocytosis, thrombocytopenia and pancytopenia. Other side effects of chloramphenicol include hypersensitivity reactions and Gray baby syndrome.

2. The dose of lithium given should aim to achieve a plasma level of ~0.7–1.0 mmol/L. Early signs of toxicity can be seen at plasma levels of ~1.5 mmol/L of lithium. Features of lithium toxicity include blurred vision, diarrhoea and vomiting, hypokalaemia, drowsiness, ataxia, coarse tremors, dysarthria, hyperextension, seizures, psychosis, coma and shock.

3. The presentation of the patient is suggestive of hypothyroidism which is a feature seen on long term use of lithium.

4. Carbamazepine is an antiepileptic drug used as 1st line in partial seizures. Its toxic effects include hyponatraemia which is the cause of confusion in this patient. Other toxic effects include rash, nausea, diplopia, dizziness, fluid retention and blood dyscrasias.

Theme 28: Diagnosis in haematology

1. Chronic lymphocytic leukaemia has 0–IV staging and is seen in > 40 years age. Male : Female ratio is 2:1. It is due to monoclonal proliferation of small lymphocytes (B cell). Patients may present with bleeding infection, enlarged rubbery nontender lymph nodes, splenomegaly, weight loss and anorexia. Patients have a normocytic normochromic anaemia with positive coombs test. Auto-immune haemolytic anaemia can be seen in CLL. Treatment is with chemotherapy–chlorambucil. Radiotherapy is given for enlarged lymph nodes or splenomegaly.

2. Chronic myeloid leukaemia has 3 phases viz Chronic, Accelerated and Blast transformation phase. It is seen mostly in the middle aged and affects males more than females. Patients may present with bleeding, bruising, spleno-megaly, hepatomegaly, fever and weight loss. Investigations show ↑ WCC, ↑ Platelets, ↑ Urate, ↑ Alk PO$_4$ase, ↓ LAP and Philadel-phia chromosome (its absence is a poor prog-nostic factor). Treatment is with hydroxyurea in chronic phase and allogenic bone marrow transplantation.

3. Autoimmune haemolytic anaemia is due to warm or cold antibodies. Warm AHA presents as acute or chronic anaemia for which steroids with/without splenectomy is the treatment. Cold AHA constitute chronic anaemia made worse by cold and therefore patients are to be kept warm.

Theme 29: Diagnosis of urinary obstruction

1. Benign prostatic hypertrophy is a common problem. Decrease in urinary flow is associated with increased frequency, urgency and voiding difficulty. Treatment involves mainly surgical (e.g. TURP, TUIP, TULIP, Retropubic prostatectomy) and in some cases medical (e.g. α blockers, 5 α reductase inhibitors) approach.

2. This is a patient with transitional cell car-cinoma which may arise in the bladder, ureter or renal pelvis. It is seen after 40 years of age with 4 times predilection towards males. Smoking, cyclophosphamide, azo dyes, β naphthalene and schistosomiasis are risk factors. Patients may present with painless haematuria, dysuria, urinary tract obstruction, frequency or urgency.

3. This is a case of prostatic carcinoma. Prostatic carcinoma is the 2nd most common malig-nancy in men. Incidence increases with age and is associated with increased levels of testosterone and a positive family history. Patients may present with nocturia, hesitancy, poor stream or urinary obstruction. Weight loss and bone pain are suggestive of metastasis. PR examination may reveal hard, irregular prostate gland. Diagnosis is by measuring serum prostate specific antigen levels and doing transrectal USG and biopsy.

Theme 30: Investigation in malignancies

1. This is a case of prostatic carcinoma. Prostatic carcinoma is the 2nd most common malignancy in men. Incidence increases with age and is associated with increased levels of testosterone and a positive family history. Patients may present with nocturia, hesitancy, poor stream or urinary obstruction. Weight loss and bone pain are suggestive of metastasis. PR examination may reveal hard, irregular prostate gland. Diagnosis is by measuring serum prostate specific antigen levels and doing transrectal USG and biopsy. Treatment options for local disease include radical prosta-tectomy, radiotherapy and waiting and watching serial PSA levels. For metastatic disease hormonal drugs e.g. Gonadotropin releasing analogues and analgesia are the options. Radiotherapy can be given to patients with bony metastasis presenting with backache.

2. Severe backache in this patient is due to bony metastasis for which radiotherapy is given. A bone scan is required to look for other sites of metastasis as well. Bony metastasis is usually through haematogenous route in prostatic carcinoma.

3. Prostatic carcinoma can spread locally via the lymph nodes to seminal vesicles, bladder and rectum. Obstruction due to the carcinoma can be a cause of chronic renal failure which would be seen on abdominal (or renal) ultrasound as small kidneys.

Theme 31: Diagnosis of Acid–Base disturbances

1. This is a case of metabolic alkalosis in which there is an increase in the pH along with incre-ase in HCO_3^-. Various causes for metabolic alkalosis include vomiting (especially severe and projectile, as in this patient), hypokalaemia (either due to diuretic use or simply vomiting) burns or due to ingestion of base.

2. Hypokalaemia is defined as K^+ level < 2.5 mmol/L. It presents with muscle weakness, hypotonia, tetany and cardiac arrhythmias. ECG changes include inverted T waves and prominent U waves. The causes of hypo-kalaemia include villous adenoma of rectum and diarrhoea, as in this patient. Other causa-tive factors are diuretics, vomiting, Cushing's syndrome, Conn's syndrome, renal tubular failure and steroid use. Treatment includes oral or IV supplements of potassium and treating the cause.

3. This is a patient with respiratory acidosis in which there, is a decrease in the pH along with increase in CO_2 levels. Any lung, neuro-muscular or physical cause of respiratory failure such as pneumonia, pulmonary embo-lism (as in this case), pulmonary oedema, asthma, emphysema, ARDS, Guillian Barrè syndrome, diaphragmatic paralysis etc can cause respiratory acidosis. The PaO_2 levels are generally low and patient would need O_2 therapy. In patients with COPD, O_2 needs to be judiciously given as too much O_2 can make matters worse.

4. The presentation of the patient suggests the diagnosis of renal failure. Most likely this patient suffers from chronic renal failure as the signs of anaemia and dry skin are present in the patient. But the presence of anaemia, decreased calcium or increased phosphates may not help distinguish ARF from CRF, though their absence suggests ARF.

Theme 32: Management of asthma

1. Asthma implies reversible obstruction of the airways. Patient may present with wheeze dyspnoea or cough. It may be life threatening if peak flow < 33%, presence of cyanosis, silent chest, fatigue or exhaustion, agitation, decrease level of consciousness. Steps in management: (i) T by occasional β agonists (ii) Add inhaled steroids or cortons (sodium cromoglycate) (iii) Add inhaled salmeterol or increased dose of steroid (iv) Try oral theophylline/salmeterol or inhaled ipratropium (v) Add prednisolone tablets. In case of severe asthma give high flow 100% O_2 → Nebulized salbutamol→Oral prednisolone→ Amino-phylline→Hydrocortisone with nebulized, ipratropium→Oximetry and CXR→Treat any pneumonia→Repeat nebulizer as needed→ Take to ITU if peak flow continues to fall.

2. As explained above.

3. Asthma implies reversible obstruction of the airways. Patient may present with wheeze dyspnoea or cough. It may be life threatening if peak flow < 33%, presence of cyanosis, silent chest, fatigue or exhaustion, agitation, decrease level of consciousness. Management of asthma in adults is slightly different from that in paediatric age group. Management steps: (i) Occasional inhaled $β_2$ agonists (ii) Add inhaled steroid (iii) increase dose of inhaled steroid or try long acting inhaled $β_2$ agonist e.g. salmeterol (iv) Add $\geq$ 1 of the following:

   a. Inhaled long acting $β_2$ agonist
   b. modified release theophylline
   c. Inhaled ipratropium
   d. Oral $β_2$ agonist
   e. High dose inhaled bronchodilator or cromoglycate

   (v) Add oral prednisolone.

4. The precipitating factor, according to the presentation of the patient is cat's fur therefore the allergen should be avoided.

5. The precipitating factor, according to the presentation of the patient is smoke therefore smoking should be avoided near the child.

Theme 33: Management of cancer pain

1. The analgesic 'ladder' consists broadly of three steps. Step I includes non-opioid analgesics like aspirin, paracetamol and NSAIDs. Step II includes weak opioids such as codeine, dihydrocodeine and dextropropoxyphene. Step III includes strong opioids such as morphine, diamorphine and hydromorphine. The presentation in the patient is suggestive of bony metastasis in which even strong opioids are usually ineffective for pain relief. Radiotherapy is the mainstay in such patients for pain relief. 8–30 Gy dosage is delivered in 1, 2, 5 or 10 fractions.

2. This is a patient with hypercalcaemia, due to multiple myeloma. A single dose of pamidronate (biphosphonate) will lower calcium levels over 2–3 days. They inhibit osteoclast activity and so bone resorption.

3. A patient of carcinoma breast with pain in the elbow is suggestive of metastasis. In such patients NSAIDs will not be able to provide symptomatic relief. Strong opioids are required to relieve patients of such pains.

Theme 34: Management of shingles

1. Ophthalmic herpes is the infection of 1st branch of Trigeminal nerve. Pain, tingling or numbness around the eye may precede a blistering rash. Nose tip involvement means involvement of the nasociliary branch of trigeminal nerve. This is also known as Hutchinson's sign. Treatment is with Aciclovir 800 mg 5 times daily PO for a week.

2. All patients of herpes who have ophthalmic involvement, motor involvement, are aged > 50 years and who are immunocompromised require treatment. Aciclovir should be given as early as possible. As the patient is immuno-compromised in this case, Aciclovir 10 mg/kg/8 hourly is given IV for 10 days.

3. Patients with herpes who develop herpetic neuralgia require oral analgesics or low dose amitriptyline for control of pain. Patients with post herpetic neuralgia may require carbamazepine, phenytoin or capsaicin cream.

4. As explained above.

Theme 35: Management of meningitis

1. The presentation of the child, with fever and rash over his whole body is suggestive of meningococcal meningitis. Diagnosis is by visualization of Gram negative cocci in pairs. But any rash with signs of meningism is to be treated as meningococcal until proved otherwise. Benzylpenicillin is the drug of choice for meningococcal meningitis. Infact not giving benzylpenicillin in this case may be counted as negligence.

2. Lumbar puncture is done for the diagnosis of meningitis unless contraindications for LP are present.

CSF examination	Pyogenic	Tubercular	Viral (aseptic)
1. Appearance	Turbid	Fibrin web	Clear
2. Predominant cell	Neutrophils	Mononuclear	Mononuclear
3. Cell counts/mm3	90–1000+	10–1000	50–1000/
4. Glucose	< ½ plasma	<½ plasma	>½ plasma
5. Protein	> 1.5	1–5	< 1

3. A trip to SE Asia in this case is suggestive of tubercular aetiology for meningitis. The CSF examination in such patients will be diagnostic.

4. Raised ICP can present as headache, irritability, drowsiness, vomiting, fits, listlessness, bradycardia, hypertension, Cheyne–Stokes respiration and papilloedema. Raised ICP is a contraindication for lumbar puncture therefore do a CT scan of the head first to rule out mass lesion or hydrocephalus.

Theme 36: Resuscitation–immediate management post trauma

1. Rattly breath sounds in this patient suggests that the airway is not clear which could be due to secretions or a sternoclavicular fracture. In this condition the patients' airway needs to be cleared.

2. Femoral shaft fracture can lead to blood loss of upto 1–1.5 litres. The presentation of thigh deformity, ecchymosis, tachycardia, hypotension and pallor are all suggestive of acute and severe blood loss due to femoral fracture. Therefore the patient requires immediate IV access and blood transfusion.

3. The site of the injury and the presentation of the patient suggests a ruptured spleen. Splenic rupture can present as shock, abdominal tenderness and distension, left shoulder tip pain and with overlying rib fractures. The extent of blood loss in this patient is also severe as is apparent from her BP recording and cold peripheries. Therefore the patient in this case also requires IV access and blood transfusion.

4. GCS of 3 implies no response to pain, no verbalization and no eye opening. The patient can be declared dead at this score if other signs of brain death are evident. In this case scenario, as there is no mention of such signs, we presume the patient is in coma. Indications for ventilation include a GCS of ≤ 8, $PaO_2 < 9$ kPa in air, $PaCO_2 > 6$ kPa, spontaneous hyperventilation and respiratory irregularity.

5. One of the causes of raised ICT is head injury. Patients with raised ICT may present with headache, drowsiness, falling pulse and rising BP (Cushing's reflex), coma, Cheyne–stokes respiration and pupil changes. CT scan of the head is a baseline investigation in such cases to exactly define and grade the severity of raised ICT.

Theme 37: Complications of myocardial infarction

1. Bradycardia and heart block are common post MI complications. Patients may have (i) sinus bradycardia requiring atropine IV (ii) 1st degree AV block requiring close observation (iii) Wenckebach block (iv) Mobitz type II block which should be paced (v) complete AV block requiring a pacemaker and (vi) Bundle branch block requiring pacing.

2. Tachyarrhythmias are also a common post MI complication. The patient in this case is of ventricular tachycardia. Hypokalaemia, hypoxia and acidosis predispose to such complications. Lignocaine is given if the patient is haemodynamically stable. If that fails, a DC shock and then procainamide are tried.
   Note: In atrial fibrillation the pulse is irregularly irregular and the pulse rate is > 150 bpm.

3. Pericarditis can be present in post MI patients as such and also as a part of Dressler's syndrome which includes recurrent pericarditis, pleural effusions, fever, anaemia and raised ESR. Patients with pericarditis complain of central chest pain relieved by sitting forwards. Their ECG will show a saddle shaped ST elevation and treatment is with NSAIDs.

4. Mitral regurgitation after an MI may be mild due to minor papillary muscle dysfunction or severe due to chordal or papillary muscle rupture. Patients may present with a pansystolic murmur and/or pulmonary oedema.

5. Severe pulmonary oedema can be due to left ventricular failure especially post MI or ischaemic heart disease. Patients will present with dyspnoea, orthopnoea, distress, pallor, sweatiness, tachycardia, pink frothy sputum, wheeze (cardiac asthma), pulsus alternans, raised JVP, fine lung crepts and gallop rhythm.

Theme 38: Psychiatry: Diagnosis

1. Alzheimer's dementia is the most common form of dementia in UK. Suspect AD in any enduring, acquired deficit of memory and cognition. Onset may be from 40 years though it may be seen earlier in patients suffering from Down's syndrome. On histological examination plaques with neurofibrillary tangles and cortical β-amyloid protein are found. On MRI an increased cortical atrophy in the medial temporal lobe can be seen. In stage I of AD there is falling memory and spatial disorientation. In stage II the personality disintegrates and in stage III the patient is apathetic, wasted and bedridden.

2. The key feature in delirium is impaired consciousness with onset over hours to days. Patient is likely to be disoriented, sometimes agitated. If there is no past history of psychiatric illness and the patient is in the setting of a general hospital, a confusional state is particularly likely if the symptoms are worse at the end of the day. It can be due to certain drugs such as benzodiazepines, opiates, anticonvulsants, digoxin, surgery or trauma. Management requires finding and treating the cause.

3. As explained above.

4. Korsakoff's psychosis implies decreased ability to acquire new memories e.g. after Wernicke's encephalopathy. It is due to thiamine deficiency especially seen in alcoholics. Patients confabulate to fill in the gaps in the memory. Urgent thiamine amine needs to be administered to prevent irreversible Korsakoff's syndrome. 200–300 mg thiamine is given PO per day and later a maintenance dose of 25 mg PO per day.

5. Schizophrenia is a common mental disorder which typically presents in adulthood with delusions, hallucinations and disordered thought. The 1st rank symptoms seen in ~70%

of patients are (i) Thought insertion (as in this patient) (ii) Thought broadcast (iii) Thought withdrawal (iv) Passivity (v) Hearing voices commenting on the actions of the patients (vi) Primary delusions (vii) Somatic hallucinations.

Theme 39: Prevention of bleeding

1. The site of injury is suggestive of a cut in the radial or possibly ulnar vessels. External pressure over the site and elevation of the part should control bleeding. Formal surgical repair can be undertaken later. One should not use tourniquet as it may augment ischaemic damage.

2. The presentation of the woman in this case is suggestive of injury to her radial or possibly ulnar artery. The mention of pallor is further suggests massive blood loss. The patient would immediately require an IV access and blood transfusion. Once stabilized, the lady should be referred to a psychiatrist.

3. The presentation of the man in this case is suggestive of an internal bleed due to splenic injury. The signs of pallor, tachycardia and hypotension clearly indicate shock in the patient. This patient would also require an immediate IV access and blood transfusion to stabilise his condition. Laparotomy is indicated even if the patient is not stabilized.

Theme 40: Pre-operative investigation

1. A pre-operative CXR is required in all those patients with known cardiorespiratory disease, pathology or symptoms or if the patient is > 65 years age. Since the patient has already got a normal chest X-ray, the anaesthetist would like to know about her functional lung volumes for which spirometry is required. In obstructive defects such as asthma and COPD, FEV_1 is reduced more than FVC and the FEV_1/FVC ratio is < 80%.

2. Blood sugar measurements are done pre-operatively in most of the patients. It especially becomes utmost important in patients who are diabetic. In patients who have IDDM, one should aim for a level of 7–11 mmol/L of blood sugar level during surgery. In patients who have NIDDM, a fasting blood sugar level should be checked on the morning of the surgery and at the time of premedication. If the level is > 15 mmol/L insulin is used either IV or subcutaneous sliding scale.

Fingerprick glucose	IV soluble insulin	SC Insulin
<2	None	None
2–5	No insulin	No insulin
5–10	1 unit/hour	2 units/hour
10–15	2 units/hour	5 units/hour
15–20	3 units/hour	7 units/hour
> 20	an urgent diabetologist review if > 20 mmol/L	

3. Syncope can be due to a cardiovascular or CNS cause. Since the patient is a known case of IHD an ECG would be required. The ECG has shown a LBBB in the patient. Ischaemic heart disease is one of the causes of LBBB. The presentation of the patient in this case suggests a syncopal attack due to ischaemic episode. Hence an angiography would be required to actually image the anatomy of the heart and flow in its blood vessels.

4. Carditis is one of the major criteria in patients with rheumatic fever. Patients with carditis may have tachycardia, mitral or aortic regurgitation murmurs, Carey Coombs' murmur, pericardial rub, CCF, cardiomegaly and conduction defects. Sometimes an apical systolic murmur is the only sign. Patients with rheumatic fever, posted for surgery, require an ECG as the first investigation. Since it is not mentioned in the options, echocardiogram should be done in this patient. .

5. A pre-operative CXR is required in all those patients with known cardiorespiratory disease, pathology or symptoms or if the patient is > 65 years age.

Section B

TESTING TIME

He slept beneath the room,
He basked beneath the sun,
He lived a life of going to do,
And died with nothing done.

— Jones Albery

Now that you are through with the first half of this book, sit back and ask yourself the following questions:

- **Did you solve the question papers as you do in an exam, or did you just read through it as a text?**
- **Do you think you are getting more questions wrong than you can afford?**

Make a note of the themes and topics where you err, and read them from the recommended text books. Never let a problem become an excuse. You can not succeed unless you find the cause of your mistakes and rectify them. And do not consider your short comings as your failure. For they are only temporary hurdles that teach you a lesson and help you improve upon yourself. If you don't make these mistakes here, you are likely to make them in the exam.

As Roosevelt had said, "The only man who makes no mistakes is the man who never does anything. Don't be afraid of mistakes, provided you don't make the same one twice".

It is the latter which is impardonable. Consider each question you get wrong here, as a question you would attempt correctly in the exam. Learn from your mistakes.

There are six mock test papers for practice. The questions have been collected from the GMC question bank. Each test paper is followed by answersheets similar to the ones you would see during the exam. Time yourself, read the instructions carefully and attempt the paper as you would attempt your PLAB exam.

Only when you've completed the 200 questions in 3 hours, can you take a break and cross-check your answers.

Now go Ahead
And All the Best!

Theme 1: Haematemesis

Options:

a. Acute gastritis
b. Peptic ulcer
c. Mallory–Weiss tear
d. Carcinoma of stomach
e. Arteriovenous malformations
f. Peptic oesophagitis
g. Haemobilia
h. Aorta cuteric fistula
i. Carcinoma of the pancreas

For each presentation below, choose the SINGLE most appropriate diagnosis from the above list of options. Each option may be used once, more than once, or not at all.

1. A 15 year old girl with recently diagnosed acute rheumatic fever presents with vomiting of bright red blood and giddiness.
2. A 50 year old smoker with episodes of epigastric discomfort for the last four years. The discomfort varies during the day and sometimes awakens him at night. It lasts for a few weeks and then disappears for months.
3. A 63 year old man with vague diffuse epigastric pain, diabetes and thrombo-phlebitis. Recently diagnosed to have steatorrhoea.
4. A 50 year old woman with a recent ERCP for evaluation of jaundice.
5. A 60 year old man who has recently undergone surgery for abdominal aortic aneurysm.

Theme 2: Choice of contraception

Options:

a. POP
b. Condoms
c. IUCD
d. Condoms + OCPs
e. COCPs
f. Mirena coil
g. Depot progestagen injection
h. Natural method
i. Diaphragm
j. Spermicidal jellies
k. Vasectomy
l. Fallopian tube ligation

For each presentation below, choose the SINGLE most appropriate method of contraception from the above list of options. Each option may be used once, more than once, or not at all.

6. A 40 year old woman who is multipara and has menorrhagia wants a contraception which can also help her for menorrhagia.

7. A 25 year old with type I DM and nephropathy wants a suitable contraception.

8. A 30 year old woman with heavy periods and stable relationship.

9. An 18 year old student who is sexually active and has multiple partners.

10. A 25 year old woman with 3 children is in a stable relationship. She had recent pelvic infection and history of DVT. She finds difficult to remember her medications.

Theme 3: Causes of constipation

Options:

a. Colorectal carcinoma
b. Hirschprung's disease
c. Diverticulosis
d. Adverse effect of medication
e. Multiple sclerosis
f. Autonomic neuropathy
g. Irritable bowel syndrome
h. Fissure in ano
i. Hypothyroidism
j. Crohn's disease
k. Parkinson's disease

For each presentation below, choose the SINGLE most appropriate cause of constipation from the above list of options. Each option may be used once, more than once, or not at all.

11. A 60 year old male presents with altered bowel habits, weight loss of around 20 lbs over past 3 months. On examination he is pale and has a palpable mass in LIF.

12. A 20 year old man has been constipated since childhood. He opens his bowels once or twice a week and has noticed faecal soiling.

13. A 45 year old woman presents with constipation, weight gain and menorrhagia. She has bradycardia and dry skin.

14. A 50 year old woman fractured her femur. She is admitted to the hospital and complains of increasing constipation since a week.

15. A 25 year old woman presents with abdominal pain and distension which is relieved by passing wind. She also complains of altered bowel habits. She has history of similar episodes in the past also. Examination was unremarkable.

Theme 4: Developmental milestones

Options:

a. Two months
b. Six months
c. Ten months
d. Eleven months
e. Five months
f. One year
g. One and half year
h. Two years
i. Three years
j. Four years
k. Five years
l. Six years

For each presentation below, choose the SINGLE most appropriate age at which it first ocurs from the above list of options. Each option may be used once, more than once, or not at all.

16. Copies a circle.
17. Says Mama or Dada.
18. Drinks from a cup.
19. Stands holding on to the furniture.
20. Tower of 8 cubes.
21. Removes clothes.
22. Reaches out for objects.

Theme 5: Diagnosis of fractures and dislocations

Options:

a. Calcaneal fracture
b. Colle's fracture
c. Anterior shoulder dislocation
d. Posterior shoulder dislocation
e. Navicular fracture
f. Humeral shaft fracture
g. Supracondylar fracture of the humerus
h. Monteggia's fracture
i. March fracture
j. Galeazzi fracture
k. Greenstick fracture
l. Spiral fracture of the tibia
m. Fracture of the proximal fibula

For each presentation below, choose the SINGLE most appropriate diagnosis from the above list of options. Each option may be used once, more than once, or not at all.

23. A 33 year old man, with a history of epilepsy, presents to casualty following a fit. He is now unable to move his right arm and shoulder. He supports the arm in internal rotation with the other hand.
24. A 26 year old woman sustains a twisiting injury to her left leg while skiing. She has mid-calf swelling and tenderness and is unable to bear weight.
25. A 10 year old girl falls and sustains an injury to her right arm. The forearm is stiff, and the hand is deformed. She is only able to extend her fingers when her wrist is passively flexed.
26. A 28 year old marathon runner complains of pain in the second toe. He ran his last marathon a week ago.
27. A 16 year old girl falls onto her outstretched hand. She complains of pain and decreased mobility of her right wrist. On examination, she is tender in the anatomical snuffbox.

Theme 6: Diagnosis of pelvic pain

Options:

a. Ectopic pregnancy
b. Ovarian cyst
c. Diverticulitis
d. Appendicitis
e. Endometriosis
f. Inflammatory bowel disease
g. Degenerating fibroid
h. Septic abortion
i. PID
j. Ovarian hyperstimulation
k. Pelvic adhesions

For each presentation below, choose the SINGLE most appropriate diagnosis from the above list of options. Each option may be used once, more than once, or not at all.

28. A 35 year old women presents with pelvic pain 10 days after delivery.
29. A 20 year old women presents with unilateral pelvic pain, fever, IUCD in situ and 6 weeks amenorrhoea.
30. A 25 year old women presents with pelvic pain. She is afebrile. On examination she has a palpable abdominal mass.
31. A 25 year old woman presents with bilateral, pelvic pain, IUCD in situ, fever and slight vaginal bleed. Her LMP was 3 weeks ago.
32. A 15 year old girl presents with pelvic pain. She had an appendicectomy done 4 months ago.

Theme 7: Principles of the duties of a doctor registered with the General Medical Council

Options:

a. Make the care of your patient your first concern
b. Treat every patient politely and considerately
c. Respect patients dignity and privacy
d. Listen to patients and respect their views
e. Give patients information in a way they can understand
f. Respect the right of patients to be fully involved in decisions about their care
g. Keep your professional knowledge and skills up to date
h. Recognise the limits of your professional competence
i. Be honest and trustworthy
j. Respect and protect confidential information
k. Make sure that your personal beliefs do not prejudice your patients' care
l. Act quickly to protect patients from risk if you have good reason to believe that your colleague may not be fit to practise
m. Avoid abusing your position as a doctor
n. Work with colleagues in the ways that best serve patients' interests

For each presentation below, choose the SINGLE most appropriate principle from the above list of options. Each option may be used once, more than once, or not at all.

33. A 23 year old Indian woman requests a female doctor to perform a pelvic examination.
34. A 55 year old man who is being admitted for a total knee replacement states that he is a jehovah's witness and therefore refuses any blood products.
35. A 16 year old girl informs you that she may be pregnant, and her parents are unaware.
36. A 28 year old man is offered the choice of

whether he would like to receive interferon injections for multiple sclerosis.

37. A 65 year old diabetic sees you for a neurological option and asks if you would renew his insulin prescription as a favour.

Theme 8: Management of heart failure

Options:

a. ACE inhibitors
b. Digoxin
c. Aortic valve replacement
d. Thiazide diuretics
e. Heart transplant
f. IV frusemide
g. Nitrates (oral)
h. Nitrates (IV)
i. Thiamine (IV)
j. Pericardiocentesis

For each presentation below, choose the SINGLE most appropriate management from the above list of options. Each option may be used once, more than once, or not at all.

38. A 15 year old boy is examined and found to have severe congestive cardiac failure.

39. A 40 year old man with cardiac failure is found to have a palpable thrill in the right second intercostal space, which radiates to the neck.

40. A 50 year old man with suspected heart failure has a blood pressure of 90/60 mmHg and pulse rate of 110 beats/min. Chest X-ray shows a globular heart.

41. A 50 year old suspected alcoholic has biventricular cardiac failure. He has deranged liver function tests.

42. A 60 year old female in cardiac failure wants long term treatment for her conditions. Echocardiography shows global hypokinesia and loss of contractility.

Theme 9: Abnormalities of water and electrolyte balance

Options:

a. Addison's disease
b. Conn's syndrome
c. Diabetes insipidus
d. RTA
e. Salmonella enteritis

For each set of biochemical values below, choose the SINGLE most appropriate diagnosis from the above list of options. Each option may be used once, more than once, or not at all.

	Na	K	HCO3
43	136	2.8	18
44	149	2.6	30
45	128	5.6	22
46	130	2.5	8
47	160	5.6	18

Theme 10: Investigations in substance abuse

Options:

a. Dexamethasone suppression test
b. Electrocardiogram
c. Electroencephalogram
d. Full blood count
e. Gamma–glutamyl transpeptidase
f. Genetic analysis
g. MRI brain
h. Serum toxicology screen
i. Thyroid function tests
j. Treponema pallidum haemagglutination assay
k. Urine drug screen

For each presentation below, choose the SINGLE most appropriate investigation from the above list of options. Each option may be used once, more than once, or not at all.

48. A 32 year old woman with bipolar affective disorder is brought to A & E department comatose. She is apyrexial and has no focal neurological deficit.

49. A 45 year old man presents with low mood and tremor, worse first thing in the morning.

50. A 25 year old nurse presents with a history of alcoholism. Her partner says that after an argument she took some medication after which she is behaving strangely, very agitated, profusely sweating, and with tremors and episodes of diarrhoea.

51. A 50 year old patient says that he had brief spells of dizziness and palpitations since he has started his new medication. He also vomited twice and had trouble coming to the A & E because his vision is compounded with coloured haloes.

52. A 65 year old man presents with progressive dementia, spastic paraparesis and seizures. He also has small irregular pupils that accommodate but do not react to light.

Theme 11: Diagnosing diseases

Options:

a. Rubella
b. Landau Barré syndrome
c. Landau Kleffner syndrome
d. Cystinuria
e. Homocystinuria
f. Phenylketonuria
g. Hirschsprung's disease
h. Coeliac disease
i. Fifth disease
j. Measles
k. Infectious mononucleosis
l. Hypothyroidism
m. Cri-du-chat syndrome

For each presentation below, choose the SINGLE most appropriate diagnosis from the above list of options. Each option may be used once, more than once, or not at all.

53. A Chinese woman of 34 year presents to you with her 5 year old son. She says that her child was speaking normally till about 3 year, thereafter he has been increasingly aloof and does not talk. On examination the child is mute. Auditory evoked response is normal bilaterally. The baby has mongoloid features. There have been two episodes of generalized convulsions in the past not associated with fever.

54. A child presents to you with history of convulsions. On examination white opacity is found in the eyes. The hair is thin and breaks easily. The urine biochemistry shows an abnormality for proteins.

55. A child presents with alternating diarrhoea and constipation. On examination abdominal distension is present. The child is in the 70th percentile of his weight for age.

56. A young adult man presents with flushed cheeks and rashes on his forearms. He complains of intermittent joint pain for the past 2 weeks. Cervical lymphadenopathy is present. The monospot test is positive.

57. An infant is brought to you with poor feeding. On examination the muscle tone is decreased. The baby has a peculiar cry. He is a full term baby delivered per vaginum. The mother is healthy and antenatal history is uneventful.

Theme 12: Management of ankle injuries

Options:

a. Elastic bandage and physiotherapy
b. External fixation
c. External fixation and wound debridement
d. MUA (manipulation under anesthesia) and POP
e. ORIF (open reduction and external fixation)
f. POP immobilization
g. Suture repair

For each presentation below, choose the SINGLE most appropriate management from the above list of options. Each option may be used once, more than once, or not at all.

58. A 26 year old man complains of sudden pain at the back of the heel and his calf while playing squash. He has calf tenderness and unable to stand on his toes. X-rays are normal.

59. 54 year old woman sustains injury on her left ankle whilst stepping dnt the kitchen ladder. She has swelling and tenderness over the lateral aspect of her an ankle. X-ray shows undisplaced fracture in distal fibula.

60. A 23 year old motorcyclist involved in a RTA has a compound open fracture of the left tibia and extending into the ankle.

61. A 31 year old footballer sustains an injury over her right ankle in a tackle. Swelling and tenderness over the medial and the lateral aspect of the ankle are positive. X-ray show displaced fracture in the distal fibula with evidence of talar shift.

62. A 43 year old cleaner falls off the ladder injuring his left heel. X-ray confirms extra-articular fracture calcaneum.

Theme 13: Investigations of hypertension

Options:

a. 24 hour ambulatory BP
b. 24 hour ambulatory ECG
c. Abdominal ultrasound scan
d. Carotid ultrasound scan
e. CT scan of thorax and abdomen
f. Echocardiogram
g. Magnetic resonance imaging of abdomen
h. Pulmonary arteriogram
i. Renal biopsy
j. Urine catecholamines
k. Urine free cortisol measurement

For each presentation below, choose the SINGLE most appropriate investigation .from the above list of options. Each option may be used once, more than once, or not at all.

63. A 58 year old woman with a 6 year history of essential hypertension presents after a sudden loss of vision in the left eye. This resolved after 30 minutes.

64. A 77 year old man comes to the Emergency department because he is feeling unwell, 2 weeks after starting treatment for systolic hypertension and headaches. He does not now the name of the drug which his GP prescribed, but his blood pressure was checked by the practice nurse for several hours after the first dose.

65. A 78 year old woman underwent hysterectomy 10 days ago. She now presents with breathlessness on minimal exertion. Her chest X-ray shows interstitial pulmonary oedema.

66. A 33 year old man with no family history of hypertension is seen in outpatient clinic. His blood pressure is 162/76 mmHg and the pulse 98 beats/minute. After 5 minutes of rest the BP is 148/80 mmHg and his pulse 72 beats/minute.

67. A 62 year old man has poorly controlled hypertension despite 4 antihypertensive drugs. His renal function (urea, creatinine) is normal but he has proteinuria.

Theme 14: Pathologic features of bowel disease

Options:

a. Ulcerative colitis
b. Crohn's disease
c. Whipple's disease
d. Hirschprung's disease
e. Coeliac disease
f. Cystic fibrosis
g. Diverticulosis
h. Colorectal carcinoma
i. Primary biliary cirrhosis
j. Colonic polyposis

For each feature below, choose the SINGLE most appropriate diagnosis from the above list of options. Each option may be used once, more than once, or not at all.

68. Segmental lesions.
69. Fistulae.
70. Periodic acid–Schiff (PAS)–positive macrophages in the lamina propria.
71. Megacolon.
72. Crypt abscesses.

Theme 15: Investigations and treatment in gynaecology and obstetrics

Options:

a. Ethinyl estradiol and levonorgestrel
b. Smear after 6 months
c. Sacrohysteropexy
d. Total hysterectomy with bilateral salpingo-oophorectomy
e. Marsupialization
f. Sacrocolpopexy
g. IUCD
h. Manchester operation
i. Pessary
j. Colposcopy
k. Antibiotics
l. Cord compression
m. Uterine rupture
n. Rubella
o. Chloroquine
p. Mendelson's syndrome
q. Placenta praevia
r. Mefloquine
s. Threatened abortion
t. Toxoplasmosis

For each presentation below, choose the SINGLE most appropriate investigation/ treatment from the above list of options. Each option may be used once, more than once, or not at all.

73. A 54 year old obese lady presents with vaginal discharge and scanty bleeding. Her periods stopped 2 year back and she has been on tamoxifen for last 5 year. The speculum examination is normal.

74. A 26 year old lady comes to you 4 days after an unprotected sex. She says that she does not wants a pregnancy at this stage of her career. She wants an emergency contraception.

75. A 73 year old lady comes with complains of something coming down her vagina along with frequency and slight passage of urine when she coughs. She has a history of chronic bronchitis.

76. A 43 year old smoker presents with vaginal discharge and post coital bleeding. On smear examination borderline nuclear abnormality is seen.

77. A 37 year old lady with history of gonorrhoea in the past, now presents with the complaints of such a severe pain that she cannot even sit down. On examination hugely swollen and red labia is seen.

Theme 16: Differential diagnosis of injuries

Options:

a. Ruptured aortic aneurysm
b. Ruptured oesophagus
c. Rib fracture with splenic rupture
d. Rupture of diaphragm
e. Cardiac contusion
f. Pneumothorax
g. Vertebral fracture
h. Haemothorax

For each presentation below, choose the SINGLE most appropriate diagnosis from the above list of options. Each option may be used once, more than once, or not at all.

78. A 50 year old male patient presents with retrosternal pain, dysphagia and surgical emphysema.

79. A 30 year old male patient after an RTA presents with hypotension and dullness to percussion over left lung base.

80. A 30 year old male patient after an RTA presents with pleuritic pain over left lower lung and hypotension.

81. A 30 year old male patient after an RTA presents with bowel sounds beneath right scapular angle.

82. A 50 year old male patient presents with left sided chest pain and tachycardia after blunt thorax trauma.

Theme 17: Diagnostic neurological signs

Options:

a. Friedrich's ataxia
b. Cerebellar ataxia
c. Dystonia
d. Myotonia
e. Muscular dystrophy
f. Hepatolenticular degeneration
g. Myasthenia gravis
h. Parietal lobe lesion
i. Myoclonus
j. De JaVu
k. Hemiballismus
l. Orofacial dyskinesia

For each presentation below, choose the SINGLE most appropriate diagnostic sign from the above list of options. Each option may be used once, more than once, or not at all.

83. A 15 year old who is started on carbamazepine treatment has difficulty maintaining gait.

84. A young man started on neuroleptic medication. Within a few days he develops stiff neck and has trouble closing his mouth.

85. A man develops difficulty in letting go when he shakes hands.

86. An 8 year old boy has difficulty getting up from lying position.

87. An elderly man has been on long term metoclopramide therapy. His wife complains that he can't stop chewing.

Theme 18: Differential diagnosis of abdominal conditions

Options:

a. Sigmoid carcinoma
b. Angiodysplasia of colon
c. Ulcerative colitis
d. Crohn's disease
e. Caecal carcinoma
f. Meckel's diverticulum
g. Appendicitis

For each presentation below, choose the SINGLE most appropriate diagnosis .from the above list of options. Each option may be used once, more than once, or not at all.

88. A 65 year old man presents with a 6 month history of a change in bowel habit, an iron deficiency anaemia and bright red rectal bleeding. There is no abdominal distension. His past history includes a lateral sphincterotomy eight years ago.

89. A 35 year old man presents with profuse rectal bleeding and diarrhoea for past two days. He has had no previous abdominal pain. His abdomen is noted to be mildly distended. There has been a previous similar episode with back and joint pain.

90. A 67 year old lady complains of lower abdominal discomfort. She is noted to have fatigue and lethargy for the past 6 months. In addition, she has noticed that she is more short of breath and that she is opening her bowels twice a day, whereas normally she opens her bowels on alternate days. Although she does not admit to any rectal bleeding, she is found to have an iron deficiency anaemia.

Theme 19: Blood supply to the brain

Options:

a. Basilar artery
b. Anterior cerebral artery
c. Superior cerebral artery
d. Posterior cerebral artery
e. Anterior communicating artery
f. Middle cerebral artery
g. Circle of Willis
h. Posterior communicating artery
i. Anterior inferior cerebellar artery
j. Spinal artery
k. Posterior inferior cerebellar artery

For each neurological area below, choose the SINGLE most appropriate artery from the above list of options. Each option may be used once, more than once, or not at all.

91. Broca's area of speech.
92. Trigeminal nerve nucleus in the medulla oblongata.
93. Visual cortex.
94. Leg area in the motor cortex.
95. Anterior aspect of the pons.

Theme 20: Management of arrhythmias

Options:

a. Carotid sinus massage
b. Adenosine
c. Lignocaine
d. Sotalol
e. Emergency DC version
f. Amiodarone
g. Digoxin
h. CAC12
i. Disopyramide
j. Elective DC cardioversion
k. Flecainide

For each presentation below, choose the SINGLE most appropriate management from the above list of options. Each option may be used once, more than once, or not at all.

96. A 50 year old man was admitted with acute anterior MI. 2 hours after thrombolysis with tPA he suddenly complains of feeling faint. On examination pulse is 145/min, BP 100/40 mmHg. Cardiac monitor shows long run of VT.

97. A young woman 30 weeks pregnant, presents in the A&E complaining of dizziness. On examination her ECG shows re-entrant tachycardia. She had one such episode in the past which resolved spontaneously and presently she is not taking any medication.

98. A 30 year old comes woman with history of palpitations for the past six months. Her ECG shows a shortened PR interval and delta waves. Holter monitor shows evidence of paroxysmal SVT.

99. A 65 year old man with renal failure being treated with CAPD presents with abdominal pain for the last two days. On examination his temperature is 99.8 F. He has also noted that the dialisate is cloudy after exchange. He suddenly deteriorates with broad complex tachycardia. The BP is 75/40 mmHg.

100. A 70 year old male collapsed on surgical ward following a left hemicolectomy. He has a very weak carotid pulse and BP cannot be recorded. Cardiac monitor shows broad complex tachycardia and the pulse rate is 160/min.

Theme 21: Diagnosis of chromosomal disorders

Options:

a. Cri-du-chat syndrome
b. Turner's syndrome
c. Down's syndrome
d. Edward syndrome
e. Patau's syndrome
f. Klinefelter's syndrome
g. Noonan's syndrome
h. Marfan's syndrome
i. Kartagener's syndrome
j. Kallman's syndrome

For each presentation below, choose the SINGLE most appropriate syndrome from the above list of options. Each option may be used once, more than once, or not at all.

101. Abnormal ear and facies, flared fingers, growth deficiency and rocker bottom feet.
102. Short stature, webbed neck, normal intelligence, cubitus valgus and infertility.
103. Cleft lip and palate, polydactyly, scalp defects, mental deficiency, microphthalmia.
104. Microcephaly, dysmorphic features, mental retardation and abnormal cry.
105. Mental deficiency, hypotonia, duodenal atresia, simian crease, Brushfield's spots on iris and mongoloid facies.

Theme 22: The natural history of joint disease

Options:

a. Ankylosing spondylitis
b. Tendinitis of long head of biceps
c. Gout
d. Tennis elbow
e. Osteoarthritis of the hip
f. Psoriatic arthritis
g. Reiter's disease
h. Prolapsed intervertebral disc
i. Rheumatoid arthritis
j. Sjögren's syndrome
k. Rotator cuff tear
l. Painful arc syndrome
m. Systemic lupus erythematosus

For each presentation below, choose the SINGLE most appropriate condition from the above list of options. Each option may be used once, more than once, or not at all.

106. A condition, which affects females more than males and which can be associated with a 'butterfly rash'.
107. Intermittent acute attacks of a severe asymmetrical monoarthritis over a period of several years with symptom free intervals.
108. Pain is felt in the anterior shoulder and is extrinsically worse on forced contraction of the biceps.
109. Patients complain of joint pain and stiffness, especially in distal interphalangeal joints. It may be associated with oncholysis.
110. The condition may follow an episode of yersinia gastroenteritis.

Theme 23: The management of acute severe asthma

Options:

a. 100% oxygen and nebulized steroids
b. Oral prednisolone
c. Ipratropium bromide
d. 100% oxygen and nebulized salbutamol
e. Paralysis with sodium thiopentone
f. Hyperbaric oxygen
g. Adrenaline (subcutaneous)
h. IV hydrocortisone and oral prednisolone
i. IV prednisolone and oral hydrocortisone
j. Skin desensitisation
k. Chlorpheniramine
l. Histamine
m. Do peak expiratory flow rate.

For each presentation below, choose the SINGLE most appropriate management from the above list of options. Each option may be used once, more than once, or not at all.

111. A 16 year old known asthmatic is brought into the A&E severely breathless. She is unable to complete a 3 word sentence.

112. A 17 year old known asthmatic is brought to the A&E department severely breathless. Her respiratory rate is 48 breaths/min. $CO_2 = 8$ kPa, Pa $O_2 = 6$ kPa.

113. Commonly used in the management of status asthmaticus following adequate oxygenation and bronchodilator therapy.

114. A 13 year old boy is brought to the A&E department with a grossly swollen face and difficulty in breathing following a bee sting.

115. May be useful in the management of worsening status asthmaticus.

Theme 24: The diagnosis of the red eye

Options:

a. Acute glaucoma
b. Trachoma
c. Trauma
d. Uveitis
e. Conjunctivitis
f. Spontaneous subconjunctival haemorrhage
g. Scleritis
h. Foreign body
i. Endophthalmitis
j. Dacroadenitis
k. Dacrocystitis

For each presentation below, choose the SINGLE most appropriate diagnosis from the above list of options. Each option may be used once, more than once, or not at all.

116. A 65 year old patient present to his GP with sudden onset of redness in the left eye. There is no pain and vision is unaffected.

117. A 70 year old patient complains of severe pain in his right eye with severe deterioration of vision. He has noticed haloes around street lights for a few days before the onset of pain.

118. A seven year old North African boy gave a history of two year of discomfort, redness and mucopurulent discharge affecting both eyes. His two siblings have a similar problem.

119. A 25 year old man has a history of recurrent attacks of blurring of vision associated with redness, pain and photophobia. Both eyes have been affected in the past. His older brother is currently being investigated for severe backache.

120. A 30 year old rugby player sustained facial injuries. 12 months later he presented with a painful swelling at the left medial canthus, associated with red eye and purulent discharge.

Theme 25: Differential diagnosis of epigastric pain

Options:

a. Reflux oesophagitis
b. Myocardial infarction
c. Lower lobe pneumonia
d. Peptic ulceration
e. Crohn's disease
f. Ulcerative colitis
g. Urinary tract infection
h. Acute cholecystitis
i. Acute pancreatitis
j. Viral hepatitis
k. Urinary tract infection
l. Hirchsprung's disease
m. Acute intermittent porphyria

For each presentation below, choose the SINGLE most appropriate diagnosis from the above list of options. Each option may be used once, more than once, or not at all.

121. An obese 45 year old man complains of a burning retrosternal pain, which is aggravated by drinking hot chocolate.

122. A 34 year old man returned from a holiday in Thailand three weeks ago. He feels weak and unable to go to work. On examination he has a tender epigastrium and a tinge of jaundice.

123. A 28 year old man complains of epigastric pain associated with water brash .He admits to 6 month history of nocturnal cough.

124. A 46 year old woman complains of an epigastric pain exacerbated by eating large meals and relieved by hunger.

125. A 29 year old woman with a 4-month history of steatorrhoea and easy fatigability complains of epigastric pain. He smokes 10 cigarettes a day.

Theme 26: Diagnosis of skin pathology

Options:

a. Pemphigus vulgaris
b. Pemphigoid
c. Porphyria cutanea tarda
d. Psoriasis
e. Impetigo
f. Pityriasis versicolor
g. Acne roseacea
h. Erythema nodosum
i. Erythema multiforme
j. Erythema marginatum
k. Acne vulgaris
l. Erythema chronicum migrans
m. Erythema ab igne
n. Erythrodermic migraine
o. Toxic epidermal necrolysis

For each presentation below, choose the SINGLE most appropriate diagnosis from the above list of options. Each option may be used once, more than once, or not at all.

126. A 13 year old boy complains of a non-pruritic rash characterized by papules and pustules affecting his face and upper chest. His voice has just started to deepen with sparse groin hair. He has no other complaints.

127. A 34 year old man presents with a swollen erythematous nose. On examination he is seen to have papules and telangiectasia in his face. Prior to this he had experienced flushing after drinking alcohol and spicy food.

128. A 78 year old man taking frusemide for nephrotic syndrome is seen in the dermatology clinic. He is found to have tense blisters covering the whole of his body except the oral mucosa. Skin biopsy is done and it reveals multiple linear IgG and C3 deposits along the basement membrane.

129. A 34 year old woman presents with red lesions on her elbows and submammary

areas. On examination, she is found to have extensive pitting and onycholysis of her nails.

130. A 32 year old woman presents with flaccid blisters all over the body with extensive oral mucosa involvement. Skin biopsy reveals intercellular IgG with a 'crazy-packing' effect. She is being treated for migraine.

Theme 27: The differential diagnosis of generalized lymphadenopathy

Options:

a. Cytomegalovirus disease
b. Tuberculosis
c. Infectious mononucleosis
d. Syringobulbia
e. Toxoplasmosis
f. Sarcoidosis
g. HIV infection
h. Myeloma
i. Chronic granulomatous disease
j. Syringomyelia
k. Brucellosis
l. Cryptococcus neoformans

For each presentation below, choose the SINGLE most appropriate diagnosis from the above list of options. Each option may be used once, more than once, or not at all.

131. A 34 year old sheep farmer from Cumbria presents with a 2 month history of an undulating fever, joint pain, weight loss and constipation. On further questioning he is found to be depressed with marked generalized lymphadenopathy.

132. A 23 year old university student complains of a sore throat, fever, and general malaise. On examination, numerous petechiae are seen on the palate.

133. A 33 year old homosexual man presents with a 3-month history of a productive cough associated with two episodes of haemoptysis. He admits to losing 3 kg of weight. On examination, he is found to have generalized lymphadenopathy.

134. A 32 year old man presents with confusion. A computed tomography scan of the head shows multiple ring enhancing lesions. He is being treated for HIV infection and on examination generalized lymphadenopathy is found.

Theme 28: Diagnosis of acute vomiting in children

Options:

a. Acute appendicitis
b. Cyclical vomiting
c. Duodenal atresia
d. Gastro-oesophageal disease
e. Gastroenteritis
f. Meconium ileus
g. Mesenteric adenitis
h. Meningitis
i. Overfeeding
j. Pancreatitis
k. Psychogenic vomiting
l. Pyloric stenosis
m. Urinary tract infection
n. Whooping cough

For each presentation below, choose the SINGLE most appropriate diagnosis from the above list of options. Each option may be used once, more than once, or not at all.

135. A three day old breast fed infant is vomiting after each feed. An abdominal X-ray demonstrated a 'double bubble'.

136. A six week old breast-fed boy has had projectile vomiting after each feed for the past two weeks. He is now lethargic, dehydrated and tachypnoiec.

137. A four month old baby boy is thriving, but has persistent vomiting, which is occasionally bloodstained and is associated with crying.

138. An eight year old girl shows signs of moderate dehydration. She has vomited all fluids for 24 hours and the vomit isn't bile stained. Her abdomen is now soft and non-tender. She has had two similar episodes in the past year.

139. A 12-week-old thriving baby is vomiting after every feed. She is developmentally normal and is fed by the bottle at 280 ml/kg/day.

Theme 29: Poisoning: Treatment

Options:

a. Atropine
b. Flumazenil
c. Dicobalt edetate
d. Specific antibody fragments
e. Antitoxin
f. Desferrioxamine
g. Naloxone
h. Phytomenadione
i. FFP and vitamin K
j. NAC
k. IV sodium bicarbonate
l. Hyperbaric O_2
m. Supportive care only
n. IV methylene blue
o. Procyclidine

For each presentation below, choose the SINGLE most appropriate treatment from the above list of options. Each option may be used once, more than once, or not at all.

140. A 35 year old woman has taken a bottle full of atenolol tablets.

141. A 5 year old girl has taken a bottle full of iron tablets.

142. A 30 year old man has chronic psychiatric illness. He is on neuroleptic medication. He presents with opisthotonus and torticollis.

143. A 10 year old student took 100 tabs of aspirin. He is now sweating, hyperventilating and vomiting. He has tachycardia with BP 102/60.

144. An 18 year old girl has taken her father's warfarin. She is not actively bleeding.

Theme 30: Liver disease in pregnancy

Options:

a. Hyperemesis gravidarum
b. Intrahepatic cholestasis
c. Biliary tract disease
d. Drug induced hepatitis
e. Viral hepatitis
f. Acute fatty liver of pregnancy
g. Pre-eclampsia and eclampsia
h. HELLP syndrome

For each presentation below, choose the SINGLE most appropriate diagnosis from the above list of options. Each option may be used once, more than once, or not at all.

145. A 24 year old woman with six weeks of amenorrhoea and persistent nausea and vomiting especially on awakening in the morning. Examination reveals mild dehydration and a tinge of icterus. Investigations reveal total bilirubin 3.0 mg/dl with direct fraction 2.1 mg/dl and SGPT 110 iu/L.

146. A 33 year old woman 36 weeks pregnant with her fourth child presenting with nausea, vomiting, right upper quadrant pain, jaundice and oliguria. Examination reveals disorientation with asterixis. She has multiple bruises at venepuncture sites. Investigation reveals SGPT 300 iu/L, bilirubin of 12 mg/dl with direct 9 mg/dl, random sugar 60 mg/dl and prolonged PT and APTT. Her serum ammonia is 2 times the normal. Her creatinine is 4.0 mg/dl. USG reveals a hypoechoic liver.

147. A 28 year old woman with 30 weeks of gestation presenting with upper abdominal pain, oedema and headache. Examination reveals pitting oedema of both lower limbs, BP of 140/100 and mild disorientation. Investigations show SGPT 196 iu/L, bilirubin 3.0 mg/dl and 2+ proteinuria.

148. A 32 year old woman presents 2 days after emergency LSCS at 34 weeks of gestation. Her relatives have noticed progressive yellowing of the eyes and she complains of oliguria. Examination reveals a BP of 140/90, oedema of feet and bruising. Her bilirubin is 8.0 mg/dl with direct fraction 6.0 mg/dl, SGPT is 340 iu/L, Hb is 8.0 gm/dl with 8% reticulocytes, platelets are 80000 and smear shows schistocytes. Her LDH is 380 iu/L.

149. A 26 year old woman with 28 weeks gestation develops fever, right pleuritic chest pain and cough with haemoptysis. She is treated with erythromycin estolate for a presumed pneumonia.

Theme 31: Sudden upper abdominal pain

Options:

a. Acute myocardial infarction
b. Pulmonary embolus to a lower lobe
c. Perforated peptic ulcer
d. Penetrating peptic ulcer
e. Acute pancreatitis
f. Mesenteric artery occlusion
g. Biliary colic
h. Acute rupture of oesophagus
i. Diabetic ketoacidosis
j. Pneumonia

For each presentation below, choose the SINGLE most appropriate diagnosis from the above list of options. Each option may be used once, more than once, or not at all.

150. A 70 year old hypertensive, diabetic man has previous history of myocardial infarction. He has sudden onset of abdominal pain, nausea and vomiting.
151. A 28 year old diagnosed case of hereditary spherocytosis.
152. A 43 year old alcoholic male with prolonged retching and vomiting following a heavy alcoholic binge.
153. A 40 year old hypertensive, smoker who is also diagnosed to have peptic ulcer disease. He presents with epigastic pain and diaphoresis. The pain is not relieved with antacids. It does not radiate to the back. Examination reveals a soft abdomen.
154. Epigastic pain of sudden onset in a 68 year old dowager hospitalized for a fracture hip. The pain is aggravated by deep breathing.

Theme 32: Clinical features of acute poisoning

Options:

a. Sympathomimetics
b. Organophosphorus
c. Opiate analgesics
d. Salicylates
e. Ethylene glycol
f. Volatile solvents
g. Benzodiazepines
h. Tricyclic antidepressants
i. Methanol
j. Anti-psychotics

For each presentation below, choose the SINGLE most appropriate poisoning agent from the above list of options. Each option may be used once, more than once, or not at all.

155. Blindness, pulmonary oedema, metabolic acidosis, shock, hyperglycaemia.
156. Coma, hypotension, reduced muscle tone and reflexes, hypoventilation.
157. Dysphagia, dysphoria, trismus, oculogyric crisis, torticollis.
158. Coma, small pupils, hypoventilation.
159. Hypersalivation, bronchorrhoea with bronchospasm, perspiration, bradycardia, urination, pin-point pupils with neuromuscular paralysis.

Theme 33: Types of emboli

Options:

a. Thrombus emboli
b. Fat emboli
c. Amniotic fluid emboli
d. Malignant emboli
e. Atheromatous emboli
f. Septic emboli
g. Paradoxical emboli
h. Fibrin emboli
i. Bone fragment emboli
j. Air emboli

For each presentation below, choose the SINGLE most appropriate type of emboli from the above list of options. Each option may be used once, more than once, or not at all.

160. A 32 year old in her third trimester of pregnancy presents with chest pain and dyspnoea increasing in severity over the last 24 hours. She has no lower limb pain or swelling.

161. A 28 year old with known congenital heart disease develops small, tender subcutaneous nodules in the pulp of the digits. On examination nodules were red and tender. The patient was noted to have splenomegaly and a new heart murmur.

162. A novice deep sea diver rises too rapidly to the surface on a training dive. That same day he develops confusion and seizures. Fundoscopy is done to help reach a diagnosis.

163. A young man is involved in a traffic accident in which he sustained severe comminuted fractures of the right femur. Three days following the accident he develops seizures.

164. A patient with deep venous thrombosis was complicated by cerebral and extremity emboli. On echocardiography he was noted to have a patent foramen ovale.

Theme 34: Treatment of poisoning

Options:

a. Desferrioxamine
b. Naloxone
c. Glucagon
d. N-acetylcysteine
e. Hyperbaric oxygen
f. Activated charcoal
g. Atropine
h. Haemodialysis
i. Supportive treatment
j. Dicobalt edetate
k. Gastric lavage

For each presentation below, choose the SINGLE most appropriate treatment from the above list of options. Each option may be used once, more than once, or not at all.

165. A 37 year old man is admitted within 1 hour of accidentally ingesting liquid paraquat. He complains of diarrhoea and painful mouth ulcers.

166. A 15 year old girl presents with sweats and hyperventilation after taking a large number of salicylate tablets. She has severe metabolic acidosis.

167. A 26 year old woman collapses after a massive overdose of atenolol. So far, she has not responded to intravenous atropine and remains in cardiogenic shock.

168. A pregnant 30 year old woman is found drowsy in her rented flat. She complains of severe nausea for the last 3 hours. Her carboxyhaemoglobin level is 41%.

169. A 25 year old man is delirious and hyperpyrexial after taking a tablet at a dancing club. He is hyper-reflexic, and has a serum sodium of 130mmol/L.

Theme 35: Adverse effects of medications

Options:

a. Amiodarone
b. Bendrofluazide
c. Carbimazole
d. Nifedipine
e. Hydralazine
f. Amitriptyline
g. Enalapril
h. Phenytoin
i. Simvastatin
j. Clonidine
k. Prednisolone
l. Bleomycin
m. Lithium
n. Metformin
o. Third generation cephalosporin

For each presentation below, choose the SINGLE most appropriate causative medication from the above list of options. Each option may be used once, more than once, or not at all.

170. A 40 year old woman presents with a greyish discolouration of her skin. She also mentions that she has become prone to sunburn even after moderate exposure.

171. A 70 year old man presents with progressive shortness of breath. On examination he has bilateral basal crepitations and his CXR reveals lung fibrosis. He is on treatment for squamous cell carcinoma of lung.

172. A 70 year old woman presents with impaired vision, cold intolerance and constipation. She is on medication for PSVT.

173. A 40 year old man presents with swollen, painful gums that bleed on brushing.

174. A 80 year old woman presents with profuse offensive diarrhoea. She has been on treatment for the past 5 days for UTI.

Theme 36: Paraesthesia and weakness in lower limbs

Options:

a. Meralgia paraesthetica
b. Lateral popliteal nerve lesion
c. Peripheral neuropathy
d. Lumbar disc herniation
e. Subacute combined degeneration of cord
f. Tabes dorsalis
g. Multiple sclerosis
h. Poliomyelitis

For each presentation below, choose the SINGLE most appropriate diagnosis from the above list of options. Each option may be used once, more than once, or not at all.

175. A 50 year old man complains of tight bands around her lower limbs. He feels electric shock like sensation moving down his legs when his neck is flexed.

176. A 50 year old woman complains of tingling in the outer aspect of her thigh which is felt on sitting and worse on standing. She mentions that the pain is gone once she lies down.

177. A 60 year old man complains of numbness in his legs. He has a sensory loss in 'stocking' fashion, extensor plantar response, brisk knee jerks and absent ankle jerks.

178. A 40 year old man complains of numbness in outer aspect of his right foot along with weakness of the foot. On examination he is found to have foot drop.

179. A 60 year old man complains of lancinating pain in his legs. He also has an unsteady gait and unresponsive pupils to light.

180. A 45 year old bricklayer complains of pain and pins and needle down the back of his right thigh. He also complains of similar set of complaints in the lateral aspect of the right leg and foot.

Theme 37: Causes of headache

Options:

a. Tension headache
b. Cervical nerve root irritation
c. Migraine
d. Cluster headaches
e. Sinusitis
f. Depression
g. SAH
h. Glaucoma
i. Head injury
j. Meningitis

For each presentation below, choose the SINGLE most appropriate cause of headache from the above list of options. Each option may be used once, more than once, or not at all.

181. A 50 year old teacher describes throbbing headache associated with difficulty in focusing on the paper while writing notes.

182. A 40 year old woman complains of headache during which areas of her scalp become tender.

183. A 40 year old woman complains of recurrent episodes of headache which are very severe in intensity. She also complains of a watery eye.

184. A 30 year old divorced woman complains of headache which she describes as a 10 lb weight kept on her head.

185. A 60 year old lady complains of headache and loss of appetite. She also complains of generalized weakness, lethargy, aches and pains in her body.

Theme 38: Investigation in thyroid diseases

Options:

a. FNAC
b. T_3
c. T_4
d. TSH
e. Thyroglobulin
f. Ultrasound
g. Thyroid scan
h. Autoantibody titres
i. Do nothing

For each presentation below, choose the SINGLE most appropriate investigation from the above list of options. Each option may be used once, more than once, or not at all.

186. A 52 year old man presents with an irregular swelling in front of the neck.

187. A 13 year old girl presents with diffuse swelling which moves with deglutition.

188. A 40 year old woman with a swelling in front of the neck and complains of palpitations and diarrhoea.

189. A 35 year old woman presents a thyroid with swelling. On thyroid scan, a single nodule is seen.

190. A 40 year old woman has come for assessment. She is presently on treatment for hypothyroidism with thyroxine.

Theme 39: Cause of epistaxis

Options:

a. Trauma
b. HTN
c. Nasal polyposis
d. Coagulopathy
e. Anticoagulant overdose
f. Nasopharyngeal angiofibroma
g. Carcinoma maxillary antrum
h. Orf
i. Septal perforation
j. Sarcoidosis

For each presentation below, choose the SINGLE most appropriate cause of epistaxis from the above list of options. Each option may be used once, more than once, or not at all.

191. A 50 year old man working in a chrome factory for the past 2 decades presents with whistling sound on speaking.
192. An 80 year old man with history of epistaxis since 2 hours.
193. A 55 year old man who is involved in furniture making for the past 2 decades presents with recurrent epistaxis and anaesthesia of left cheek.
194. A 50 year old sheep farmer presents with epistaxis. He also has history of similar episodes of epistaxis in the past 2 year.
195. A 45 year old man presents with epistaxis. He has just underwent surgery for prosthetic valve replacement.

Theme 40: Choice of antibiotics

Options:

a. Zidovudine
b. Amoxicillin and gentamycin
c. Clindamycin
d. IV ampicillin
e. Rifampicin
f. Penicillin V
g. Benzylpenicillin
h. Trimethoprim
i. Metronidazole
j. Ciprofloxacin
k. Mefloquine
l. Chloroquine and proguanil
m. Amoxicillin

For each presentation below, choose the SINGLE most appropriate antibiotic from the above list of options. Each option may be used once, more than once, or not at all.

196. A 5 year old boy presents with sickle cell disease.
197. A mother brings her 5 year old child and is worried that his best friend is suffering from meningococcal meningitis.
198. A 30 year old woman presents with urinary frequency and dysuria. She has no loin pain and is otherwise normal.
199. A 50 year old man admitted, is being treated for pneumonia. He develops profuse yellow brown diarrhoea.
200. A 25 year old mother develops neck stiffness, fever, headache and purpuric rash. Her son is on treatment for meningococcal meningitis.

ANSWERS

1. **(a)** Acute gastritis
2. **(b)** Peptic ulcer
3. **(i)** Carcinoma of the pancreas
4. **(g)** Haemobilia
5. **(h)** Aorta cuteric fistula
6. **(f)** Mirena coil
7. **(a)** POP
8. **(e)** COCPs
9. **(b)** Condoms
10. **(j)** Spermicidal jellies
11. **(a)** Colorectal carcinoma
12. **(b)** Hirschprung's disease
13. **(i)** Hypothyroidism
14. **(d)** Adverse effect of medication
15. **(g)** Irritable bowel syndrome
16. **(i)** Three years
17. **(f)** One year
18. **(g)** One and half year
19. **(c)** Ten months
20. **(i)** Three years
21. **(h)** Two years
22. **(e)** Five months
23. **(d)** Posterior shoulder dislocation
24. **(l)** Spiral fracture of the tibia
25. **(g)** Supracondylar fracture of the humerus
26. **(i)** March fracture
27. **(e)** Navicular fracture
28. **(e)** Endometriosis
29. **(a)** Ectopic pregnancy
30. **(b)** Ovarian cyst
31. **(i)** PID
32. **(k)** Pelvic adhesions
33. **(d)** Listen to patients and respect their views
34. **(k)** Make sure that your personal beliefs do not prejudice your patients' care
35. **(j)** Respect and protect confidential information
36. **(f)** Respect the right of patients to be fully involved in decisions about their care
37. **(h)** Recognise the limits of your professional competence
38. **(b)** Digoxin
39. **(c)** Aortic valve replacement
40. **(j)** Pericardiocentesis
41. **(i)** Thiamine (IV)
42. **(e)** Heart transplant
43. **(d)** RTA
44. **(b)** Conn's syndrome
45. **(a)** Addison's disease
46. **(e)** Salmonella enteritis
47. **(c)** Diabetes insipidus
48. **(h)** Serum toxicology screen
49. **(i)** Thyroid function tests
50. **(e)** Gamma–glutamyl transpeptidase
51. **(b)** Electrocardiogram
52. **(j)** Treponema pallidum haemagglutination assay
53. **(c)** Landau Kleffner syndrome
54. **(e)** Homocystinuria
55. **(g)** Hirschsprung's disease
56. **(j)** Measles
57. **(l)** Hypothyroidism
58. **(g)** Suture repair
59. **(f)** POP immobilization
60. **(c)** External fixation and wound debridement
61. **(e)** ORIF (open reduction and external fixation)
62. **(f)** POP immobilization
63. **(d)** Carotid ultrasound scan
64. **(c)** Abdominal ultrasound scan
65. **(f)** Echocardiogram
66. **(a)** 24–hour ambulatory BP

67. (i) Renal biopsy
68. (b) Crohn's disease
69. (b) Crohn's disease
70. (c) Whipple's disease
71. (d) Hirschprung's disease
72. (a) Ulcerative colitis
73. (j) Colposcopy
74. (g) IUCD
75. (i) Pessary
76. (b) Smear after 6 months
77. (e) Marsupialization
78. (b) Ruptured oesophagus
79. (h) Haemothorax
80. (c) Rib fracture with splenic rupture
81. (d) Rupture of diaphragm
82. (e) Cardiac contusion
83. (b) Cerebellar ataxia
84. (c) Dystonia
85. (d) Myotonia
86. (e) Muscular dystrophy
87. (l) Orofacial dyskinesia
88. (a) Sigmoid carcinoma
89. (c) Ulcerative colitis
90. (e) Caecal carcinoma
91. (f) Middle cerebral artery
92. (a) Basilar artery
93. (d) Posterior cerebral artery
94. (b) Anterior cerebral artery
95. (a) Basilar artery
96. (c) Lignocaine
97. (a) Carotid sinus massage
98. (d) Sotalol
99. (h) CAC12
100. (e) Emergency DC version
101. (d) Edward syndrome
102. (b) Turner's syndrome
103. (e) Patau's syndrome
104. (a) Cri-du-chat syndrome
105. (c) Down's syndrome
106. (m) Systemic lupus erythematosus
107. (c) Gout
108. (b) Tendinitis of long head of biceps
109. (f) Psoriatic arthritis
110. (g) Reiter's disease
111. (d) 100% oxygen and nebulized salbutamol
112. (d) 100% oxygen and nebulized salbutamol
113. (h) IV hydrocortisone and oral prednisolone
114. (g) Adrenaline (subcutaneous)
115. (e) Paralysis with sodium thiopentone
116. (f) Spontaneous subconjunctival haemorrhage
117. (a) Acute glaucoma
118. (b) Trachoma
119. (d) Uveitis
120. (k) Dacrocystitis
121. (a) Reflux oesophagitis
122. (j) Viral hepatitis
123. (a) Reflux oesophagitis
124. (d) Peptic ulceration
125. (e) Crohn's disease
126. (k) Acne vulgaris
127. (g) Acne roseacea
128. (b) Pemphigoid
129. (d) Psoriasis
130. (a) Pemphigus vulgaris
131. (k) Brucellosis
132. (c) Infectious mononucleosis
133. (b) Tuberculosis
134. (e) Toxoplasmosis
135. (c) Duodenal atresia
136. (l) Pyloric stenosis
137. (d) Gastro-oesophageal disease
138. (b) Cyclical vomiting
139. (i) Overfeeding
140. (a) Atropine
141. (f) Desferrioxamine
142. (o) Procyclidine
143. (k) IV sodium bicarbonate
144. (h) Phytomenadione
145. (a) Hyperemesis gravidarum
146. (f) Acute fatty liver of pregnancy
147. (g) Pre-eclampsia and eclampsia
148. (h) HELLP syndrome

149. **(d)** Drug induced hepatitis
150. **(f)** Mesenteric artery occlusion
151. **(g)** Biliary colic
152. **(h)** Acute rupture of oesophagus
153. **(a)** Acute myocardial infarction
154. **(b)** Pulmonary embolus to a lower lobe
155. **(i)** Methanol
156. **(g)** Benzodiazepines
157. **(j)** Anti-psychotics
158. **(c)** Opiate analgesics
159. **(b)** Organophosphorus
160. **(a)** Thrombus emboli
161. **(f)** Septic emboli
162. **(j)** Air emboli
163. **(b)** Fat emboli
164. **(g)** Paradoxical emboli
165. **(f)** Activated charcoal
166. **(h)** Haemodialysis
167. **(c)** Glucagon
168. **(e)** Hyperbaric oxygen
169. **(f)** Activated charcoal
170. **(f)** Amitriptyline
171. **(l)** Bleomycin
172. **(a)** Amiodarone
173. **(d)** Nifedipine
174. **(o)** Third generation cephalosporin

175. **(g)** Multiple sclerosis
176. **(a)** Meralgia paraesthetica
177. **(e)** Subacute combined degeneration of cord
178. **(b)** Lateral popliteal nerve lesion
179. **(f)** Tabes dorsalis
180. **(d)** Lumbar disc herniation
181. **(c)** Migraine
182. **(b)** Cervical nerve root irritation
183. **(d)** Cluster headaches
184. **(a)** Tension headache
185. **(f)** Depression
186. **(g)** Thyroid scan
187. **(f)** Ultrasound
188. **(b)** T_3
189. **(a)** FNAC
190. **(d)** TSH
191. **(j)** Septal perforation
192. **(b)** HTN
193. **(g)** Carcinoma maxillary antrum
194. **(c)** Nasal polyposis
195. **(e)** Anticoagulant overdose
196. **(f)** Penicillin V
197. **(e)** Rifampicin
198. **(h)** Trimethoprim
199. **(i)** Metronidazole
200. **(g)** Benzylpenicillin

Full Name

Test Centre/Date

- Use pencil only • Make heavy marks that fill the lozenge completely
- Write your candidate number in the top row of the box to the right **and** fill in the appropriate lozenge below each number
- Given **one** answer only for each question

Do not Write in this space

Do not Write in this space

Do not Write in this space

Two

Mock Test Paper

Theme 1: Pathologic features of bowel disease

Options:

a. Ulcerative colitis
b. Crohn's disease
c. Whipple's disease
d. Hirschprung's disease
e. Coeliac disease
f. Cystic fibrosis
g. Diverticulosis
h. Colorectal carcinoma
i. Primary biliary cirrhosis
j. Colonic polyposis

For each pathological features below, choose the SINGLE most appropriate diagnosis from the above list of options. Each option may be used once, more than once, or not at all.

1. Granulomas.
2. Superficial ulceration.
3. Transmural inflammation.
4. Pseudo-polyps of regenerating mucosa.
5. Bronchiectasis.

Theme 2: Thyroid carcinoma: Diagnosis

Options:

a. Papillary
b. Follicular
c. Lymphoma
d. Anaplastic
e. Medullary
f. Teratoma
g. Sarcoma
h. Melanoma

For each presentation below, choose the SINGLE most appropriate diagnosis from the above list of options. Each option may be used once, more than once, or not at all.

6. A 20 year old man presents with 1 cm swelling adjacent to thyroid gland. A focal swelling of the thyroid is also noted. He complains of night sweats and has lost 10 lbs weight in past 6 months. He also has swelling in the groin and axillae.

7. A 70 year old man presents with a woody hard swelling of right lobe of his thyroid. He also complains of hoarseness in his voice. The swelling is growing rapidly in size.

8. A 45 year old woman presents with a lump in the thyroid gland. She has family history of MEN and has experienced diarrhoea. She undergoes thyroidectomy with ipsilateral modified block dissection of the neck.

9. A 50 year old woman presents with a solitary lump in the thyroid which has spread haematogenously to the lung and bone. No nodes are involved. On histological examination capsular invasion and vascular spread of the tumour is noted.

10. An 18 year old boy presents with a swelling adjacent to thyroid gland. On examination a focal swelling of the thyroid is also noted, although his TFTs are found to be normal.

Theme 3: Tumour markers

Options:

a. α fetoprotein
b. CA 19-9
c. CA 125
d. CEA
e. HCG
f. NSE
g. PLAP
h. PSA
i. Calcitonin
j. S-100
k. None of the above
l. Thyroglobulin
m. Urinary metanephrines
n. 5-HIAA

For each malignancy below, choose the SINGLE most appropriate tumour marker from the above list of options. Each option may be used once, more than once, or not at all.

11. Ovarian carcinoma.
12. Carcinoma head of pancreas.
13. Medullary thyroid carcinoma.
14. Hepatocellular carcinoma.
15. Ductal carcinoma of the breast.

Theme 4: Choice of antibiotics

Options:

a. Zidovudine
b. Amoxicillin and gentamycin
c. Clindamycin
d. IV ampicillin
e. Rifampicin
f. Penicillin V
g. Benzylpenicillin
h. Trimethoprim
i. Metronidazole
j. Ciprofloxacin
k. Mefloquine
l. Chloroquine and proguanil
m. Amoxicillin

For each presentation below, choose the SINGLE most appropriate antibiotic from the above list of options. Each option may be used once, more than once, or not at all.

16. A 40 year old abbatoir worker presents with an ulcer over his hand which forms a black eschar.

17. A 30 year old man develops profuse diarrhoea. He has been on amoxicillin for the past week for his chest infection.

18. A 30 year old pregnant woman who has an HIV positive status wants minimum risk of transmitting the infection to her fetus.

19. A 30 year old Irish man wants to travel to India for 2 weeks. He wants prophylactic medication to avoid contracting malaria.

20. An 18 year old boy with rheumatic heart disease is due for a dental extraction. He is allergic to penicillin.

Theme 5: Diagnosis of skin conditions

Options:

a. Pityriasis rosea
b. Pityriasis versicolor
c. Erythema multiforme
d. Eczema
e. Hereditary angioedema
f. Leprosy
g. Necrotizing fasciitis
h. Tinea corporis
i. Secondary syphilis
j. Lichen planus
k. Pemphigus
l. Psoriasis
m. Dermatitis herpetiformis

For each presentation below, choose the SINGLE most appropriate diagnosis from the above list of options. Each option may be used once, more than once, or not at all.

21. A 25 year old woman with history of small erythematous patch over her chest which disappeared. A week later patches are noted on her front and back which are brown in colour, macular, discrete and itchy.

22. A 30 year old African lady presents with depigmented patches of skin on her shins. They are painless with decreased skin sensation.

23. A 25 year old man presents with erythematous papules over the dorsum of his hands and on arms. There is a central pallor within these papules.

24. A 35 year old man presents which painless rash on his trunk. He has a number of pink scaly circular lesions with central clearing which are itchy and measure around 4 cm each.

25. A 22 year old woman presents with swellings of her limbs associated with purpura and breathlessness. She has had similar set of problems over most of her life.

Theme 6: Diagnosis of sudden visual loss

Options:

a. Cataract
b. Central retinal artery occlusion
c. Acute glaucoma
d. Cerebral embolism
e. Cerebral embolism
f. Chronic simple glaucoma
g. Hypertensive encephalopathy
h. Polymyalgia rheumatica
i. Retinal detachment
j. Temporal arteritis
k. Uveitis

For each presentation below, choose the SINGLE most appropriate diagnosis from the above list of options. Each option may be used once, more than once, or not at all.

26. A 40 year old lady has recurrent episodes of an acutely painful red eye with reduced vision.

27. A 70 year old smoker suddenly notices markedly reduced vision in one eye. He cannot read any letter on the visual acuity chart, but can count fingers. The fundus looks pale.

28. A 90 year old woman notices sudden increased visual impairment. She is found to have homonymous hemianopia.

29. A 45 year old lady complains of sudden loss of vision in one eye. She describes the incident like a curtain coming down.

30. An 80 year old lady has had a painful scalp and headache for three weeks and is generally unwell. She presents with an acute onset of blindness in the left eye.

Theme 7: Investigations and treatment in gynaecology and obstetrics

Options:

a. Ethinyl estradiol and levonorgestrel
b. Smear after 6 months
c. Sacrohysteropexy
d. Total hysterectomy with bilateral salpingo-oophorectomy
e. Marsupialization
f. Sacrocolpopexy
g. IUCD
h. Manchester operation
i. Pessary
j. Colposcopy
k. Antibiotics
l. Cord compression
m. Uterine rupture
n. Rubella
o. Chloroquine
p. Mendelsons syndrome
q. Placenta praevia
r. Mefloquine
s. Threatened abortion
t. Toxoplasmosis

For each presentation below, choose the SINGLE most appropriate investigation/ treatment from the above list of options. Each option may be used once, more than once, or not at all.

31. A lady with 34 weeks of gestation comes for her routine checkup. The foetal heart rate is noted to be around 100 bpm.

32. A pregnant lady presents in a state of shock with severe bleeding per vaginam. The uterus is not tender and the fetal heart rate is within normal limits.

33. A pregnant lady had fever, rash and eosinophilia. She was started on spiramycin for it.

Theme 8: Investigation and management of scrotal swellings

Options:

a. Ultrasound scan of scrotum
b. Surgical exploration
c. Reassurance
d. Aspiration
e. Mid stream urine for microscopy and/or culture
f. Biopsy
g. Analgesia
h. Doppler ultrasound of scrotum
i. Computed tomography (CT) scan of scrotum
j. Clotting studies
k. Urethral swab
l. Antibiotics
m. Urine cytology
n. Herniotomy

For each presentation below, choose the SINGLE most appropriate investigation/ management from the above list of options. Each option may be used once, more than once, or not at all.

34. A 12 year old boy presents with a tender, red swollen scrotum. He has already been given analgesia by his general practitioner.

35. A young boy with acute lymphoblastic leukaemia is given chemotherapy. He now develops a right testicular swelling.

36. A 70 year old man comes in to have his right testicular hydrocele aspirated. A day after the procedure, he develops a scrotal swelling on the right.

37. A 6 year old boy presents with bilateral scrotal swelling. He had suffered from mumps two week prior to presentation.

38. A 13 year old boy presents with bilateral pain and testicular swelling, after cycling.

Theme 9: Association of systemic diseases and skin lesions

Options:

a. Erythema chronicum migrans
b. Erythema multiforme
c. Pretibial myxoedema
d. Dermatitis herpetiformis
e. Livedo reticularis
f. Dermatomyositis
g. Bazin's disease
h. Dermatitis artefacta
i. Alopecia areata
j. Mycosis fungoides
k. Bowen's disease
l. Paget's disease
m. Rodent ulcer
n. Cafe-au-lait spots

For each pathology below, choose the SINGLE most appropriate skin lesion from the above list of options. Each option may be used once, more than once, or not at all.

39. Addison's disease.
40. Cutaneous T-cell lymphoma.
41. Coeliac disease.
42. Hyperthyroidism.
43. Tuberculosis.

Theme 10: Diagnosis of infections

Options:

a. Lyme disease
b. Brucellosis
c. Infective endocarditis
d. Listeriosis
e. Psittacosis
f. Typhoid fever
g. Infectious mononucleosis
h. Legionnaire's disease
i. Tularaemia
j. Tuberculosis

For each presentation below, choose the SINGLE most appropriate diagnosis from the above list of options. Each option may be used once, more than once, or not at all.

44. A 34 year old man gets bitten on his hand by a rat. A few days later he develops enlarged and tender localized cervical and axillary lymphadenopathy on the same side as the bite. The bite becomes rapidly red and painful and undergoes necrosis. He also complains of generalized fever, headache and fatigue.

45. A 22 year old male has a gradual onset of cough, night sweats, vomiting and weight loss. On his chest X-ray there is a density which enlarges the left hilum. It occupies the site of the apico-posterior segment of the left upper lobe. There is a lobulated left para-tracheal density.

46. Five days after a working journey in France, a 42 year old male smoker begins to feel ill with malaise, general aches, a headache, and a dry cough. He rapidly develops diffuse and acute renal failure. Investigations reveal a thrombocytopenia.

47. A mother notes that her eight year old son has mild weight loss and a prolonged low grade fever over about two weeks. On examination he is found to have cervical lymphadenopathy and splenomegaly.

48. While working with a missions organisation in Africa a doctor is asked to see a 28 year old male with fresh bleeding per rectum. The man gives a history of increasing fever, headache and constipation. On inspection he is noted to have a relatively slow pulse rate and pinkish spots are seen on his abdomen.

49. A pregnant woman and her husband develop fever, muscle aches and severe diarrhoea about three weeks after eating a soft cheese given to them as a present from a guest. Her baby is later born at term with septicaemia and becomes acutely unwell.

Theme 11: Investigations of the unconscious patient

Options:

a. Blood cultures
b. Blood gases
c. Brain stem death tests
d. Carboxyhaemoglobin level
e. Computed tomography of head
f. Cardiac monitoring
g. Lumbar puncture
h. Serum glucose
i. Thyroid function tests
j. Toxicology screen
k. Urea and electrolytes

For each presentation below, choose the SINGLE most appropriate investigation from the above list of options. Each option may be used once, more than once, or not at all.

50. A 47 year old woman is found collapsed in her home. Examination reveals meningism and bilateral upgoing plantars.

51. A 67 year old man with severe chronic obstructive pulmonary disease was brought to Casualty department by ambulance. His breathing and conscious level seems much worse with oxygen during the ambulance journey, although his oxygen saturation on pulse oximetry is 90%.

52. A middle–aged couple is found comatosed in their caravan by their teenaged son, who woke up in the middle of the night with nausea and vomiting. All three of them had been well before they went to sleep.

53. A 45 year old man collapses in the ward. Examination reveals cardiorespiratory arrest.

54. A 56 year old diabetic is found unresponsive at home by her neighbour. She is presently being treated for urinary tract infection. There is no focal neurological deficit on examination.

Theme 12: Management of ischaemic limb

Options:

a. Stop smoking, do exercise
b. Amputation
c. Angiography
d. Duplex scan
e. IV vasodilator
f. Chemical sympathectomy
g. Angioplasty
h. Calcium channel blockers
i. Antibiotics

For each presentation below, choose the SINGLE most appropriate management from the above list of options. Each option may be used once, more than once, or not at all.

55. A 40 year woman with history of angina complains of sudden pain, pale, pulseless, lower limb. She can hardly move her foot.

56. A 45 year man has been suffering from intermittent claudication and it is getting worse now.

57. A 53 year man with history of femoral–popliteal reconstruction on the left leg. On examination progressive cellulitis, ulcers on the shin and no dorsalis pedis pulses are noted.

58. A 45 year smoker complain of pain in calf walking up hill 400 yards. On examination absent dorsalis pedis. Other P's are normal.

59. A 25 year old man after RTA with fructure of tibia/fibula. There appears to be no palpation of pulse in the foot.

Theme 13: Diagnosis of eye diseases

Options:

a. Acute glaucoma
b. Acute iritis
c. Amaurosis fugax
d. Cataract
e. Pituitary tumour
f. Retinitis pigmentosa
g. Subconjunctival haemorrhage
h. Temporal arteritis
i. Thyroid associated opthalmopathy
j. Viral conjunctivitis
k. Behcet's disease
l. Cavernous sinus thrombosis
m. Graves' disease
n. Multiple sclerosis
o. Ophthalmic herpes zoster
p. Pancoast tumour
q. Reiter's syndrome
r. Sjögren's syndrome
s. Syphilis
t. Wegener's granulomatosis

For each presentation below, choose the SINGLE most appropriate diagnosis from the above list of options. Each option may be used once, more than once, or not at all.

60. A 27 year old girl presents with unilateral proptosis, weight loss, palpitations and increased appetite.

61. A 75 year old lady complains of a temporary loss of vision 'like a curtain coming down'.

62. A 60 year old man presents with pain and blurring of vision in his right eye. His right pupil is fixed and dilated.

63. A 15 month old child diagnosed with whooping cough presents with a red eye.

64. A 50 year old man presents with early morning headaches and visual field defects.

Theme 14: Poisoning: Treatment

Options:

a. Atropine
b. Flumazenil
c. Dicobalt edetate
d. Specific antibody fragments
e. Antitoxin
f. Desferrioxamine
g. Naloxone
h. Phytomenadione
i. FFP and vitamin K
j. NAC
k. IV sodium bicarbonate
l. Hyperbaric O_2
m. Supportive care only
n. IV methylene blue
o. Procyclidine

For each presentation below, choose the SINGLE most appropriate treatment from the above list of options. Each option may be used once, more than once, or not at all.

65. An 18 year old girl took 30 paracetamol tablets and is brought to A & E now.

66. A 20 year old woman becomes very agitated and sweaty in a night club. She is febrile and has tachycardia and dilated pupils. Her BP is 190/110.

67. A 30 year old man has been brought to A & E with shock and seizures. On examination his breath smells of bitter almonds.

68. A 45 year old man has been on painkiller. He accidently overdosed himself and is now brought to A&E with breathing difficulty and dilated pupils.

69. A 30 year old man presents with diplopia, blurred vision and paralysis and has low GCS. He says that he took canned food last night.

Theme 15: Principles of the dutes of a doctor registered with the General Medical Council

Options:

a. Make the care of your patient your first concern

b. Treat every patient politely and considerately

c. Respect patients dignity and privacy

d. Listen to patients and respect their views

e. Give patients information in a way they can understand

f. Respect the right of patients to be fully involved in decisions about their care

g. Keep your professional knowledge and skills up to date

h. Recognise the limits of your professional competence

i. Be honest and trustworthy

j. Respect and protect confidential information.

k. Make sure that your personal beliefs do not prejudice your patients' care

l. Act quickly to protect patients from risk if you have good reason to believe that your colleague may not be fit to practise

m. Avoid abusing your position as a doctor

n. Work with colleagues in the ways that best serve patients' interests

For each presentation below, choose the SINGLE most appropriate principle from the above list of options. Each option may be used once, more than once, or not at all.

70. There is a lunch-time teaching session, but a patient on the ward is experiencing chest pain.

71. Your patient reports feeling of depression. You seek a psychiatric opinion.

72. You asked a patient to undress to examine the abdomen. You remember to cover the patient's groin.

73. You are asked to examine a patient at his bedside. You remember to pull the curtain around the bed to ensure privacy.

74. You see an overworked colleague struggle with his duties. You intervene and offer assistance.

Theme 16: Drug of first choice in management of schizophrenia

Options:

a. Sertindole
b. Chlorpromazine
c. Orphenadrine
d. Biperidine
e. Tetrabenazine
f. Fluphenazine
g. Clozapine
h. Haloperidol
i. Clonazepam
j. Benzhexol
k. Phenelzine
l. Lofepramine
m. Mianserin
n. Protryptiline

For each pathology below, choose the SINGLE most appropriate drug from the above list of options. Each option may be used once, more than once, or not at all.

75. Drug of 1st choice in patients suffering from akathesia.
76. Drug of 1st choice for maintainance therapy.
77. Drug of 1st choice in resistant schizophrenia.
78. Drug of 1st choice in acute positive symptoms.
79. Drug of 1st choice in patients having acute negative symptoms.
80. Drug of 1st choice in patients with tardive dyskinesia.

Theme 17: Differential diagnosis of diarrhoea

Options:

a. Ulcerative colitis
b. Laxative abuse
c. Pseudomembranous colitis
d. Viral gastroenteritis
e. Campylobacter infection
f. Shigella dystentery
g. Amoebic dystentery
h. Irritable bowel syndrome
i. Colorectal carcinoma

For each presentation below, choose the SINGLE most appropriate diagnosis from the above list of options. Each option may be used once, more than once, or not at all.

81. A healthy 20 year old man has an acute diarrhoeal disease characterized by bloody stool, crampy abdominal pain and low grade fever. His symptoms resolve spontaneously in 5 days and do not recur.
82. A healthy 20 year old man has an acute onset of bloody diarrhoea, crampy abdominal pain, and fever. His symptoms persists for several weeks.
83. A 30 year old woman develops severe watery diarrhoea, 2 weeks after undergoing antibiotic therapy for pelvic inflammatory disease. Procto-sigmoidoscopy shows plaque-like lesions covering the mucosa.
84. A 30 year old woman complains of chronic watery diarrhoea. Stool examination shows an osmolarity of 300 mEq/dl, Na concentration of 30 mEq/dl and a K concentration of 45 mEq/dl. Shortly after she is hospitalized for evaluation and begun on a 48-hour fast, her diarrhoea disappears.

Theme 18: Eye diseases

Options:

a. Malignant melanoma of eye
b. Holmes-Adie pupil
c. Proliferative retinopathy
d. Toxic amblyopia
e. Methanol poisoning
f. Psychogenic
g. CMV retinopathy
h. Syphilis
i. Senile macular degeneration
j. Cortical blindness
k. Retinitis pigmentosa
l. Retinoblastoma
m. Optic neuritis

For each presentation below, choose the SINGLE most appropriate diagnosis from the above list of options. Each option may be used once, more than once, or not at all.

85. A 34 year old man with long history of smoking and alcohol presents with blurring of vision. His wife has noted that he cant differentiate between red and green colours now.

86. A 32 year old male with some blurring of vision and pain on eye movements.

87. A soldier returned from Vietnam now complains of some visual problems. On fundoscopy there are pale areas with haemorrhages below the fovea.

88. A 38 year old male with meiosis and irregular pupils. His pupils respond to accommodation but not to light.

89. A 65 year old women blind on testing but denies that there is any problem with her eyesight.

Theme 19: Causes of gout

Options:

a. Chronic renal failure
b. Diuretics
c. Ethambutol
d. Hyperparathyroidism
e. Lesch-Nyhan syndrome
f. Myeloma
g. Polycythaemia
h. Psoriasis
i. Pyrazinamide
j. Sarcoidosis
k. Waldenstrom's macroglobulinaemia

For each presentation below, choose the SINGLE most appropriate cause of gout from the above list of options. Each option may be used once, more than once, or not at all.

90. A 12 year old boy presents with gouty arthritis, spasticity and choreoathetosis. He has a several year history of worsening behavioural problems, particularly with self-mutilation.

91. A 76 year old man complains of a painful right knee, tiredness and weight loss. His ESR was markedly elevated, serum IgM 17gm/l, and bone marrow biopsy showed plasmacytoid lymphocytes.

92. A normally fit 56 year old Caucasian male develops gout after several weeks of anti-tubercular treatment. His night sweats have resolved and his dry cough has eased considerably.

93. A 76 year old woman with type II respiratory failure secondary to severe chronic obstructive pulmonary disease, presents with pain in her right ankle and 1st metatarsophalangeal joint. Her medication consists of a number of inhalers and steroid tablets.

94. A 75 year old man with controlled hypertension presents with recurrent attacks of gout.

Theme 20: Developmental milestones

Options

a. 1 month
b. 2 months
c. 4 months
d. 6 months
e. 8 months
f. 10 months
g. 1 year
h. 18 months
i. 2 years
j. 3 years
k. 4 years
l. 5 years

For each presentation below, choose the SINGLE most appropriate age at which it first occurs from the above list of options. Each option may be used once, more than once, or not at all.

95. Just stands, walks using a table's support.
96. Holds head steady, when sitting reaches out, rolls over.
97. Jumps,can stand on one foot.
98. Can walk backwards.
99. Kicks a ball, overarm bowling.

Theme 21: Management of meningitis

Options:

a. Benzylpenicillin
b. Ceftriaxone
c. Netilmicin
d. Ampicillin and Gentamycin
e. Symptomatic treatment
f. Ampicillin only

For each pathogen below, choose the SINGLE most appropriate drug from the above list of options. Each option may be used once, more than once, or not at all.

100. Neisseria meningitides.
101. Haemophilus influenzae.
102. Streptococcus pneumoniae.
103. E.coli.
104. Group β haemolytic streptococci.
105. Listeria monocytogenes.
106. Viruses.

Theme 22: The natural history of endometrial carcinoma

Options:

a. 5-6 year
b. <5%
c. 10-12 year
d. 2-3 year
e. 5 year
f. 50-60 year
g. 35-45 year
h. <2%
i. 10-20%
j. 7 year
k. 10 year
l. 5-10%
m.2-3 months

For each presentation below, choose the SINGLE most appropriate time or time interval from the above list of options. Each option may be used once, more than once, or not at all.

107. The peak age of presentation of endometrial carcinoma.

108. The times scale within which 80% of patients with recurrent disease will present following the treatment of a Stage I tumour.

109. Within this period, up to 80% of patients will be alive following radiotherapy for Stage I cancer of the endometrium.

110. The percentage of women who commonly present with both cervical and endometrial carcinoma.

111. The percentage of women with stage IV cancer of the endometrium who will be alive after 5 year following surgical removal.

Theme 23: The clinical management of hypertension in pregnancy

Options:

a. Magnesium hydroxide
b. Oral antihypertensive
c. Oral diuretic
d. Recheck blood pressure in seven days
e. Renal function tests
f. Retinoscopy
g. 24 hour urinary protein
h. A period of observation for blood pressure
i. Complete neurological examination
j. Fetal ultrasound
k. Immediate Caesarean section
l. Induction of labour
m.Intravenous antihypertensive
n. Intravenous benzodiazepines
o. Low dose aspirin

For each presentation below, choose the SINGLE most appropriate action from the above list of options. Each option may be used once, more than once, or not at all.

112. At 34 weeks, an 80 kg woman complains of persistent headaches and "flashing lights". There is no hyper-reflexia and her BP is 155/100 mmHg. Urinalysis is negative but she has digital oedema.

113. At 33 weeks, a 19 year old primigravida is found to have BP of 145/100 mmHg. At her first visit at 12 weeks the BP was 145/90 mmHg. She has no proteinuria, but she is found to have oedema to her knees.

114. At an antenatal clinic visit at 38 weeks gestation, a 38 year old multigravida has BP of 140/95 mmHg. She has no proteinuria and is otherwise well.

115. A 29 year old woman has an uneventful first pregnancy to 31 weeks. She is then admitted as an emergency with epigastric pain. During the first 3 hours her BP rises from 150/100 to 170/119 mmHg. On

dipstick she is found to have 3+ proteinuria. The fetal cardiotocogram is normal.

116. A 32 year old woman in her second pregnancy presents to her GP at 12 weeks gestation. She was mildly hypertensive in both of her previous pregnancies. Her BP is 150/100 mmHg. Two weeks later, at the hospital antenatal clinic, her BP is 155/95 mmHg.

Theme 24: Investigation of post-operative complications

Options:

a. Chest X-ray
b. Abdominal ultrasound
c. Echocardiography
d. ECG
e. Computed tomography (CT) scan of the abdomen
f. Serum amylase
g. Coeliac axis angiography
h. Sigmoidoscopy
i. Barium enema
j. Double contrast enema
k. Laparotomy

For each presentation below, choose the SINGLE most appropriate investigation from the above list of options. Each option may be used once, more than once, or not at all.

117. A 67 year old man complains of a retro-sternal chest pain associated with increased sweating lasting 45 minutes. He is recovering from pancolectomy.

118. A 67 year old man is recovering from laparoscopic cholecystectomy. He is tachy-pnoeic and is found to have a tender abdomen .He complains of a cough associated with chest pain.

119. Four hours after surgery to repair a ruptured abdominal aneurysm, a 78 year old woman complains of difficulty in breathing and severe abdominal pain radiating to her back. Her blood pressure is 100/70 mmHg.

120. A 34 year old woman presents with abdominal pain, vomiting and constipation. She had a total abdominal hysterectomy 3 weeks ago.

Theme 25: The management of diarrhoea in children

Options:

a. Metronidazole
b. Gluten free diet
c. No action
d. Soya milk
e. Lactose free milk
f. Pancreatic enzyme supplements
g. Vitamin D
h. High fibre diet
i. Breast milk allergy
j. Praziquantel
k. Niclosamide
l. Benzylpenicillin (IV)
m. Steroids (in moderation)

For each presentation below, choose the SINGLE most appropriate treatment from the above list of options. Each option may be used once, more than once, or not at all.

121. A 2 year old girl is brought to the A&E department by her mother who says that she has diarrhoea. She describes the stool as looking like 'peas and carrots'.

122. A 4 year old girl is brought to the A&E department by her mother who has noticed that she dislikes bright lights. In addition, the child has a 6 hour history of diarrhoea and increasing drowsiness.

123. A 12 year girl whose height is on the 20th centile complains of diarrhoea, with stools that are difficult to flush away. She is found to have anti-endomyseal antibodies.

124. A 7 month old baby boy has had 7 episodes of diarrhoea. The mother associates all the episodes with the introduction of cow's milk since weaning. The mother is a known asthmatic.

125. A 13 year old girl from Northern Ireland complains of diarrhoea. She is found to have iron deficiency anaemia and a high titre of anti-reticulin and α-gliadin antibodies. She denies any history of gastrointestinal upsets after eating rice, soya or potatoes.

Theme 26: The management of genital prolapse and incontinence

Options:

a. Tension free vaginal tape (TVT)
b. Vaginal pessary
c. Anterior colporrhaphy
d. Posterior colporrhaphy
e. Bilateral salpingo-oophorectomy
f. Pelvic floor exercises
g. Lose weight
h. Total abdominal hysterectomy
i. Oestrogen cream
j. Mirena coil (progesterone containing IUCD)
k. Vaginopexy
l. Urodynamic studies
m. Bladder drill
n. Cystoscopy
o. Oxybutinin
p. Vaginal hysterectomy

For each presentation below, choose the SINGLE most appropriate treatment from the above list of options. Each option may be used once, more than once, or not at all.

126. A 56 year old woman presents with a 2 month history of urinary incontinence. Because of her inconsistent history, you are unsure whether this is genuine stress incontinence or detrusor instability.

127. A 34 year para 7 + 1 with glaucoma presents with urinary incontinence. She is found to have detrusor instability. She dislikes surgery.

128. A 35 year para 2 presents with urinary incontinence. She is found to have genuine stress incontinence. She is put on conservative treatment without much success.

129. A 67 year old woman presents with Grade II uterine prolapse. She also complains of urinary incontinence and is found have to a cystocele.

130. A fit 65 year old woman presents with uterine procidentia. She has 5 healthy children born from 2 different fathers.

131. A frail 57 year old woman presents with Grade I uterine prolapse. She also complains of hot flushes and excessive sweating.

Theme 27: Medical statistics

Options:

a. Stillbirth
b. Early neonatal death
c. Pe rinatal mortality
d. Perinatal mortality rate
e. Late neonatal death
f. Post neonatal death
g. Stillbirth rate
h. Perinatal death rate
i. Late neonatal death rate
j. Infant death

For each presentation below, choose the SINGLE most appropriate statement from the above list of options. Each option may be used once, more than once, or not at all.

132. Death at age 28 days and over, but under one year.
133. This term is used to define the number of stillbirths, plus deaths in the first week after birth per a thousand live births.
134. Any fetus born with no signs of life, after 24 weeks' gestation.
135. Death from age 7 days to 27 completed days of life.
136. This denotes death in the first week after birth.
137. Death at age under one year.
138. A 56 year old woman who is 3 year post-menopausal complains of per vaginal bleeding not associated with sexual inter-course. Her Body Mass Index (BMI) is 32.
139. A 39 year old woman had a total abdominal hysterectomy following rupture during delivery. She now complains of excessive sweating, weight loss and palpitations.

Theme 28: Investigation of a patient with haemoptysis

Option:

a. Computed tomography
b. Fibre optic bronchoscopy
c. Fine needle aspiration
d. Mediastinoscopy
e. Mediastinotomy
f. Magnetic resonance imaging (MRI)
g. Pulmonary angiogram
h. Selective arteriogram
i. Sputum culture
j. Sputum cytology
k. Thoracoscopy
l. Ventilation perfusion scan
m. CXR

For each pathology below, choose the SINGLE most appropriate definitive investigation from the above list of options. Each option may be used once, more than once, or not at all.

140. Bronchial carcinoid.
141. Carcinoma of the right main bronchus.
142. Pulmonary embolism.
143. Lobar pneumonia.
144. Bronchiectasis.
145. Tuberculosis.

Theme 29: Dysphagia

Options:

a. Pseudobulbar palsy
b. Motor neurone disease
c. Myasthenia gravis
d. Scleroderma
e. Dermatomyositis
f. Diffuse oesophageal spasm
g. Achalasia
h. Gastro-oesophageal reflux with stricture
i. Carcinoma of oesophagus
j. Plummer–Vinson syndrome

For each presentation below, choose the SINGLE most appropriate cause of dysphagia from the above list of options. Each option may be used once, more than once, or not at all.

146. A 60 year old man presents with progressive difficulty in chewing, swallowing and talking. Examination reveals wasting and fasciculation of the tongue and muscles of the limbs. Electromyography shows changes of chronic partial denervation.

147. A 25 year old woman with SLE presents with difficulty in swallowing, double vision, and drooping of her eyelids. Her symptoms worsen before her menstrual periods.

148. A 66 year old woman with ovarian cancer presents with recent onset rash. She complains of dysphagia and difficulty climbing stairs. Muscle biopsy reveals necrosis of muscle fibres.

149. A 32 year old woman with progressive difficulty in opening her mouth, dysphagia and episodes of painful burning in her hands.

150. A 45 year old man with progressive dysphagia to solid foods. He has had a long history of chest discomfort 30-60 minutes after meals.

Theme 30: Diagnosing medical conditions

Options:

a. Cirrhosis
b. Congestive heart failure
c. Constrictive pericarditis
d. Nephrotic syndrome
e. Protein losing enteropathy
f. Mesothelioma
g. Secondary carcinomatosis
h. Tuberculous peritonitis
i. Myxoedema
j. Systemic lupus erythematosus

For each presentation below, choose the SINGLE most appropriate diagnosis from the above list of options. Each option may be used once, more than once, or not at all.

151. A 43 year old male presents with anasarca, shortness of breath and loss of lean body mass. Examination reveals a raised JVP that increases on inspiration and an extra diastolic sound. He has a past history of tuberculosis.

152. A 53 year old woman presents with fatigue, hoarse voice and paraesthesia in both hands. Investigations reveal a macrocytic anaemia and hyponatraemia.

153. A 70 year old retired pipe fitter presents with 3 month history of progressive shortness of breath and swelling of the abdomen.

154. A 26 year old woman presents with fever, malaise, migratory arthralgia and rash. Investigations reveal an anaemia, thrombocytopenia and proteinuria.

155. A 64 year old man comes with fever, weight loss and night sweats. Examination reveals fluid in the abdomen. Analysis of the fluid shows a lymphocytic exudate with an increased adenosine deaminase level.

Theme 31: Firm nodular liver

Options:

a. Chronic alcohol abuse
b. Chronic viral hepatitis
c. Autoimmune chronic active hepatitis
d. Haemochromatosis
e. Wilson's disease
f. α_1 Antitrypsin deficiency
g. Primary biliary cirrhosis
h. Sclerosing cholangitis
i. Budd Chiari syndrome
j. Congestive cardiac failure

For each presentation below, choose the SINGLE most appropriate cause of liver disorder from the above list of options. Each option may be used once, more than once, or not at all.

156. A 54 year old man presenting with weakness, lassitude, weight loss, generalized pigmentation and loss of libido. Examination reveals hepatomegaly, loss of body hair, splenomegaly and bilateral knee joint swelling. His random blood sugar is 430 mg/dl.

157. A 29 year old female presents with resting and intention tremors, stiffness and dysphagia. Examination reveals greenish deposits at the limbus of the cornea and hepatomegaly.

158. A 33 year old female on the pill presents with a 30 day history of progressive ascites, jaundice, right upper quadrant pain and oedema of feet. Her SGOT is 967 and SGPT 1285.

159. A 20 year old female with a six month history of jaundice, fever, malaise, arthralgias, and dryness of mouth and eyes. Investigations reveal SGOT 836, SGPT 962, serum globulin 4.09/dl and serologic evaluation for infection with hepatitis B,C,D, is negative.

160. A 33 year old male smoker presenting with progressive dyspnoea and jaundice. Examination reveals hepatomegaly and hyperinflation of the chest with increased resonance to percussion especially in the lower zones.

Theme 32: Palliative care

Options:

a. Hyoscine
b. Octreotide
c. SL Buprenorphine
d. Diamorphine
e. External beam
f. Midazolam
g. Cholestyramine
h. Cyclizine
i. Haloperidol
j. Dexamethasone

For each presentation below, choose the SINGLE most appropriate management from the above list of options. Each option may be used once, more than once, or not at all.

161. A 55 year old man with oesophageal carcinoma and total dysphagia has pain due to bony metastases. He is unable to swallow any medication and finds morphine causing unacceptable drowsiness.

162. A 58 year old man has profuse watery diarrhoea from an inoperable small bowel tumour.

163. A 62 year old woman with carcinoma of the pancreas complains bitterly of pruritus, which does not respond to anti-histamines. She is jaundiced.

164. A 45 year old woman with metastatic breast cancer is getting increasingly agitated and complains of headache and weakness in her left leg. On examination she has increased tone and brisk reflexes in the leg.

Theme 33: Headache: Selection of diagnostic tests

Options:

a. CT head
b. MRI brain
c. Lumbar puncture
d. ESR
e. S. calcium level
f. Cervical spine X-ray
g. Sinus X-ray
h. Skull X-ray
i. No tests required
j. Temporal artery biopsy

For each presentation below, choose the SINGLE most appropriate diagnostic test from the above list of options. Each option may be used once, more than once, or not at all.

165. A 59 year old woman presents with severe left-sided headache for three days. Her left temporal artery is tender and pulseless.

166. A 24 year old woman complains of headaches every four weeks. She started taking the oral contraceptive pill four months ago and her headaches are getting worse. The headaches last up to two days and she is unable to work during that time.

167. An 18 year old man presents with a 24-hour history of severe right frontal headache and nasal congestion. He is tender over his right forehead.

168. Three days ago, a 40 year old builder was hit by a plank while he was at work. He did not lose consciousness at the time and has no amnesia, but he vomited once. He is now complaining of increasing headache, dizziness and poor concentration. He says that he is worried about returning to work.

169. A 35 year old woman complains of increasing headache over a two-month period. The headache is worse in the morning and on bending forwards. She has also noticed some difficulty in writing but

had put this down to being distracted by the headache.

170. A 20 year old man complains of a severe generalized headache and photophobia for two days. He has a low-grade fever, sore throat and mild neck stiffness. He has no neurological signs or rashes.

Theme 34: Diagnosis of cardiovascular diseases in children

Options:

a. Kawasaki disease
b. Hereditary angioedema
c. Congenital nephrotic syndrome
d. Myocarditis
e. Pericarditis
f. Primary pulmonary hypertension
g. Juvenile rheumatoid arthritis
h. Acute rheumatic fever
i. Congestive heart failure
j. Toxic synovitis
k. Aortic stenosis
l. Systemic lupus erythematosus
m. Paroxysmal atrial tachycardia
n. Mitral stenosis

For each presentation below, choose the SINGLE most appropriate diagnosis from the above list of options. Each option may be used once, more than once, or not at all.

171. A 10 year old boy presents with stridor. He has history of recurrent swelling of the hands and feet with abdominal pain and diarrhoea. His sister also suffer from similar attacks.

172. A 6 year old girl presents with spiking fevers. On examination, she has spindle-shaped swellings of the finger-joints.

173. A 12 year old boy presents with polyarthritis and abdominal pain. He had a sore throat a week ago. On examination, he is noted to have an early blowing diastolic murmur at the left sternal edge.

174. A 10 year old boy presents to casualty following a seizure during gym. On examination, he has a loud systolic ejection murmur with a thrill.

175. A 12 year old girl prsents with pallor, dyspnoea, and pulse rate of 190/min. She is noted to have cardiomegaly and hepatomegaly.

Theme 35: The management of traumatic injuries

Options:

a. Peritoneal lavage
b. Observation and angiography
c. Closed thoracotomy-tube drainage
d. Pressure dressing
e. Cricothyroidotomy
f. Nasogastric tube suction and observation
g. Surgical repair of the flexor digitorum profundus tendon
h. Urgent surgical exploration
i. Debridement and repair
j. Endotracheal intubation
k. Needle pericardiocentesis
l. Fasciotomy

For each presentation below, choose the SINGLE most appropriate management from the above list of options. Each option may be used once, more than once, or not at all.

176. A 23 year old man presents to A & E having been stabbed in the neck. He complains of difficulty swallowing and talking. He has no stridor, On examination, there is a small penetrating wound with diffuse neck swelling.

177. A 12 year old boy presents with a hand injury sustained while playing rugby and attempting to catch the ball. On examination, he is unable to bend the tip of his right middle finger.

178. A 35 year old woman is brought into A & E acutely short of breath. Her respiratory rate is 50/min. She was involved in a road traffic accident. She has no breath sound on the left. Her trachea is deviated to the right.

179. An 18 year old man sustains a stab wound to the right thigh. On examination, he has a large haematoma over the thigh and weak distal pulses. He is unable to move his foot and complains of pins and needles in his foot.

180. A 30 year old woman involved in a head-on car collision presents with diffuse abdominal pain. Upright chest X-ray shows elevation of the diaphragm with a stomach gas bubble in the left lower lung field.

Theme 36: Dermatology

Options:

a. Crust
b. Scale
c. Macule
d. Vesicle
e. Papule
f. Nodule
g. Bullae
h. Pustule
i. Urticaria

For each presentation below, choose the SINGLE most appropriate description from the above list of options. Each option may be used once, more than once, or not at all.

181. Deeply set lump in the skin.
182. Flat spot which differs in colour as compared to the surrounding skin.
183. Horny cells loosened from skin surface.
184. Blister filled with purulent material.
185. Blister filled with clear fluid.

Theme 37: Causes of lump in scrotum

Options:

a. Inguinal hernia
b. Epididymal cyst
c. Hydrocele
d. Tuberculosis of epididymis
e. Testicular tumour
f. Spermatocele
g. Varicocele
h. Orchitis

For each presentation below, choose the SINGLE most appropriate cause from the above list of options. Each option may be used once, more than once, or not at all.

186. A 30 year old man with cystic lump in the scrotum. Testes cannot be felt separately from the swelling which transilluminates well.
187. A 40 year old retired weight lifter complains of a swelling in his scrotum. On examination one cannot get above the swelling.
188. A 30 year old man with a hard, painless lump in his scrotum. Testes cannot be felt separately from the swelling. He noticed the swelling after an injury to the scrotum.
189. A 40 year old presents with a swelling which is cystic and felt separately from the testes. The lump transilluminates slightly.
190. A 40 year old presents with a lump in one side of his scrotum. It is hard, thickened and separately felt from the testes.

Theme 38: Investigation of diarrhoea

Options:

a. Barium enema
b. Bone marrow biopsy
c. Echocardiography
d. Clostridium
e. Karyotyping
f. Serum gastrin estimation
g. Upper gastro-oesophagoscopy
h. Thyroid function tests
i. X-ray PNS
j. Sigmoidoscopy
k. Serum B_{12} level
l. Jejunal biopsy
m. Coomb's test
n. None required

For each presentation below, choose the SINGLE most appropriate investigation from the above list of options. Each option may be used once, more than once, or not at all.

191. A 58 year old female presents with recurrent jaundice. Her haemoglobin is 8.5 gm% and MCV is 125 fL.

192. A 45 year old man comes with weight loss, heat intolerance and diarrhoea. His sleeping pulse is 100/minute and he is febrile.

193. A 52 year old man presents with alternating diarrhoea and constipation. He is anaemic and has lost 10 lbs in the past 3 months. His stool guaiac test is positive.

194. A 20 year old man developed maxillary sinusitis. He was prescribed amoxicillin for 10 days. He has developed bloody diarrhoea from day 7.

195. A 45 year old man comes with abdominal pain and diarrhoea. His endoscopy was done which has shown multiple ulcers in the oesophagus and stomach.

Theme 39: Diagnosis of psychiatric illness

Options:

a. Depression
b. General anxiety
c. Obsessive compulsive disorder
d. Panic attacks
e. Manic depressive psychosis
f. Schizophrenia.
g. Claustrophobia
h. Agoraphobia
i. Post traumatic stress disorder.

For each presentation below, choose the SINGLE most appropriate diagnosis of from the above list of options. Each option may be used once, more than once, or not at all.

196. A 25 year old female patient gets scared suddenly and starts hyperventilating. There are no obvious precipitating factors.

197. A 35 year old male patient has a habit of checking doors repeatedly to see if they are locked.

198. A 52 year old male just returned to the UK. He has witnessed his family getting killed in a car accident and hence fears going out of the house. He also feels that he can not cope and has developed suicidal tendencies.

199. A 35 year old male suddenly stops while talking and complains that his thoughts are being removed by somebody.

200. A 40 year old woman is scared to go out. Whenever she does, she comes back sweating and drinks water to relieve anxiety.

ANSWERS

1. **(b)** Crohn's disease
2. **(a)** Ulcerative colitis
3. **(b)** Crohn's disease
4. **(a)** Ulcerative colitis
5. **(f)** Cystic fibrosis
6. **(c)** Lymphoma
7. **(d)** Anaplastic
8. **(e)** Medullary
9. **(b)** Follicular
10. **(a)** Papillary
11. **(c)** CA 125
12. **(b)** CA 19-9
13. **(i)** Calcitonin
14. **(a)** α fetoprotein
15. **(k)** None of the above
16. **(e)** Rifampicin
17. **(i)** Metronidazole
18. **(a)** Zidovudine
19. **(l)** Chloroquine and proguanil
20. **(c)** Clindamycin
21. **(a)** Pityriasis rosea
22. **(f)** Leprosy
23. **(h)** Tinea corporis
24. **(c)** Erythema multiforme
25. **(e)** Hereditary angioedema
26. **(k)** Uveitis
27. **(b)** Central retinal artery occlusion
28. **(d)** Cerebral embolism
29. **(i)** Retinal detachment
30. **(j)** Temporal arteritis
31. **(l)** Cord compression
32. **(q)** Placenta praevia
33. **(t)** Toxoplasmosis
34. **(e)** Mid stream urine for microscopy and/or culture
35. **(f)** Biopsy
36. **(b)** Surgical exploration
37. **(c)** Reassurance
38. **(b)** Surgical exploration
39. **(i)** Alopecia areata
40. **(j)** Mycosis fungoides
41. **(d)** Dermatitis herpetiformis
42. **(c)** Pretibial myxoedema
43. **(g)** Bazin's disease
44. **(i)** Tularaemia
45. **(j)** Tuberculosis
46. **(h)** Legionnaire's disease
47. **(g)** Infectious mononucleosis
48. **(f)** Typhoid fever
49. **(d)** Listeriosis
50. **(e)** Computed tomography of head
51. **(b)** Blood gases
52. **(d)** Carboxyhaemoglobin level
53. **(f)** Cardiac monitoring
54. **(h)** Serum glucose
55. **(g)** Angioplasty
56. **(a)** Stop smoking, do exercise
57. **(c)** Angiography
58. **(d)** Duplex scan
59. **(c)** Angiography
60. **(i)** Thyroid associated opthalmopathy
61. **(c)** Amaurosis fugax
62. **(a)** Acute glaucoma
63. **(j)** Viral conjunctivitis
64. **(e)** Pituitary tumour
65. **(j)** NAC
66. **(m)** Supportive care only
67. **(c)** Dicobalt edetate
68. **(g)** Naloxone
69. **(e)** Antitoxin
70. **(a)** Make the care of your patient your first concern
71. **(n)** Work with colleagues in the ways that best serve patients' interests
72. **(c)** Respect patients dignity and privacy
73. **(c)** Respect patients dignity and privacy

74. **(l)** Act quickly to protect patients from risk if you have good reason to believe that your colleague may not be fit to practise
75. **(c)** Orphenadrine
76. **(f)** Fluphenazine
77. **(g)** Clozapine
78. **(b)** Chlorpromazine
79. **(a)** Sertindole
80. **(e)** Tetrabenazine
81. **(e)** Campylobacter infection
82. **(a)** Ulcerative colitis
83. **(c)** Pseudomembranous colitis
84. **(b)** Laxative abuse
85. **(d)** Toxic amblyopia
86. **(m)** Optic neuritis
87. **(g)** CMV retinopathy
88. **(h)** Syphilis
89. **(j)** Cortical blindness
90. **(e)** Lesch-Nyhan syndrome
91. **(k)** Waldenstrom's macroglobulinaemia
92. **(i)** Pyrazinamide
93. **(g)** Polycythaemia
94. **(b)** Diuretics
95. **(g)** 1 year
96. **(c)** 4 months
97. **(j)** 3 years
98. **(h)** 18 months
99. **(i)** 2 years
100. **(a)** Benzylpenicillin
101. **(b)** Ceftriaxone
102. **(a)** Benzylpenicillin
103. **(c)** Netilmicin
104. **(a)** Benzylpenicillin
105. **(d)** Ampicillin and Gentamycin
106. **(e)** Symptomatic treatment
107. **(f)** 50-60 year
108. **(d)** 2-3 year
109. **(e)** 5 year
110. **(h)** <2%
111. **(h)** <2%
112. **(b)** Oral antihypertensive
113. **(d)** Recheck blood pressure in seven days
114. **(h)** A period of observation for blood pressure
115. **(m)** Intravenous antihypertensive
116. **(b)** Oral antihypertensive
117. **(d)** ECG
118. **(a)** Chest X-ray
119. **(b)** Abdominal ultrasound
120. **(e)** Computed tomography (CT) scan of the abdomen
121. **(c)** No action
122. **(l)** Benzylpenicillin (IV)
123. **(b)** Gluten free diet
124. **(e)** Lactose free milk
125. **(b)** Gluten free diet
126. **(l)** Urodynamic studies
127. **(m)** Bladder drill
128. **(a)** Tension free vaginal tape (TVT)
129. **(c)** Anterior colporrhaphy
130. **(p)** Vaginal hysterectomy
131. **(i)** Oestrogen cream
132. **(f)** Post neonatal death
133. **(h)** Perinatal death rate
134. **(g)** Stillbirth rate
135. **(e)** Late neonatal death
136. **(b)** Early neonatal death
137. **(j)** Infant death
138. **(j)** Infant death
139. **(h)** Perinatal death rate
140. **(b)** Fibre optic bronchoscopy
141. **(b)** Fibre optic bronchoscopy
142. **(l)** Ventilation perfusion scan
143. **(m)** CXR
144. **(a)** Computed tomography
145. **(i)** Sputum culture
146. **(b)** Motor neurone disease
147. **(c)** Myasthenia gravis
148. **(e)** Dermatomyositis
149. **(d)** Scleroderma
150. **(h)** Gastro-oesophageal reflux with stricture
151. **(c)** Constrictive pericarditis
152. **(i)** Myxoedema

153. **(f)** Mesothelioma
154. **(j)** Systemic lupus erythematosus
155. **(h)** Tuberculous peritonitis
156. **(d)** Haemochromatosis
157. **(e)** Wilson's disease
158. **(i)** Budd Chiari syndrome
159. **(c)** Autoimmune chronic active hepatitis
160. **(f)** α_1 Antitrypsin deficiency
161. **(c)** SL Buprenorphine
162. **(b)** Octreotide
163. **(g)** Cholestyramine
164. **(e)** External beam
165. **(d)** ESR
166. **(i)** No tests required
167. **(g)** Sinus X-ray
168. **(h)** Skull X-ray
169. **(a)** CT head
170. **(c)** Lumbar puncture
171. **(b)** Hereditary angioedema
172. **(g)** Juvenile rheumatoid arthritis
173. **(h)** Acute rheumatic fever
174. **(k)** Aortic stenosis
175. **(i)** Congestive heart failure
176. **(h)** Urgent surgical exploration
177. **(g)** Surgical repair of the flexor digitorum profundus tendon
178. **(c)** Closed thoracotomy-tube drainage
179. **(h)** Urgent surgical exploration
180. **(h)** Urgent surgical exploration
181. **(f)** Nodule
182. **(c)** Macule
183. **(b)** Scale
184. **(h)** Pustule
185. **(d)** Vesicle
186. **(c)** Hydrocele
187. **(a)** Inguinal hernia
188. **(e)** Testicular tumour
189. **(b)** Epididymal cyst
190. **(d)** Tuberculosis of epididymis
191. **(k)** Serum B_{12} level
192. **(h)** Thyroid function tests
193. **(j)** Sigmoidoscopy
194. **(d)** Clostridium
195. **(f)** Serum gastrin estimation
196. **(d)** Panic attacks
197. **(c)** Obsessive compulsive disorder
198. **(i)** Post traumatic stress disorder
199. **(f)** Schizophrenia
200. **(h)** Agoraphobia

General Medical Council PLAB Test Part 1

Full Name

Test Centre/Date

- Use pencil only • Make heavy marks that fill the lozenge completely
- Write your candidate number in the top row of the box to the right **and** fill in the appropriate lozenge below each number
- Given **one** answer only for each question

Do not Write in this space

Do not Write in this space

Do not Write in this space

151 (A) (B) (C) (D) (E) (F) (G) (H) (I) (J) (K) (L) (M) (N) (O) (P) (Q) (R) (S) (T) 151
152 (A) (B) (C) (D) (E) (F) (G) (H) (I) (J) (K) (L) (M) (N) (O) (P) (Q) (R) (S) (T) 152
153 (A) (B) (C) (D) (E) (F) (G) (H) (I) (J) (K) (L) (M) (N) (O) (P) (Q) (R) (S) (T) 153
154 (A) (B) (C) (D) (E) (F) (G) (H) (I) (J) (K) (L) (M) (N) (O) (P) (Q) (R) (S) (T) 154
155 (A) (B) (C) (D) (E) (F) (G) (H) (I) (J) (K) (L) (M) (N) (O) (P) (Q) (R) (S) (T) 155
156 (A) (B) (C) (D) (E) (F) (G) (H) (I) (J) (K) (L) (M) (N) (O) (P) (Q) (R) (S) (T) 156
157 (A) (B) (C) (D) (E) (F) (G) (H) (I) (J) (K) (L) (M) (N) (O) (P) (Q) (R) (S) (T) 157
158 (A) (B) (C) (D) (E) (F) (G) (H) (I) (J) (K) (L) (M) (N) (O) (P) (Q) (R) (S) (T) 158
159 (A) (B) (C) (D) (E) (F) (G) (H) (I) (J) (K) (L) (M) (N) (O) (P) (Q) (R) (S) (T) 159
160 (A) (B) (C) (D) (E) (F) (G) (H) (I) (J) (K) (L) (M) (N) (O) (P) (Q) (R) (S) (T) 160
161 (A) (B) (C) (D) (E) (F) (G) (H) (I) (J) (K) (L) (M) (N) (O) (P) (Q) (R) (S) (T) 161
162 (A) (B) (C) (D) (F) (G) (H) (I) (J) (K) (L) (M) (N) (O) (P) (Q) (R) (S) (T) 162
163 (A) (B) (C) (D) (E) (F) (G) (H) (I) (J) (K) (L) (M) (N) (O) (P) (Q) (R) (S) (T) 163
164 (A) (B) (C) (B) (E) (F) (G) (H) (I) (J) (K) (L) (M) (N) (O) (P) (Q) (R) (S) (T) 164
165 (A) (B) (C) (D) (E) (F) (G) (H) (I) (J) (K) (L) (M) (N) (O) (P) (Q) (R) (S) (T) 165
166 (A) (B) (C) (D) (E) (F) (G) (H) (I) (J) (K) (L) (M) (N) (O) (P) (Q) (R) (S) (T) 166
167 (A) (B) (C) (D) (E) (F) (G) (H) (I) (J) (K) (L) (M) (N) (O) (P) (Q) (R) (S) (T) 167
168 (A) (B) (C) (D) (E) (F) (G) (H) (I) (J) (K) (L) (M) (N) (O) (P) (Q) (R) (S) (T) 168
169 (A) (B) (C) (D) (E) (F) (G) (H) (I) (J) (K) (L) (M) (N) (O) (P) (Q) (R) (S) (T) 169
170 (A) (B) (C) (D) (E) (F) (G) (H) (I) (J) (K) (L) (M) (N) (O) (P) (Q) (R) (S) (T) 170
171 (A) (B) (C) (D) (E) (F) (G) (H) (I) (J) (K) (L) (M) (N) (O) (P) (Q) (R) (S) (T) 171
172 (A) (B) (C) (D) (E) (F) (G) (H) (I) (J) (K) (L) (M) (N) (O) (P) (Q) (R) (S) (T) 172
173 (A) (B) (C) (D) (E) (F) (G) (H) (I) (J) (K) (L) (M) (N) (O) (P) (Q) (R) (S) (T) 173
174 (A) (B) (C) (D) (E) (F) (G) (H) (I) (J) (K) (L) (M) (N) (O) (P) (Q) (R) (S) (T) 174
175 (A) (B) (C) (D) (E) (F) (G) (H) (I) (J) (K) (L) (M) (N) (O) (P) (Q) (R) (S) (T) 175
176 (A) (B) (C) (D) (E) (F) (G) (H) (I) (J) (K) (L) (M) (N) (O) (P) (Q) (R) (S) (T) 176
177 (A) (B) (C) (D) (E) (F) (G) (H) (I) (J) (K) (L) (M) (N) (O) (P) (Q) (R) (S) (T) 177
178 (A) (B) (C) (D) (E) (F) (G) (H) (I) (J) (K) (L) (M) (N) (O) (P) (Q) (R) (S) (T) 178
179 (A) (B) (C) (D) (E) (F) (G) (H) (I) (J) (K) (L) (M) (N) (O) (P) (Q) (R) (S) (T) 179
180 (A) (B) (C) (D) (E) (F) (G) (H) (I) (J) (K) (L) (M) (N) (O) (P) (Q) (R) (S) (T) 180
181 (A) (B) (C) (D) (E) (F) (G) (H) (I) (J) (K) (L) (M) (N) (O) (P) (Q) (R) (S) (T) 181
182 (A) (B) (C) (D) (E) (F) (G) (H) (I) (J) (K) (L) (M) (N) (O) (P) (Q) (R) (S) (T) 182
183 (A) (B) (C) (D) (E) (F) (G) (H) (I) (J) (K) (L) (M) (N) (O) (P) (Q) (R) (S) (T) 183
184 (A) (B) (C) (D) (E) (F) (G) (H) (I) (J) (K) (L) (M) (N) (O) (P) (Q) (R) (S) (T) 184
185 (A) (B) (C) (D) (E) (F) (G) (H) (I) (J) (K) (L) (M) (N) (O) (P) (Q) (R) (S) (T) 185
186 (A) (B) (C) (D) (E) (F) (G) (H) (I) (J) (K) (L) (M) (N) (O) (P) (Q) (R) (S) (T) 186
187 (A) (B) (C) (D) (E) (F) (G) (H) (I) (J) (K) (L) (M) (N) (O) (P) (Q) (R) (S) (T) 187
188 (A) (B) (C) (D) (E) (F) (G) (H) (I) (J) (K) (L) (M) (N) (O) (P) (Q) (R) (S) (T) 188
189 (A) (B) (C) (D) (E) (F) (G) (H) (I) (J) (K) (L) (M) (N) (O) (P) (Q) (R) (S) (T) 189
190 (A) (B) (C) (D) (E) (F) (G) (H) (I) (J) (K) (L) (M) (N) (O) (P) (Q) (R) (S) (T) 190
191 (A) (B) (C) (D) (E) (F) (G) (H) (I) (J) (K) (L) (M) (N) (O) (P) (Q) (R) (S) (T) 191
192 (A) (B) (C) (D) (E) (F) (G) (H) (I) (J) (K) (L) (M) (N) (O) (P) (Q) (R) (S) (T) 192
193 (A) (B) (C) (D) (E) (F) (G) (H) (I) (J) (K) (L) (M) (N) (O) (P) (Q) (R) (S) (T) 193
194 (A) (B) (C) (D) (E) (F) (G) (H) (I) (J) (K) (L) (M) (N) (O) (P) (Q) (R) (S) (T) 194
195 (A) (B) (C) (D) (E) (F) (G) (H) (I) (J) (K) (L) (M) (N) (O) (P) (Q) (R) (S) (T) 195
196 (A) (B) (C) (D) (E) (F) (G) (H) (I) (J) (K) (L) (M) (N) (O) (P) (Q) (R) (S) (T) 196
197 (A) (B) (C) (D) (E) (F) (G) (H) (I) (J) (K) (L) (M) (N) (O) (P) (Q) (R) (S) (T) 197
198 (A) (B) (C) (D) (E) (F) (G) (H) (I) (J) (K) (L) (M) (N) (O) (P) (Q) (R) (S) (T) 198
199 (A) (B) (C) (D) (E) (F) (G) (H) (I) (J) (K) (L) (M) (N) (O) (P) (Q) (R) (S) (T) 199
200 (A) (B) (C) (D) (E) (F) (G) (H) (I) (J) (K) (L) (M) (N) (O) (P) (Q) (R) (S) (T) 200

Sample

Three

Mock Test Paper

Theme 1: Poisoning: Treatment

Options:

a. Atropine
b. Flumazenil
c. Dicobalt edetate
d. Specific antibody fragments
e. Antitoxin
f. Desferrioxamine
g. Naloxone
h. Phytomenadione
i. FFP and vitamin K
j. NAC
k. IV sodium bicarbonate
l. Hyperbaric O_2
m. Supportive care only
n. IV methylene blue
o. Procyclidine

For each presentation below, choose the SINGLE most appropriate treatment from the above list of options. Each option may be used once, more than once, or not at all.

1. A 20 year old man was caught stealing an aerosol can. He is agitated and complains of blurred vision and headache. He has slurred speech with ataxic gait. He also appears cyanosed.

2. A 25 year old man in an attempt to commit suicide has taken a bottle full of diazepam. He complains of difficulty in breathing.

3. An 18 year old girl has taken her father's warfarin. She is actively bleeding.

4. A 25 year old man was rushed to A & E after he was found to be moribund. He took tinned chicken soup the last night.

5. A 55 year old man was found in his car with a hose leading from exhaust pipe through a window into his car. He is brought to A & E in drowsy state. He has extensor plantars and brisk reflexes.

Theme 2: Management of raised blood pressure

Options:

a. Lisinopril
b. Timetaphan camsilate
c. Imipramine followed by propranolol
d. Verapamil
e. Nifedipine
f. Propranolol
g. Sodium nitroprusside
h. Terazosin
i. Methyldopa
j. Hydralazine hydrochloride
k. Sotalol
l. Propranolol followed by phenoxybenzamine
m. Betaxolol
n. Digoxin
o. Glibenclamide
p. Phenoxybenzamine followed by propranolol

For each presentation below, choose the SINGLE most appropriate medication from the above list of options. Each option may be used once, more than once, or not at all.

6. A frail 65 year old man presents with difficulty in starting micturition associated with poor stream .He has no history of weight loss and denies any dysuria. On examination blood pressure of 130/90 mmHg is found.

7. A 34 year old known diabetic with chronic renal failure is examined and found to have a blood pressure of 150/100 mmHg.

8. A 70 year old woman complains of a chronic temporal headache associated with blurring of vision .She reports a history of seeing 'rings' of colour around lights especially at night. Her blood pressure is found to be 135/90 mmHg.

9. A 55 year old company executive complains of palpitations and episodes of feeling dizzy. A 24 hour ECG tracing reveals episodes of atrial fibrillation which come and go at various times, lasting only 2-3 seconds each time.

10. A 26 year old gravida 3 para 1 + 1 is found to have a blood pressure of 150/100 mmHg at 30 weeks gestation on routine antenatal screening.

11. A 45 year old man has been treated for panic attacks by his GP for over 6 months without much improvement. He complains of excessive sweating, flushing and diarrhoea. On examination he is found to have a blood pressure of 160/110 mmHg. In the outpatients clinic the following day he is found to have a glycosuria and a blood pressure of 130/80 mmHg.

Theme 3: Skin disease in children

Options:

a. Erythema chronicum migrans
b. Erythema infectiosum
c. Erythema multiforme
d. Erythema nodosum
e. Exanthema subitum
f. Purpura fulminans
g. Tinea corporis

For each presentation below, choose the SINGLE most appropriate condition from the above list of options. Each option may be used once, more than once, or not at all.

12. A nine month old child is non-specifically unwell for three days with a fever. The rash subsides and the child breaks out in a maculo-papular rash over its body.

13. Following a course of Septrin for a bacterial infection, a 5 year old child breaks out in a widespread macular rash with target lesions.

14. A 4 year old boy has a runny nose and mild fever and develops bright red cheeks and reticular rash on the forearms.

15. Following a tick bite on holiday in a forested area, a 7 year old boy develops an erythematous macule at the site of the bite which then spreads into an annular lesion with a clear central area.

Theme 4: Treatment of acute breathlessness

Options:

a. IV adrenaline
b. Mechanical ventilation
c. Refer to psychiatrist
d. Rebreathe into paper bag
e. Heparin
f. Diuretics.
g. Heimlich manoeuvre
h. Nebulized salbutamol
i. Chest drain
j. IM adrenaline
k. Forced alkaline diuresis
l. IV aminophylline

For each presentation below, choose the SINGLE most appropriate treatment from the above list of options. Each option may be used once, more than once, or not at all.

16. A 25 year old man presents with breathlessness, wheeze and flushing. He has hoarseness of voice and stridor. His lips and tongue are swollen.

17. A 25 year old woman presents to A&E drowsy and tired. Her husband says she has an asthmatic attack. On examinaton she is cyanosed with a silent chest.

18. A 40 year old man became suddenly breathless whilst eating chicken. He has marked stridor and is choking and drooling saliva.

19. A 21 year old woman presents with sudden onset breathlessness, palpitations and anxiety. She also complains of tingling around her lips. She is having tachycardia and her O_2 saturation is normal.

20. A 55 year old known asthmatic presents with history of worsening breathlessness since 1 day. On examination there is reduced expansion on the right side and trachea is deviated to the left.

Theme 5: The management of thromboembolic conditions

Options:

a. Spiral computed tomography
b. Low dose subcutaneous heparin
c. Chest X-ray
d. Subcutaneous dose of LMW heparin upto 15000U/12 hourly
e. Warfarin
f. Abciximab
g. TED (thrombo-embolic deterrent) stockings.
h. Glyceryl trinitrate
i. Acetylsalicylic acid
j. Streptokinase
k. Fresh frozen plasma
l. Loading dose of 5000U (unfractionated heparin)
m. Cefotaxime (IV)
n. Aspirin and Heparin

For each presentation below, choose the SINGLE most appropriate action from the above list of options. Each option may be used once, more than once, or not at all.

21. A 33 year old woman who has just flown in to the UK from California (USA) complains of calf pain. While passing stool at Gatwick Airport, he suddenly gets breathless and coughs up blood. He is rushed to the nearby Crawley hospital where a Ventilation-Perfusion scan and femoral venography are done with equivocal results.

22. A 67 year old man suffers an acute loss of consciousness, associated with weakness of the left arm and leg CT scan done in A&E reveals no haemorrhagic areas.

23. An obese 34 year old woman on Depoprovera (contraceptive) is recovering from surgery to fix an intra-medullary nail for a mid-shaft fracture of the femur she sustained while ice-skating.

24. A 24 year old woman, who has been taking the oral contraceptive pill for 2 months, presents with a 2 day history of cough, producing 'rusty' sputum and fever. Further history was unremarkable.

25. A 31 year old woman with a history of two mid-trimester abortions is found to have anti-cardiolipin antibodies. Further tests reveal lupus anticoagulant antibodies but no anti-nuclear antibodies are seen. She has an ESR of 3mm/hr.

Theme 6: Causes of pneumonia

Options:

a. Chalmydia psittaci
b. Staphylococcus aureus
c. Streptococcus pneumoniae
d. Mycoplasma pneumoniae
e. Legionella pneumoniae
f. Mycobacterium tuberculosis
g. Haemophilus influenzae
h. Chlamydia trachomatis
i. Pneumocystis carinii

For each presentation below, choose the SINGLE most appropriate causative organism from the above list of options. Each option may be used once, more than once, or not at all.

26. A young male homosexual with Kaposi's sarcoma complains of a dry cough associated with increasing breathlessness.

27. A 22 year old girl who works in a pet shop complains of fever and a dry cough associated with increasing breathlessness.

28. A 30 year old woman has just returned from a holiday in Cyprus. She complains of dry cough, fever and general malaise. A chest X-ray shows patchy consolidation.

29. A 56 year old smoker with chronic obstructive airway disease develops a fever. He reports bringing up green phlegm.

30. A 40 year old homeless alcoholic presents with a chronic productive cough. He reports 3 episodes of seeing red streaks in the sputum. Chest X-ray shows a cavitating lesion in the right lower zone.

Theme 7: Diagnosis of abdominal pain

Options:

a. Acute appendicitis
b. Diverticular disease
c. Abdominal aortic aneurysm
d. Perforated peptic ulcer
e. Crohn's disease
f. Ulcerative colitis
g. Acute pancreatitis
h. Chronic active hepatitis
i. Acute pancreatitis
j. Pseudo-obstruction
k. Acute cholecystitis
l. Acute diverticulitis

For each presentation below, choose the SINGLE most appropriate diagnosis from the above list of options. Each option may be used once, more than once, or not at all.

31. An 80 year old lady with stable angina presents with massive abdominal distension 10 days following a total hip replacement.

32. A 55 year old man presents with left-sided colicky iliac fossa pain, change in bowel habits and rectal bleeding. A thickened mass is palpated in the region of the sigmoid colon. His full blood count is normal.

33. A 50 year old man presents with severe epigastric pain radiating to the back. He is noted to have some bruising in the flanks.

34. A 40 year old lady presents with anorexia, abdominal pain, and increasing jaudice. She is asthmatic and takes methyldopa for hypertension.

35. A 25 year old man presents with colicky periumbical pain, which shifts to the right iliac fossa, fever and loss of appetite.

Theme 8: Causes of headache

Options:

a. Meningitis
b. Migraine headache
c. Cluster headache
d. Tension headache
e. Subarachnoid haemorrhage
f. Sinusitis
g. Benign intracranial hypertension
h. Cervical spondylosis
i. Giant cell arteritis
j. Otitis media
k. Transient ischaemic attack

For each presentation below, choose the SINGLE most appropriate cause of headache from the above list of options. Each option may be used once, more than once, or not at all.

36. A 35 year old obese female presents with headache and diplopia. On examination, she has papilloedema. She is alert with no focal symptoms and signs.

37. A 65 year old female presents with bitemporal headache, unilateral blurry vision, and pain on combing her hair. Her ESR is elevated.

38. A 10 year old boy presents with fever, headache, left eye pain and swelling. He described his vision as blurry. He has recently recovered from a cold.

39. A 45 year old man presents with severe pain around his right eye, with eyelid swelling lasting 20 minutes. He has had several attacks during the past weeks. The attacks are worse at night.

40. A 25 year old female presents with episodes of unilateral throbbing headache, nausea, and vomiting. She states that it is aggravated by light. The episodes seem to occur prior to her menstruation.

Theme 9: Developmental milestones

Options:

a. Two months
b. Six months
c. Ten months
d. Eleven months
e. Five months
f. One year
g. One and half year
h. Two years
i. Three years
j. Four years
k. Five years
l. Six years

For each presentation below, choose the SINGLE most appropriate age at which it first occurs from the above list of options. Each option may be used once, more than once, or not at all.

41. Copies a square.
42. Walks holding on furniture.
43. Smiles responsively.
44. Drinks from a cup.
45. Smiles spontaneously

Theme 10: Clotting disorders

Options:

a. Desmopressin
b. Factor VIII concentrate
c. Factor X
d. Fresh frozen plasma
e. Folic acid
f. Gelofusin
g. Heparin
h. Steroids
i. Vitamin K
j. Warfarin

For each presentation below, choose the SINGLE most appropriate management from the above list of options. Each option may be used once, more than once, or not at all.

46. A 23 year old lady, 10 weeks pregnant, is diagnosed with a pulmonary embolism. She is allergic to warfarin.

47. A 65 year old alcoholic man is admitted with bleeding oesophageal varices. He has received 6 units of blood and has a prolonged prothrombin time.

48. A 70 year old man with prosthetic mitral valves is admitted to hospital with a 2 day history of bleeding per rectum and a INR of 6. He had been commenced on ciprofloxacin 3 days previously, to treat a urinary tract infection by his GP.

49. A 5 day old baby girl whose mother is taking anticonvulsants is admitted with unexplained bruising. Clotting profile reveals both her prothrombin and partial thromboplastin times are elevated.

50. A 7 year old boy is admitted with haemarthrosis of his left knee. This has been a recurrent since his early year. His activated partial thromboplastin time is significantly prolonged but bleeding time is normal.

Theme 11: Side-effects of drugs used in tuberculosis

Options:

a. Ciprofloxacin
b. Clarithromycin
c. Cycloserine
d. Dexamethasone
e. Ethambutol
f. Isoniazid
g. Prothionamide
h. Pyridoxime
i. Pyrazinamide
j. Rifampicin
k. Streptomycin

For each side effect below, choose the SINGLE most appropriate involved drug from the above list of options. Each option may be used once, more than once, or not at all.

51. Colour blindness.
52. Peripheral neuropathy.
53. Ototoxicity.
54. Hepatic enzyme induction.
55. Vertigo.

Theme 12: Prevention and treatment of DVT

Options:

a. Systemic heparin 30,000 units per day
b. Systemic heparin 5000 units BD
c. Compression stockings
d. Systemic fibrinolysis
e. Use caval filters
f. Cardiopulmonary bypass
g. LMW heparin
h. No treatment
i. Oral anticoagulants
j. LMW dextran

For each presentation below, choose the SINGLE most appropriate preventive measure from the above list of options. Each option may be used once, more than once, or not at all.

56. A 56 year old obese man undergoing surgery for total hip replacement.

57. A 45 year old man with previous history of peptic ulcer undergoes surgery for soft tissue sarcoma of the thigh.

58. A 45 year old female undergoes surgery for a fracture shaft femur. She develops tender swelling in the calf. An I^{131} fibrinogen uptake scan shows increased uptake.

59. A 36 year old, 45 kg female undergoes surgery for fibroadenoma.

60. A 45 year old female who has undergone surgery for a fracture shaft femur, develops repeated episodes of cough, dyspnoea and haemoptysis inspite of adequate medical treatment. V/Q scan shows perfusion defects.

Theme 13: Diagnosis of ophthalmic diseases

Options

a. Acute glaucoma
b. Acute iritis
c. Amaurosis fugax
d. Cataract
e. Pituitary tumour
f. Retinitis pigmentosa
g. Subconjunctival haemorrhage
h. Temporal arteritis
i. Thyroid associated opthalmopathy
j. Viral conjunctivitis
k. Behcet's disease
l. Cavernous sinus thrombosis
m. Graves disease
n. Multiple sclerosis
o. Ophthalmic herpes zoster
p. Pancoast tumour
q. Reiter's syndrome
r. Sjögren's syndrome
s. Syphilis
t. Wegener's granulomatosis

For each presentation below, choose the SINGLE most appropriate diagnosis from the above list of options. Each option may be used once, more than once, or not at all.

61. A 60 year old diabetic presents with gradual deterioration of vision and dazzling of view in well light places.

62. A 65 year old woman presents with tiredness, headache, blurring of vision in the left eye and is unable to comb her hair.

63. A 50 year old male presents with generalized lethargy, weight loss, eye discomfort and nasal stuffiness. Examination reveals a pulse of 70 beats per minute, mild proptosis of the left eye with diplopia on left lateral gaze and a tenderness over the nasal bridge.

64. A 72 year old female presents with severe pain in the face and right eye. Examination reveals a temperature of 36.7°C and two

small red eruptions on the right lower forehead which are exquisitely tender.

65. A 24 year old male presents acutely with pain in the left eye. Examination reveals a temperature of 39°C, redness and swelling of a completely closed left eye. On raising the eye ocular movements are universally impaired.

Theme 14: Features of pericardial pathology

Options

a. Postpericardiotomy syndrome
b. Pneumopericardium
c. Uraemic pericarditis
d. Constrictive pericarditis
e. Mesothelioma
f. Cardiac tamponade
g. Congenital pericardial defects
h. Acute viral pericarditis
i. Pericardial cysts
j. Bronchogenic carcinoma

For each presentation below, choose the SINGLE most appropriate diagnosis from the above list of options. Each option may be used once, more than once, or not at all.

66. The commonest pericardial manifestation of the Coxsackie infective agent.
67. A patient with retrosternal pain is found to have an elevated jugular venous pressure that increases with inspiration.
68. A young male is brought to casualty in a confused state. He is found to have a fall in systemic arterial pressure of greater than 20 mmHg with inspiration.
69. Malignant pericardial involvement is most likely to be secondary to this carcinoma.
70. An 18 year old has a chest X-ray as part of his pre-employment examination before joining the army. A density is seen in the cardiophrenic sulcus.

Theme 15: Diagnosis of thyroid disorders

Options:

a. Thyroglossal cyst
b. De Quervain's disease
c. Hypothyroidism
d. MEN type I
e. Simple goitre
f. Hashimoto's thyroiditis
g. Grave's disease
h. MEN type II
i. Papillary carcinoma
j. Lymphoma
k. Follicular carcinoma
l. MEN type II B

For each presentation below, choose the SINGLE most appropriate diagnosis from the above list of options. Each option may be used once, more than once, or not at all.

71. A 26 year old man presents with hypertension, bone pains, prominent mucosal neuromas involving lips, tongue, and inner aspect of the eyelids. His uncle had the same problems.

72. A 43 year old woman presents with weight loss despite good appetite, constipation, frontal headaches and metrorrhagia. She also complains of recurrent dyspepsia and peptic ulcers. Her abdominal radiography shows renal stones.

73. A 30 year old woman presents with weight gain, constipation, lethargy and flaky rash. She prefers to stay indoors even in warm weather.

74. A 19 year old student presents with a neck swelling. On examination swelling moves up with swallowing and protrusion of the tongue.

75. A 49 year old woman presents with goitre. On examination thyroid is firm and rubbery. Thyroid microsomal antibodies are positive in high titre.

Theme 16: Oral hypoglycaemic therapy: Indications and contra-indications

Options:

a. Glibenclamide
b. Orlistat-Xenical
c. Metformin
d. Acarbose
e. Gliclazide
f. Rosiglitazone
g. Repaglinide
h. Netaglinide
i. Guar Gum
j. Chlorpropamide
k. Pravastatin

For each presentation below, choose the SINGLE most appropriate drug from the above list of options. Each option may be used once, more than once, or not at all.

76. A 70 year old man with a BMI 34 complains of feeling increasingly lethargic. He has suffered with type II diabetes, treated with diet only for 2 years and his HbA_{1c} measures 9%.

77. The most appropriate drug for a 80 year old lady, with diet treated type II diabetes. Most recent HbA_{1c} is 8.9% and BMI 26. She lives on her own and complains of osmotic symptoms.

78. A 40 year old man with type II diabetes and obesity (BMI 39). His glycaemic control is moderate with HbA_{1c} 8% and no osmotic symptoms. He has successfully lost 3.6 kg in weight over the last 2 months and is on a low-fat diet. with a noticeable improvement in his home glucose monitoring.

79. A 66 year old man intolerant of metformin, with HbA_{1c} 10.6%, on glibenclamide 15 mg daily.

80. A 50 year old man with type II diabetes for 5 year. BMI 36, HbA_{1c} 9.9% complaining of thirst and lethargy. Present medication includes gliclazide 160 mg twice daily, metformin 2 grams daily.

Theme 17: Treatment of fractures and dislocations

Options:

a. Kocher's method
b. AO cannulated screws
c. Bed rest
d. Open reduction and K wire
e. Strapping
f. Reconstructive surgery with internal graft
g. Physiotherapy
h. Hemiarthroplasty
i. Dyanamic hip screw
j. THR
k. Open reduction and internal fixation

For each presentation below, choose the SINGLE most appropriate management from the above list of options. Each option may be used once, more than once, or not at all.

81. A 50 year old man presents with right hip fracture. On X-ray the fracture line is subcapital.

82. A 20 year old athelete twists his knee while skiing. On examination he has positive drawer sign with the tibia sliding anteriorly.

83. A 70 year old woman presents with left hip fracture. On X-ray the fracture line is intertrochanteric.

84. A 40 year old woman sprains her wrist. She complains of persistant pain and tenderness over the dorsum distal to the Lister's tubercle. X-ray shows a large gap between the scaphoid and the lunate. In lateral view, the lunate is tilted dorsally and the scaphoid anteriorly.

85. A 30 year old basketball player presents with severe pain in his shoulder. He is holding his arm with his opposite hand. He explains that he fell on an outstretched hand. X ray shows overlapping shadows of the humeral head and the glenoid fossa, with the head lying below and medial to the socket.

Theme 18: Fitness to drive

Options:

a. Banned to drive
b. Should not drive for 1 month
c. Should not drive for 2 months
d. Must not drive for 3 months
e. Must not drive for 1 year
f. Must not drive for 2 year
g. Must not drive for 3 year
h. Should not drive for 48 hrs
i. Should not drive for 6 weeks
j. May drive(but inform the DVLA)
k. Should not drive for 1 and a half year
l. Must not drive for 2 and half year

For each presentation below, choose the SINGLE most appropriate statement from the above list of options. Each option may be used once, more than once, or not at all.

86. A 42 year old has type II DM and taking metformin. He has no other complications or other medical problems.

87. A 26 year old has epilepsy but only has seizures during sleep.

88. An 18 year old had a wisdom tooth extraction under GA.

89. After an accident at work, a mechanic loses his sight of left eye. He is otherwise well and has 6/5 vision with a normal field on the right.

90. A 27 year old has had a heart transplant following myocarditis. She is well and taking no sedatives.

Theme 19: Karyotype abnormalities and their presentations

Options:

a. Triploidy
b. Karyotype 46XX
c. Karyotype 47 XYY
d. Di George syndrome
e. Karyotype 45 XO
f. Trisomy 18
g. Trisomy 9
h. Klinefelter's syndrome

For each presentation below, choose the SINGLE most appropriate karyotype from the above list of options. Each option may be used once, more than once, or not at all.

91. Gross fetal oedema with cystic hygroma at 16 weeks gestation with ultrasound features of female sex.
92. The uterus is large for dates, ultrasound shows a 'snowstorm' appearance and both ovaries are enlarged.
93. A major cardiac abnormality with otherwise normal ultrasound features and a normal FISH (fluorescent *in situ* hybridization) result on amniocentesis.
94. Delivery, at 18 weeks, of a fetus with severe asymmetric growth restriction, cleft palate and polydactyly.
95. A 3 year old boy with undescended testes and mild learning disorder.

Theme 20: Diagnosis of fractures

Options:

a. Anteriorly displaced radial head
b. Posteriorly displaced radial head
c. Subluxation of MCP joint of thumb with abduction
d. Thenar eminence swelling, palmar bruising and inability to move thumb
e. Pain in the area between extensor and abductor pollicis longus tendons

For each fracture below, choose the SINGLE most appropriate presentation from the above list of options. Each option may be used once, more than once, or not at all.

96. Colles fracture.
97. Smith's fracture.
98. Fracture of scaphoid bone.
99. Bennett's fracture.
100. Game keeper's thumb.

Theme 21: Cardiovascular anomalies in chromosomal disorders

Options:

a. Marfan's syndrome
b. Glycogen storage disorder
c. Down's syndrome
d. Turner's syndrome
e. Noonan's syndrome
f. William's syndrome
g. Rubella syndrome
h. Trisomy syndrome

For each anomaly below, choose the SINGLE most appropriate syndrome from the above list of options. Each option may be used once, more than once, or not at all.

101. Endocardial cushion defect.
102. Patent ductus arteriosus.
103. Aortic aneurysm.
104. Coarctation of the aorta.
105. Supraventricular aortic stenosis.
106. Hypertrophic cardiomyopathy.
107. Ventricular septal defect.
108. Pulmonary stenosis.

Theme 22: Cause of bleeding PV

Options:

a. Adenomyosis
b. Endometrial carcinoma
c. Endometriosis
d. Anovulatory cycles
e. Adenomyosis
f. Hypothyroidism
g. DUB
h. Ectopic pregnancy
i. Polycystic ovarian syndrome
j. Von Willebrand's disease
k. Vaginal carcinoma
l. Fibroid

For each presentation below, choose the SINGLE most appropriate cause of bleeding PV from the above list of options. Each option may be used once, more than once, or not at all.

109. A 35 year old African woman presents with heavy regular periods, dyspareunia and infertility.
110. A 55 year old perimenopausal woman with IDDM uses about 30–35 pads during her periods which last more than a week.
111. A 19 year old complains of heavy periods. All investigations and examination are normal.
112. A 14 year old girl who started menstruating 4 months ago.
113. A 40 year old woman with five children and a 12 week sized 'bulky' uterus.

Theme 23: The management of chronic renal failure

Options:

a. Aluminium hydroxide
b. Iron Saccharin(Iron sucrose)
c. Insulin-increased dosage
d. Insulin-reduced dosage
e. Alpha-calcidol
f. Calcitriol
g. Calcium
h. Captopril
i. Diamorphine
j. Iron dextran
k. Frusemide
l. Renal dialysis
m. 25, Cholecalciferol
n. Metoprolol
o. Paracetamol
p. Recombinant Erythropoietin
q. Calcium carbonate

For each presentation below, choose the SINGLE most appropriate management step from the above list of options. Each option may be used once, more than once, or not at all.

114. A 17 year old youth with chronic renal failure has been noted to have severe anaemia. The most cost effective first line treatment.

115. A 56 year old man with diabetes mellitus and severe renal failure (serum creatinine 400 umol/L) and a blood glucose concentration of 59 mmol/L.

116. A 46 year old woman with chronic renal failure is found to be severely anaemic. Iron therapy has been done without much success.

117. A 54 year old woman with chronic renal failure presents with markedly swollen ankles.

118. A 34 year old man with chronic renal failure is found to have a high phosphate concentration. He is on renal dialysis.

Theme 24: Management of pain in children

Options:

a. Paracetamol
b. Sweets and feed
c. Carbamazepine
d. Transcutaneous electrical nerve stimulation
e. IV morphine
f. IM opiates
g. Aspirin
h. Benzylpenicillin
i. Vincristine and doxorubicin
j. Biopsy
k. Mantoux test
l. Resuscitate and IV fluids
m. Nasogastric tube
n. 250 mg/6hr oral penicillin

For each presentation below, choose the SINGLE most appropriate definitive action from the above list of options. Each option may be used once, more than once, or not at all.

119. A 12 year old girl complains of a toothache. She is due to see her dentist in 3 days time.

120. A 13 year old girl complains a headache. 3 hours later she starts vomiting and becomes progressively drowsy.

121. A 7 year old boy with a 3-month history of flank pain is seen in the A&E department. He is found to have an abdominal mass in his left flank and haematuria on dipstick.

122. An 8 month old infant has a history of episodic intermittent crying associated with vomiting. He draws up his legs with each episode of crying. Sausage-shaped mass is felt on abdominal examination.

123. A 10 year old girl complains of abdominal pain. She has a 2-day history of sore throat and difficulty in swallowing. On examination she is found to have a macular rash covering her upper chest and a 'strawberry' tongue.

Theme 25: Diagnosis of skin conditions

Options:

a. Pityriasis rosea
b. Pityriasis versicolor
c. Erythema multiforme
d. Eczema
e. Hereditary angioedema
f. Leprosy
g. Necrotizing fasciitis
h. Tinea corporis
i. Secondary syphilis
j. Lichen planus
k. Pemphigus
l. Psoriasis
m. Dermatitis herpetiformis

For each presentation below, choose the SINGLE most appropriate diagnosis from the above list of options. Each option may be used once, more than once, or, not at all.

124. A 27 year old African woman presents with painless rash on her trunk which are multiple, scaly, pale patches measuring between 1 and 3 cm in diameter.

125. A 40 year old man presents with 12 hr history of a painful swollen arm. He also complains of pins and needles sensation in his fingers. He has fever and his arm is tender with dusky skin.

126. A 20 year old woman presents with well demarcated salmon pink patch with a silvery scaling especially on the extensor surfaces of her arm.

127. A 35 year old man presents with faint papular rash which includes his palms and soles. He has history of a painless ulcer over his penis which resolved weeks ago. He also gives history of travel to Thailand 3 months ago.

128. A 50 year old lady presents with purplish coloured flat papules over her wrist and ankles which are itchy. A fine white lacy pattern is noted over the papules.

Theme 26: Ethical practice of medicine in the United Kingdom

Options:

a. Reversal of the circumcision
b. Reversal of circumcision for catheter to be inserted and re-circumcising her
c. Trial of labour
d. Termination
e. Refusal of termination since it's illegal after 24 weeks for social reasons
f. Give her contraception
g. Withhold contraception
h. Call Police and then give her the contraception
i. Inform mother and police immediately
j. Inform the General practitioner (GP)

For each presentation below, choose the SINGLE most appropriate action from the above list of options. Each option may be used once, more than once, or not at all.

129. A 22 year Somalian primigravida who doesn't speak English presents in labour. On vaginal examination you notice a very small introitus, barely enough to admit your little finger. A CTG is done and is shows a baseline rate of 100beats/min. Your team decides, she needs an emergency caesarean section but because of the small introitus you are unable to pass the catheter to proceed to theatre.

130. A 13 year old girl demands the morning after pill. She says the condom she used with her 13 year old boyfriend split in two, while having intercourse.

131. A tearful 19 year old girl at 27 weeks of pregnancy requests a termination, saying her boyfriend has just left her and that she wouldn't want the baby to remind her of him. The boyfriend who is now in Jail is reported to have assaulted her during their stormy 2 year relationship.

Theme 27: The treatment of menopausal symptoms

Options:

a. Mirena coil (progesterone containing IUCD)
b. Oestrogen only HRT
c. Raloxifene (a selective oestrogen receptor modulator)
d. Gestrinone
e. Combined oestrogen and progesterone implant
f. Oestrogen only implant
g. Oral combined oestrogen and progesterone pill
h. Thyroid function tests
i. Continuous oestrogen and progesterone oral preparation
j. Endometrial sampling
k. Transdermal oestrogen
l. Dietary supplementation
m. Hysterectomy
n. Progesterone only pill
o. Vaginal oestrogens
p. KY gel (lubricant)
q. Exercise

For each presentation below, choose the SINGLE most appropriate treatment from the above list of options. Each option may be used once, more than once, or not at all.

132. A 58 year old smoker with a past history of mild deep vein thrombosis is 2 year post-menopausal. She complains of vaginal dryness and dyspareunia. She denies any flushes.

133. A 55 year old woman who is 1 year post-menopausal complains of excessive sweating, palpitations and hot flushes. She wants a preparation that won't make her bleed every month.

134. A 33 year old model had abdominal radio-therapy 6 months ago. She now complains of hot flushes and vaginal dryness. She wants treatment that will fit in with her busy lifestyle.

Theme 28: Antibiotic prophylaxis of surgical patients

Options:

a. Angiography
b. Bronchoscopy
c. Colles' fracture
d. Dental treatment of a cardiac patient
e. Dislocated shoulder
f. Emergency appendicectomy
g. Heart valve replacement
h. Sigmoid colectomy
i. Splenectomy
j. Thyroidectomy

For each presentation below, choose the SINGLE most appropriate indication from the above list of options. Each option may be used once, more than once, or not at all.

135. Three days of intravenous broad-spectrum antibiotics beginning with induction of anaesthesia.

136. 3g of amoxicillin one hour before the procedure.

137. Clear fluids (per oral) and two sachets of sodium picosulphate on the day before the operation plus some broad-spectrum IV antibiotics at induction of anaesthesia.

138. Long term administration of Penicillin V and pneumococcal vaccine.

139. One dose of metronidazole at induction of anaesthesia.

Theme 29: Thyroid conditions: Diagnosis

Options:

a. Primary atrophic hypothyroidism
b. Hashimoto's thyroiditis
c. Iodine deficiency
d. Antithyroid drugs
e. Subacute thyroiditis
f. Hypoparathyroidism
g. Hypopituitarism
h. Amiodarone
i. Previous radioiodine

For each presentation below, choose the SINGLE most appropriate diagnosis from the above list of options. Each option may be used once, more than once, or not at all.

140. A 23 year old male with a history of severe neck pain and dysphagia three months ago. The pain would radiate to the ears. His ESR was 66 at the time of the neck pain.

141. A 40 year old woman with progressive thyroid swelling which is diffuse and non-tender. She has high titres of thyroid anti-peroxidase and anti microsomal antibodies.

142. A 64 year old male with history of heart disease presents with pigmentation of the skin and symptoms of hypothyroidism.

143. A 52 year old man presents with cold intolerance, postural giddiness and bumping into objects especially on the right. Examination reveals pallor, loss of body hair and bilateral papilloedema—right more than left.

144. A 16 year old boy with detected hypothyroidism since the last 12 years. He has frequent numbness and tingling in the hands and feet and perioral paraesthesiae. Examination reveals short stature, short 3rd and 4th metacarpals and mild mental retardation.

Theme 30: Headache

Options:

a. Tension headache
b. Migraine
c. Cluster headache
d. Encephalitis
e. Subarachnoid haemorrhage
f. Intracranial tumour
g. Temporal arteritis
h. Meningitis
i. Glaucoma
j. Pseudotumour cerebri

For each presentation below, choose the SINGLE most appropriate cause of headache from the above list of options. Each option may be used once, more than once, or not at all.

145. A middle aged man with recurrent severe nocturnal headaches accompanied by severe eye pain, watering from the eyes and nasal congestion. The pain lasts about 2 hours and returns the next night. The pain recurs for about a week and then disappears for months.

146. A 15 year old girl with headaches for the last 15 days. She now presents with very severe headache for 1 day and on examination has a complete left ophthalmoplegia.

147. A 32 year old HIV positive woman with progressive headache for the past 2 months. Examination reveals papilloedema.

148. A 35 year old obese woman on the OCPs presents with progressive headache for the last 3 months. She gives history of visual obscuration and examination reveals an enlarged blind spot, papilloedema and impaired visual acuity.

149. A 17 year old male with severe headache, altered sensorium and vomiting. He has had fever, cough and a rash for the last 4 days.

Theme 31: Shortness of breath (SOB)

Options:

a. Acute myocardial infarction
b. Myocarditis
c. Arrhythmia
d. Pulmonary embolism
e. Pneumonia
f. Pneumothorax
g. Pleural effusion
h. Anaemia
i. Psychogenic
j. Primary pulmonary hypertension

For each presentation below, choose the SINGLE most appropriate cause of SOB from the above list of options. Each option may be used once, more than once, or not at all.

150. A 72 year old lady with hip surgery for fracture neck femur four days ago.
151. A 13 year old boy with fever, rash and painful ulcers in the mouth for the last five days. Examination reveals raised JVP and a left ventricular S_3 gallop.
152. A 32 year old lady presents with paroxysms of palpitations. ECG reveals a PR interval of 0.08 seconds.
153. An asthenic twenty year old male with a history of cigarette smoking. He presents with sudden onset of dyspnoea.
154. A 28 year old female with progressive shortness of breath. Examination reveals weak pulses, CV waves in the JVP and a Graham-Steell murmur. Breath sounds are normal.

Theme 32: Causes of ear ache

Options:

a. Glossopharyngeal neuralgia
b. Mastoiditis
c. Carcinoma nasopharynx
d. Otitis media
e. Bullous myringitis
f. Cervical root irritation
g. Barotrauma
h. Otitis externa
i. Ramsay—Hunt syndrome
j. Furunculosis
k. Quinsy

For each presentation below, choose the SINGLE most appropriate cause of ear ache from the above list of options. Each option may be used once, more than once, or not at all.

155. A 55 year old businessman developed sudden onset of dull left ear pain whilst returning from India. He also has conductive hearing loss in that ear.
156. A 25 year old man has a four day history of dry cough and fever with pain in both ears. On examination, there are haemorrhagic blisters on the eardrum.
157. A 65 year old man has a two week history of left ear pain, fever and hearing loss. The pinna is pushed downwards by a painful swelling behind it.
158. A 65 year old man has a two day history of right ear pain and right facial droop. He has a few small vesicles in the right external auditory meatus.
159. A 34 year old lady comes with fever, with severe throat pain, dysphagia and left ear-ache. On examination she has swelling in left tonsillar fossa with surrounding inflammation and tenderness.

Theme 33: Tumour markers

Options:

a. α fetoprotein
b. CA 19-9
c. CA 125
d. CEA
e. HCG
f. NSE
g. PLAP
h. PSA
i. Calcitonin
j. S-100
k. None of the above
l. Thyroglobulin
m. Urinary metanephrines
n. 5-HIAA

For each condition below, choose the SINGLE most appropriate tumour marker from the above list of options. Each option may be used once, more than once, or not at all.

160. Prostate cancer.
161. Rectal cancer.
162. Papillary thyroid carcinoma.
163. Malignant melanoma.
164. Phaeochromocytoma.

Theme 34: Causes of purpura

Options:

a. Amyloidosis
b. Cushing's disease
c. Disseminated intravascular coagulation
d. Ehler–Danlos syndrome
e. Haemophilia
f. Henoch–Schönlein purpura
g. Iatrogenic
h. Idiopathic thrombocytopenic purpura
i. Paroxysmal nocturnal haemoglobinuria
j. Scurvy
k. Thrombotic thrombocytopenic purpura

For each presentation below, choose the SINGLE most appropriate cause from the above list of options. Each option may be used once, more than once, or not at all.

165. A 45 year old asthmatic has a moon-like facies and truncal obesity. He complains of easy bruising and thin skin.
166. A 35 year old woman presents with purpura, fever, haemolytic anaemia, microvascular thrombosis, renal failure and mild stroke. Blood film shows fragmented red cells and clotting screen is normal.
167. A 56 year old vagrant presents with peri-follicular skin bleeding and prolonged bleeding time.
168. A 35 year old man has hyperextensible joints and elastic skin. He also has purpura, and pseudotumours over his knees and elbows.
169. A 20 year old man presents with colicky abdominal pain, arthritis and polyarthritis following a chest infection. He also has purpura over his buttocks and legs.

Theme 35: Investigations for infectious diseases

Options:

a. Lyme disease serology
b. MRI hand
c. Hepatitis A serology
d. Hepatitis B serology
e. Viral antibodies
f. Blood film for malaria
g. Wound swab test
h. Skin prick test
i. Leptospirosis serology
j. Nail and skin scrappings

For each presentation below, choose the SINGLE most appropriate investigation from the above list of options. Each option may be used once, more than once, or not at all.

170. A 14 year old girl girl comes with a rash on thigh with central fading. She has a history of holiday in a forested area.

171. A businessman comes from Zambia with a 10 day history of rigors, fever and headache.

172. A 42 year old surfer presents with fever and jaundice.

173. A police officer is bitten by a heroine addict he catches. He presents with a deep wound on his hand at A&E.

174. A 60 year old diabetic presents with discoloured toe nails.

Theme 36: Oral lesions

Options:

a. Lichen planus
b. Measles
c. Syphilis
d. Erythema multiforme.
e. Hand foot and mouth disease
f. Monilia
g. Behcet's disease
h. Thrush

For each presentation below, choose the SINGLE most appropriate diagnosis from the above list of options. Each option may be used once, more than once, or not at all.

175. A man presents with lesion that are erosive and have a hard base. Lacy white areas are seen on the inner cheek.

176. The lesions are associated mostly with HIV infected patients.

177. Painless, 'snail track' ulcers seen in the oral mucosa.

178. Painful ulcers in the mouth, sore throat and spots on the buttocks.

179. Aphthous ulcers which are accompanied by arthritis and iritis.

Theme 37: Diagnosis of arthritis

Options:

a. Rheumatoid arthritis
b. Osteoarthritis
c. Ankylosing spondylitis
d. Rheumatic fever
e. SLE
f. Reiter's syndrome
g. Psoriatic arthritis
h. Septic arthritis

For each presentation below, choose the SINGLE most appropriate diagnosis from the above list of options. Each option may be used once, more than once, or not at all.

180. A 30 year old woman presents with sudden onset swelling of small joints of hands and feet. She also has a facial rash in a butterfly distribution.

181. A 30 year old man presents with swelling of the distal interphalangeal joints in an asymmetrical fashion. He is also noted to have pitting of nails.

182. A 30 year old man complains of swelling and pain in the joint which moves from one joint to another. He is also noted to have chorea.

183. A 25 year old man presents with stiffness in the back and painful, swollen knees and feet. He also complains of recent onset pain in the eye.

184. A 45 year old woman complains of pain and swelling in the small joints of hands and feet which are found to be inflamed. She also complains of morning stiffness.

185. A 65 year old man complains of pain in the hands which worsens on working. There are also swellings in the hands in distal interphalangeal joints.

Theme 38: Investigation of abdominal pain

Options:

a. Gastro-oesophagoscopy
b. Oral cholecystography
c. IVU
d. Blood sugar
e. Urinary porphyrins
f. Chest X-ray
g. ERCP
h. Abdominal X-ray
i. Ultrasound abdomen
j. Laparoscopy
k. Echocardiogram

For each presentation below, choose the SINGLE most appropriate investigation from the above list of options. Each option may be used once, more than once, or not at all.

186. A 45 year old man comes with history of recurrent epigastric pain in lying position. His pain has become constant now-a-days.

187. A 60 year old man presents with dizziness and perspiration. He complains of abdominal pain and backache. On examination his BP is found to be 100/70 and prominent aortic pulsation.

188. A 18 year old boy complains of right lower abdominal pain which was initially around umbilicus. Later he develops increased frequency of micturition.

189. A 45 year old obese woman complains of recurrent pain under her right lower ribs after eating fatty foods.

190. A 65 year old alcoholic presents with recurrent abdominal pain which is relieved by leaning forwards.

Theme 39: Treatment of diabetic complications

Options:

a. Ampicillin
b. Tetracycline
c. Amitriptyline
d. Coproxamol
e. Dexamethasone
f. Fludrocortisone
g. Testosterone
h. Sildenafil
i. Metoclopramide
j. Oxybutinin

For each presentation below, choose the SINGLE most appropriate drug from the above list of options. Each option may be used once, more than once, or not at all.

191. A 65 year old male has NIDDM. He complains of a feeling of light headedness. His BP was found to be 130/84 lying and 100/74 standing.

192. A 65 year female who has NIDDM complains of incontinence. Investigations reveals a dystonic bladder.

193. A 65 year old male who has NIDDM complains of reduced libido and impotence. Investigations reveal primary hypogonadism.

194. A 50 year old male diabetic complains of nausea and vomiting. Investigations have revealed gastric dilatation and reduced motility.

195. A 50 year old IDDM complains of weight loss. Hydrogen breath test reveals increased values. Gut motility is also found to be slowed.

Theme 40: Association of systemic diseases and skin lesions

Options:

a. Erythema chronicum migrans
b. Erythema multiforme
c. Pretibial myxoedema
d. Dermatitis herpetiformis
e. Livedo reticularis
f. Dermatomyositis
g. Bazin's disease
h. Dermatitis artefacta
i. Alopecia areata
j. Mycosis fungoides
k. Bowen's disease
l. Paget's disease
m. Rodent ulcer
n. Cafe-au-lait spots

For each condition below, choose the SINGLE most appropriate skin lesions from the above list of options. Each option may be used once, more than once, or not at all.

196. Polyarteritis nodosa.
197. Mycoplasma pneumoniae.
198. Lyme disease.
199. Von-Recklinghausen disease.
200. Bronchial carcinoma.

ANSWERS

1. **(n)** IV methylene blue
2. **(b)** Flumazenil
3. **(i)** FFP and vitamin K
4. **(e)** Antitoxin
5. **(l)** Hyperbaric O_2
6. **(h)** Terazosin
7. **(a)** Lisinopril
8. **(m)** Betaxolol
9. **(k)** Sotalol
10. **(i)** Methyldopa
11. **(p)** Phenoxybenzamine followed by propranolol
12. **(e)** Exanthema subitum
13. **(c)** Erythema multiforme
14. **(b)** Erythema infectiosum
15. **(a)** Erythema chronicum migrans
16. **(j)** IM adrenaline
17. **(b)** Mechanical ventilation
18. **(g)** Heimlich manoeuvre
19. **(d)** Rebreathe into paper bag
20. **(i)** Chest drain
21. **(d)** Subcutaneous dose of LMW heparin upto 15000U/12 hourly
22. **(i)** Acetylsalicylic acid
23. **(g)** TED (thrombo-embolic deterrent) stockings.
24. **(c)** Chest X-ray
25. **(e)** Warfarin
26. **(i)** Pneumocystis carinii
27. **(a)** Chalmydia psittaci
28. **(e)** Legionella pneumoniae
29. **(c)** Streptococcus pneumoniae
30. **(f)** Mycobacterium tuberculosis
31. **(j)** Pseudo-obstruction
32. **(b)** Diverticular disease
33. **(g)** Acute pancreatitis
34. **(h)** Chronic active hepatitis
35. **(a)** Acute appendicitis
36. **(g)** Benign intracranial hypertension
37. **(i)** Giant cell arteritis
38. **(f)** Sinusitis
39. **(c)** Cluster headache
40. **(b)** Migraine headache
41. **(l)** Six years
42. **(f)** One year
43. **(a)** Two months
44. **(g)** One and half year
45. **(e)** Five months
46. **(g)** Heparin
47. **(i)** Vitamin K
48. **(d)** Fresh frozen plasma
49. **(i)** Vitamin K
50. **(b)** Factor VIII concentrate
51. **(e)** Ethambutol
52. **(f)** Isoniazid
53. **(k)** Streptomycin
54. **(j)** Rifampicin
55. **(c)** Cycloserine
56. **(b)** Systemic heparin 5000 units BD
57. **(j)** LMW dextran
58. **(a)** Systemic heparin 30,000 units per day
59. **(h)** No treatment
60. **(e)** Use caval filters
61. **(d)** Cataract
62. **(h)** Temporal arteritis
63. **(n)** Multiple sclerosis
64. **(o)** Ophthalmic herpes zoster
65. **(l)** Cavernous sinus thrombosis
66. **(h)** Acute viral pericarditis
67. **(d)** Constrictive pericarditis
68. **(f)** Cardiac tamponade
69. **(j)** Bronchogenic carcinoma
70. **(i)** Pericardial cysts
71. **(l)** MEN type II B
72. **(d)** MEN type I
73. **(c)** Hypothyroidism
74. **(a)** Thyroglossal cyst
75. **(f)** Hashimoto's thyroiditis

76. **(c)** Metformin
77. **(e)** Gliclazide
78. **(b)** Orlistat-Xenical
79. **(f)** Rosiglitazone
80. **(f)** Rosiglitazone
81. **(b)** AO cannulated screws
82. **(f)** Reconstructive surgery with internal graft
83. **(i)** Dyanamic hip screw
84. **(d)** Open reduction and K wire
85. **(k)** Open reduction and internal fixation
86. **(j)** May drive(but inform the DVLA)
87. **(g)** Must not drive for 3 years
88. **(h)** Should not drive for 48 hrs
89. **(j)** May drive(but inform the DVLA)
90. **(c)** Should not drive for 2 months
91. **(e)** Karyotype 45 XO
92. **(b)** Karyotype 46XX
93. **(d)** Di George syndrome
94. **(a)** Triploidy
95. **(h)** Klinefelter's syndrome
96. **(a)** Anteriorly displaced radial head
97. **(b)** Posteriorly displaced radial head
98. **(e)** Pain in the area between extensor and abductor pollicis longus tendons
99. **(d)** Thenar eminence swelling, palmar bruising and inability to move thumb
100. **(c)** Subluxation of MCP joint of thumb with abduction
101. **(c)** Down's syndrome
102. **(h)** Trisomy syndrome
103. **(a)** Marfan's syndrome
104. **(d)** Turner's syndrome
105. **(f)** William's syndrome
106. **(b)** Glycogen storage disorder
107. **(g)** Rubella syndrome
108. **(e)** Noonan's syndrome
109. **(l)** Fibroid
110. **(b)** Endometrial carcinoma
111. **(g)** DUB
112. **(d)** Anovulatory cycles
113. **(e)** Adenomyosis
114. **(b)** Iron Saccharin(Iron sucrose)
115. **(l)** Renal dialysis
116. **(p)** Recombinant Erythropoietin
117. **(k)** Frusemide
118. **(q)** Calcium carbonate
119. **(a)** Paracetamol
120. **(h)** Benzylpenicillin
121. **(j)** Biopsy
122. **(l)** Resuscitate and IV fluids
123. **(h)** Benzylpenicillin
124. **(b)** Pityriasis versicolor
125. **(g)** Necrotizing fasciitis
126. **(l)** Psoriasis
127. **(i)** Secondary syphilis
128. **(j)** Lichen planus
129. **(a)** Reversal of the circumcision (circumcision is illegal in UK)
130. **(f)** Give her contraception
131. **(d)** Termination
132. **(p)** KY gel (lubricant)
133. **(i)** Continuous oestrogen and progesterone oral preparation
134. **(e)** Combined oestrogen and progesterone implant
135. **(g)** Heart valve replacement
136. **(d)** Dental treatment of a cardiac patient
137. **(h)** Sigmoid colectomy
138. **(i)** Splenectomy
139. **(f)** Emergency appendicectomy
140. **(e)** Subacute thyroiditis
141. **(b)** Hashimoto's thyroiditis
142. **(h)** Amiodarone
143. **(g)** Hypopituitarism
144. **(f)** Hypoparathyroidism
145. **(c)** Cluster headache
146. **(f)** Intracranial tumour
147. **(h)** Meningitis
148. **(j)** Pseudotumour cerebri
149. **(d)** Encephalitis
150. **(d)** Pulmonary embolism
151. **(b)** Myocarditis
152. **(c)** Arrhythmia

153. **(f)** Pneumothorax
154. **(j)** Primary pulmonary hypertension
155. **(g)** Barotrauma
156. **(e)** Bullous myringitis
157. **(b)** Mastoiditis
158. **(i)** Ramsay–Hunt syndrome
159. **(k)** Quinsy
160. **(h)** PSA
161. **(d)** CEA
162. **(l)** Thyroglobulin
163. **(j)** S-100
164. **(m)** Urinary metanephrines
165. **(g)** Iatrogenic
166. **(k)** Thrombotic thrombocytopenic purpura
167. **(j)** Scurvy
168. **(d)** Ehler–Danlos syndrome
169. **(f)** Henoch–Schönlein purpura
170. **(a)** Lyme disease serology
171. **(f)** Blood film for malaria
172. **(i)** Leptospirosis serology
173. **(g)** Wound swab test
174. **(j)** Nail and skin scrappings
175. **(a)** Lichen planus
176. **(h)** Thrush
177. **(c)** Syphilis
178. **(e)** Hand foot and mouth disease
179. **(g)** Behcet's disease
180. **(e)** SLE
181. **(g)** Psoriatic arthritis
182. **(d)** Rheumatic fever
183. **(c)** Ankylosing spondylitis
184. **(a)** Rheumatoid arthritis
185. **(b)** Osteoarthritis
186. **(a)** Gastro-oesophagoscopy
187. **(i)** Ultrasound abdomen
188. **(j)** Laparoscopy
189. **(i)** Ultrasound abdomen
190. **(g)** ERCP
191. **(f)** Fludrocortisone
192. **(j)** Oxybutinin
193. **(g)** Testosterone
194. **(i)** Metoclopramide
195. **(b)** Tetracycline
196. **(e)** Livedo reticularis
197. **(b)** Erythema multiforme
198. **(a)** Erythema chronicum migrans
199. **(n)** Cafe-au-lait spots
200. **(f)** Dermatomyositis

Do not Write in this space

Four

Mock Test Paper

Theme 1: Syncope

Options:

a. Vasovagal syncope
b. Antihypertensive drugs
c. Carotid sinus hypersensitivity
d. Cough induced
e. Micturition
f. Aortic stenosis
g. Atrial myxoma
h. Pulmonary hypertension
i. Sick sinus syndrome
j. Ventricular tachycardia

For each presentation below, choose the SINGLE most appropriate cause of syncope from the above list of options. Each option may be used once, more than once, or not at all.

1. A 19 year old medical student on her first day in the surgery ward. She has a fall followed by a 5 minute period of unresponsiveness. Her colleagues noticed that she went pale and was sweating profusely just before the fall.

2. A 60 year old man presents with acute exacerbation of his COPD due to an attack of influenza.

3. A 70 year old man with known benign prostatic hypertrophy, presents to the A & E with a large scalp C.L.W. His wife states that he had a fall in the bathroom.

4. An 88 year old retired farmer with history of attacks of loss of consciousness since the last 3 months. His relatives describe sudden collapse during which he becomes very pale then develops a bluish tinge to his face. This is followed by flushing and abrupt return to consciousness. The episodes last less than a minute.

5. A middle aged lady presents with fever, malaise and weight loss since 3 months. In the last week she has had 2 episodes of sudden loss of consciousness on assuming an upright posture. Cardiac examination reveals a third heart sound and a diastolic murmur.

Theme 2: Cause of bleeding PV

Options:

a. Hypothyroidism
b. Endometrial carcinoma
c. DUB
d. Anovulatory cycles
e. Adenomyosis
f. Fibroid
g. Endometriosis
h. Adenomyosis
i. Polycystic ovarian syndrome
j. Von Willebrand's disease
k. Vaginal carcinoma
l. Ectopic pregnancy

For each presentation below, choose the SINGLE most appropriate cause of bleeding PV from the above list of options. Each option may be used once, more than once, or not at all.

6. A 35 year old woman with menorrhagia since 9 months complains of weight gain and constipation. She is infertile and is cold intolerant.

7. A 35 year old woman with dymenorrhoea and deep dyspareunia. On USG examination echogenic nodules were seen in the uterosacral ligaments. PV examination reveals a fixed retroverted uterus.

8. A 35 year old woman with no obvious pathology, has dysmenorrhoea.

9. A 25 year old woman presents with dark vaginal discharge, severe abdominal pain and hypotension. Her last menstrual period was 2 months ago.

10. A 28 year old woman presents with irregular periods, marked obesity and facial acne.

Theme 3: Respiratory diseases in children

Options:

a. Laryngomalacia
b. Respiratory distress syndrome
c. Congenital diaphragmatic hernia
d. Asthma
e. Cardiac failure
f. Tetralogy of Fallot
g. Pneumonia
h. Foreign body aspiration
i. Epiglotittis
j. Bronchiolitis

For each presentation below, choose the SINGLE most appropriate diagnosis from the above list of options. Each option may be used once, more than once, or not at all.

11. A 7 year old girl was brought to the A&E with sudden onset of high fever, respiratory distress and drooling of saliva.

12. A 9 months old infant with respiratory distress has been unable to complete feeds and is sweating a lot. The infant is tachypnoeic and tachycardic.

13. A 3 months old female infant has been having noisy breathing since day 5. Wheezing is more pronounced while the child feeds and diminishes during sleep.

14. A 5 year old girl with history of bouts of respiratory distress and cough which has had a variable course over one year.

15. A 5 year old girl was brought with history of bouts of cough and breathlessness since 3 months. The episodes are not relieved by bronchodilators but the child is well in between the episodes.

Theme 4: Eponymous terms

Options:

a. CCF
b. Hereditary haemorrhagic telangiectasia
c. Jaundice
d. Pericarditis
e. Tuberculosis
f. Ataxia
g. Gastroenteritis
h. Impotence
i. Leprosy
j. Stroke
k. Vasculitis

For each pathology below, choose the SINGLE most appropriate eponymous term from the above list of options. Each option may be used once, more than once, or not at all.

16. Hansen's disease.
17. Pott's disease.
18. Osler weber rendu syndrome.
19. Dressler's syndrome.

Theme 5: Diagnosis of falls

Options:

a. Parkinson's disease
b. Impaired vision
c. Aortic stenosis
d. Vertebro basilar insufficiency
e. Cerebellar ataxia
f. Postural hypotension
g. Drop attacks
h. Peripheral neuropathy
i. Acute labyrinthitis
j. Sick sinus syndrome
k. Sensory ataxia
l. Meniere's disease

For each presentation below, choose the SINGLE most appropriate diagnosis from the above list of options. Each option may be used once, more than once, or not at all.

20. A 55 year old man presents with history of recurrent falls over the last one year or so. He has difficulty walking fast. On examination cogwheel rigidity is noted.

21. A 60 year old man complains of imbalance on standing while on the wash basin in the morning. He walks with a stamping gait. On examination Romberg test is positive.

22. A 40 year old man complains of a tendency to fall if he tries to walk fast. He also complains of a sensation of pins and needles in his feet. On examination he has ataxia with a stamping gait.

23. A 70 year old man complains of feeling giddy and falling sometimes while walking. He says he has never lost consciousness though he feels a sensation of vertigo at the time of fall.

24. A 48 year old woman presents with slurred speech, nystagmus and intention tremor. She complains of frequent falls. Her gait is seen to be wide based.

Theme 6: Diagnosis of weight loss

Options:

a. Starvation
b. Malabsorption
c. Anorexia nervosa
d. Depression
e. Hyperthyroidism
f. Atrophic gastritis
g. Dementia

For each presentation below, choose the SINGLE most appropriate diagnosis from the above list of options. Each option may be used once, more than once, or not at all.

25. An elderly man with alcoholic liver disease is found to be wasted.

26. A 50 year old man presents to A & E with a 4 month history of diarrhoea, weight loss and palpitations. On examination, there are no significant findings.

27. A 37 year old company executive has just had a company merger. She now complains of weight loss and early morning wakening.

28. A 21 year old girl presents to her GP before her forthcoming A-level exams, complaining of amenorrhoea. She has lost 18 lbs over the last 3 months.

Theme 7: Diagnosis of joint pain

Options:

a. Gout
b. Pseudogout
c. Osteoarthritis
d. Infective arthritis
e. Psoriatic arthropathy
f. Ankylosing spondylitis
g. Juvenile chronic arthritis
h. Rheumatoid arthritis
i. Reiter's syndrome
j. Felty's syndrome
k. Osteogenesis imperfecta

For each presentation below, choose the SINGLE most appropriate diagnosis from the above list of options. Each option may be used once, more than once, or not at all.

29. A 30 year old homosexual male is found to have a markedly swollen knee of one month duration and a temperature of 38°C. He says the knee has only recently become painful and also admitted to losing weight. He had no other complaints apart from a 2-month history of cough, which he attributed to his heavy smoking.

30. A 36 year old lady presents with swollen knee joint. She says they feel stiff, especially in the morning. On examination, she is found to be pyrexic and ulcers on both her legs and marked hyperpigmentation. Hb 9 g/dl, WBC, platelets are decreased and a serum albumin of 20 g/L.

31. A 45 year old obese man presented with a painful and swollen ankle. The symptoms had started gradually in the previous month. Joint fluid aspiration was done and positively birefringent crystals were found. The patient drinks alcohol but doesn't smoke.

32. A 15 year old boy complains of temporomandibular joint pain for three months. On examination, he has micrognathia, loss of neck extension and unequal lengths of the lower limbs. He is rheumatoid factor negative.

Theme 8: Trauma: Management/ diagnosis

Options:

a. Ruptured bronchus
b. Ruptured aorta
c. Ruptured oesophagus
d. Tension pneumothorax
e. Cardiac tamponade
f. Blood transfusion
g. Oral analgesia
h. Morphine (IV)
i. Strap chest
j. Ruptured spleen
k. Immobilization

For each presentation below, choose the SINGLE most appropriate management/ treatment from the above list of options. Each option may be used once, more than once, or not at all.

33. A 17 year old boy with multiple fractures is taken for open reduction. His pulse rate is 120 beats/min and BP is 100/60 mmHg.

34. A 47 year old man is involved in a road traffic accident. Chest X-ray shows a transverse fracture of the sternum. He is otherwise well.

35. A 35 year old man is brought to the A & E with a haemothorax. Bilateral chest drainage is done, but his condition fails to improve.

36. A 12 year old boy was involved in a fight in which he received a kick to his chest. He presents the following day with chest pain and is found to have 3 fractured ribs.

37. A 45 year old man who was wearing a seat belt is involved in a high-speed car accident. On X-ray, a 'widened' mediastinum is seen.

Theme 9: Overdosage management

Options

a. Acetylcysteine
b. Desferrioxamine
c. Dimercaprol
d. Ethanol
e. Flumazenil
f. Glucagon
g. Naloxone
h. Observation
i. Pralidoxime
j. Penicillamine
k. Sodium nitrite

For each presentation below, choose the SINGLE most appropriate management from the above list of options. Each option may be used once, more than once, or not at all.

38. A 50 year old female is admitted unconscious after taking an overdose of an unknown substance. The only history is from her husband who states that she has been depressed and anxious of late and has been prescribed some medication by the GP. Examination reveals a Glasgow Coma Scale of 10/15 and she responds and opens her eyes to pain. She has a pulse of 62 beats per minute which is regular, a blood pressure of 130/80 mmHg and a respiratory rate of 20/minute with a saturation of 96 per cent. The pupils are of normal size.

39. A 70 year old farmer is admitted acutely after ingesting an unknown overdose. Examination reveals a particularly anxious male who is sweaty and salivating. His temperature is 40°C and he has a blood pressure of 90/60 mmHg with a pulse of 65 beats per minute.

40. A 6 year old child is admitted after consuming her mothers ferrous sulphate tablets. She has had one haematemesis and the iron concentration is excessive.

41. A 52 year old vagrant attends casualty with hyperventilation and vomiting. He confesses to having drunk methanol.

42. A 16 year old girl is admitted after taking a paracetamol overdose with alcohol 4 hours previously. Her plasma paracetamol concentration is 120 mg/L.

Theme 10: Investigations of paediatric endocrinological and metabolic disorders

Options:

a. FBC
b. Serum electrolytes
c. Serum ADH
d. Serum GH
e. Phenylketones in urine
f. Thyroid function tests
g. Galactose in urine
h. Serum ACTH
i. High serum blood glucose
j. Low blood glucose
k. Cystine in urine
l. Plasma cortisol

For each presentation below, choose the SINGLE most appropriate investigation from the above list of options. Each option may be used once, more than once, or not at all.

43. 1 month baby with poor feeding and lethargy. On examination umbilical hernia and enlarged tongue.

44. Newborn female with enlarged clitoris and fused labia.

45. A 13 year obese girl presents with asthma, eczema and amenorrhoea. Her BP was found to be 130/80.

46. 1 month baby with vomiting, jaundice and hepatomegaly. Baby is worse after feeding.

47. An 8 year old boy with short stature complains of thirst and passes huge volume of colourless urine.

Theme 11: Milestones

Options:

a. 3 months
b. 6 months
c. 9 months
d. 12 months
e. 18 months
f. 2 years
g. 3 years
h. 4 years
i. 5 years
j. 6 years
k. 7 years

For each presentation below, choose the SINGLE most appropriate age at which it is seen from the above list of options. Each option may be used once, more than once, or not at all.

48. A child can copy a square and triangle but not a diamond.

49. A mother is concerned that the baby is not walking yet. The baby can sit unsupported, bables, holds pencil in scissor grasp, can transfer it to his mouth and between his hands.

50. A child can only copy a circle, climbs stairs one foot per step, builds tower of nine cubes.

51. A child can only copy a circle and cross, stand on 1 foot for 5 seconds and climbs up and down stairs one foot per step.

52. A mother is concerned that the baby is not talking yet, he can walk around furniture, can stand alone for few seconds, holds objects in pincer grasp.

Theme 12: Diagnosis of breast lumps

Options:

a. Carcinoma
b. Fibroadenoma
c. Cyst
d. Cyclical mastalgia
e. Breast abscess
f. Paget's disease
g. Cystosarcoma phylloides

For each presentation below, choose the SINGLE most appropriate diagnosis from the above list of options. Each option may be used once, more than once, or not at all.

53. A 72 year old lady, with a complaint of unilateral mass, in the right upper quadrant with axillary nodes which are enlarged and fixed.

54. A 21 year old lady with a firm mass in the lower quadrant. The mass is mobile and no axillary nodes are palpable.

55. A 58 year old lady comes with excoriation of skin on the nipple with bloody discharge.

56. A 52 year old patient comes with a history of a bloody discharge from the nipple on squeezing.

57. A post-partum patient with a unilateral localised swelling, accompanied by tenderness and rise in temperature.

Theme 13: Teratogenicity

Options:

a. Betamethasone
b. Norethisterone
c. Salbutamol
d. Ergometrine
e. Oxytocin
f. Prostaglandin F_2 alpha
g. Indomethacin
h. Oxytetracycline
i. Amoxicillin
j. Alcohol
k. Isotretinoin
l. Lithium
m. Valproic acid
n. Dilantin
o. Streptomycin
p. Thalidomide

For each presentation below, choose the SINGLE most appropriate involved drug from the above list of options. Each option may be used once, more than once, or not at all.

58. Ebstein's anomaly.
59. Congenital deafness, CNS and heart defects.
60. Short palpebral fissure, long philtrum and midfacial hypoplasia.
61. Oligohydraminos.
62. Pulmonary oedema.

Theme 14: The diagnosis of infertility

Options:

a. Polycystic ovary disease
b. Endometriosis
c. Adenomyosis
d. Chronic salpingitis
e. Diabetes mellitus
f. Hyperprolactinaemia
g. Hypopituitarism
h. Hyperthyroidism
i. Hypothyroidism
j. Pulmonary tuberculosis
k. Possible malignancy

For each presentation below, choose the SINGLE most appropriate diagnosis from the above list of options. Each option may be used once, more than once, or not at all.

63. A 42 year old woman complains of being unable to conceive for the past 2 years despite have regular unprotected sex. She complains of excessive sweating, frequent stools and says this explains her loss in weight over recent weeks. She denied starving herself and says she has a very good appetite. Glycosylated Hb (Hb A_{1c}) = 5%.

64. A 28 year old woman complains of infertility and is otherwise well. She had been on haloperidol to treat a schizophreniform illness she had for six year. She has a healthy 3 year old daughter.

65. A 26 year old woman complains of infertility for 3 year. She has a low libido, and has put on a lot of weight over the last couple of year. Her breasts were found to be discharging on examination.

66. A 31 year old woman complains of abdominal pain which seems to increase during her periods. Over the last year, she has noticed difficulty in breathing and chest pain associated with occasional haemoptysis,

following her periods. She has been unable to conceive. On examination she is found to have an enlarged and tender uterus. Her BMI is 20.

Theme 15: Management of haematological conditions

Options:

a. Oral ferrous sulphate
b. Parenteral iron infusion
c. Folic acid
d. Oral prednisolone
e. High dose immunoglobulins
f. Venesection
g. Venesection followed by hydroxyurea
h. Vitamin K
i. Heparin
j. Protamine sulphate
k. Cryoprecipitate
l. Secure haemostasis
m. DDAVP
n. Tranexaemic acid
o. NSAIDs
p. IV Morphine
q. SC Diamorphine with cyclizine
r. TENS
s. Activated charcoal
t. Phentolamine

For each presentation below, choose the SINGLE most appropriate management from the above list of options. Each option may be used once, more than once, or not at all.

67. A 55 year old man presented in A & E with chest pain of 2 hours duration and suspected MI. He has been well yet has developed night sweats and lost 20 lbs in last 3 months. He does not smoke nor has past history of chest problems. His Hb came out to be 22 gm/dl, PCV 0.58, WBC 20 × 10^9/L and platelets 600 × 10^9/L.

68. As a medical SHO on call, you are paged by the Surgical SpR in the late hours on Friday afternoon asking you whether he can give cryoprecipitate to his patient. He says that he just finished a bilateral herniorraphy on a 55 year old man. The left side has

been bleeding excessively and he had to tranfuse 2 units within last 45 minutes.

69. A 29 year old woman has had a D & C for long standing menorrhagia. She is now 4 days into post procedure period and is still bleeding. She is taken back to the theatre yet no abnormality could be found. She says that she had been having problems in the past with bleeding after dental extractions. Her PT, APTT and platelet count, all turn out to be normal.

70. A 72 year old man presented to medical OPD with dyspnoea, wheezing, fever and cough productive of sputum. Initial investigations are: Hb 23 gm/dl, PCV 0.62, a mild neutrophilia and platelets 200×10^9/ L. His son says that he has been smoking all his life and keeps on getting bouts of bronchitis but is otherwise well.

71. A 19 year old Afro-carribean female presented to A & E with pains in her left leg, right hip and back. She has had been on an all night rave club.

Theme 16: Diagnosis of abdominal pain

Options:

a. Amoebic liver abscess
b. Acute intermittent porphyria
c. Functional
d. Perforated peptic ulcer
e. Retrocaecal appendicitis
f. Myocardial infarction
g. Basal pneumonia
h. Acute pancreatitis
i. Acute cholecystitis
j. Pancreatic carcinoma
k. Hepatocellular carcinoma
l. Hydatid disease
m. AIDS
n. Chronic pancreatitis
o. Chronic cholecystitis
p. Pyogenic liver abscess.

For each presentation below, choose the SINGLE most appropriate diagnosis from the above list of options. Each option may be used once, more than once, or not at all.

72. A 50 year old man complains of weight loss, diarrhoea and abdominal pain and flatulence. On examination he has icterus and pedal oedema.

73. A 48 year old man presents with acute epigastric pain which radiates through to the back. On physical examination you find tenderness and guarding.

74. A 62 year old farmer complains of pain in the right hypochondrium. Examination reveals enlarged liver and USG shows fluid filled cyst.

75. A 45 year old truck driver presents with a large, tender, irregular liver. He has no appetite and has lost 2 stones of weight in the past 3 months. He was known to have Hepatitis B.

76. A 38 year old woman presents with fever and abdominal pain. On examination she is icteric and has a tender right hypochondrium.

Theme 17: Pain control

Options:

a. Paracetamol
b. Morphine
c. Diamorphine
d. Dihydrocodiene
e. Amitriptyline
f. Nerve radical destruction
g. Carbamazepine

For each presentation below, choose the SINGLE most appropriate durg from the above list of options. Each option may be used once, more than once, or not at all.

77. A 25 year old underwent excision of sebaceous gland under local anaesthesia. She uses salbutamol inhaler on regular basis.

78. A 40 year old patient requires analgesia following a total thyroidectomy.

79. A 40 year old complains of phantom limb pain following below knee amputation.

Theme 18: Endocrine tests

Options:

a. Clonidine test
b. GHRH/arginine test
c. High dose dexamethasone test
d. Insulin induced hypoglycaemia
e. LHRH test
f. Oral glucose tolerance test
g. Overnight dexamethasone test
h. Short synacthen test
i. TRH test
j. Urine catecholamines
k. Water deprivation test

For each presentation below, choose the SINGLE most appropriate test from the above list of options. Each option may be used once, more than once, or not at all.

80. A 60 year old male presents with polyuria and polydipsia. His blood pressure is 165/80. He is treated with atenolol. Urine analysis reveals glycosuria and normal urine free cortisol estimates.

81. A 55 year old male who has undergone previous pituitary surgery for a non-functional tumour presents with a long history of tiredness and weight gain. He currently is taking thyroxine, hydrocortisone, testosterone together with aspirin and atorvastatin. Two years ago he underwent angioplasty. You wish to assess his growth hormone reserve.

82. A 45 year old male is diagnosed with a non-functional pituitary tumour. You want to assess his cortisol and GH secretory function.

83. A 19 year old female presents with primary amenorrhoea and hirsutism. Phenotypically she is a normal female, but has marked hirsutism with virilization. Her karyotype is 46XX.

84. A 60 year old male complains of a 6 month history of frontal headaches. On questioning he has noticed an increase in his ring size and an enlargement in shoe size over the last 10 years.

Theme 19: The diagnosis of abdominal pain

Options:

a. Primary hypertension
b. Conn's syndrome
c. Nephroma
d. Hepatoma
e. Bladder tumour
f. Adrenal tumour
g. Bronchogenic carcinoma
h. Phaeochromocytoma
i. Adrenogenital syndrome
j. Neurofibromatosis
k. Cushing's disease
l. Medullary carcinoma thyroid
m. Diabetes mellitus
n. Hyperthyroidism

For each presentation below, choose the SINGLE most appropriate diagnosis from the above list of options. Each option may be used once, more than once, or not at all.

85. A 28 year man complains of headache, nausea and vomiting. His BP is 169/115. Fundoscopy reveals optic atrophy. Over the past year he has suffered from bouts of headaches, sweating and abdominal pain.

86. A young woman treated for persistent hypertension with diuretics has found her BP increasingly difficult to control and complains of recurrent headaches and visual loss. Sometimes going to the toilet causes her to faint.

87. A young woman complains of amenorrhoea and obesity. Over the past few years she has felt that she has aged rapidly. Her face has become full, her skin greasy and she has started using depilatory preparation.

88. A middle aged woman is found to be hypertensive on a routine check up. She also complains of headaches and visual disturbances. She has felt loss of strength,

cannot finish her gardening and goes to toilet all the time, especially at night.

89. An adolescent boy develops small breast bilaterally. He has noticed a loss of interest in his school and social life. Physical examination shows small testes and a large abdominal mass.

Theme 20: Tumour markers

Options:

a. α fetoprotein
b. CA 19-9
c. CA 125
d. CEA
e. HCG
f. NSE
g. PLAP
h. PSA
i. Calcitonin
j. S-100
k. None of the above
l. Thyroglobulin
m. Urinary metanephrines
n. 5-HIAA

For each malignancy below, choose the SINGLE most appropriate tumour marker from the above list of options. Each option may be used once, more than once, or not at all.

90. Choriocarcinoma.
91. Small cell carcinoma of lung.
92. Teratoma.
93. Seminoma.
94. Carcinoid tumour.

Theme 21: Prescribing in pregnancy

Options:

a. Bendrofluazide
b. Paracetamol
c. Methyldopa
d. Insulin
e. Carbamazepine with 5 mg/day folate
f. Captopril
g. Acamprosate
h. Reduce glibenclamide
i. Heparin and aspirin
j. Continue carbamazepine
k. Lisinopril
l. Prednisolone
m. Vigabatrin
n. Warfarin and aspirin
o. Increase glibenclamide
p. Gliclazide
q. Aspirin

For each presentation below, choose the SINGLE most appropriate prescription from the above list of options. Each option may be used once, more than once, or not at all.

95. A 40 year old diabetic on glibenclamide (10 mg/day) misses her period and requests a pregnancy test. The test is positive. Up to now her blood glucose control has been excellent.

96. A 32 year old woman is found to have a blood pressure of 150/100 mmHg at 30 weeks of pregnancy. She has no complaints.

97. A pregnant 33 year old woman, with a history of recurrent second trimester miscarriages is found to have lupus anticoagulant and anti-cardiolipin antibodies at 10 weeks of pregnancy.

98. A 28 year old woman is being treated with carbamazepine, with good results. She misses her periods and goes for a pregnancy test, which comes out to be positive.

99. A pregnant 40 year old woman complains of chronic knee joint pain and stiffness. She is found to have osteoarthritis.

Theme 22: Developmental milestones

Options:

a. 1-2 months
b. 8-9 months
c. 3-6 year
d. 5-7 months
e. 10-14 months
f. 2-3 years
g. 14-16 months
h. 18-22 months
i. 7-10 months
j. 16-20 months.

For each presentation below, choose the SINGLE most appropriate age at which it first occurs in the normal child from the above list of options. Each option may be used once, more than once, or not at all.

100. Transfers a cube from one hand to another.
101. Lifts the head when in prone position.
102. Walks holding on to furniture.
103. Drinks from the cup.
104. Builds a tower of 8 cubes.
105. Builds a tower of 2 cubes.

Theme 23: Headache: Selection of diagnostic tests

Options:

a. Mental state examination
b. Magnetic resonance imaging of cervical spine
c. Lumbar puncture
d. Intraocular pressure
e. Fundoscopy
f. Erythrocyte sedimentation rate
g. Electroencephalogram
h. Computed tomography scan of the brain
i. Carotid arteriography
j. Visual fields
k. Toxoplasma serology
l. Temporal artery biopsy
m. Skull X-ray

For each presentation below, choose the SINGLE most appropriate investigation from the above list of options. Each option may be used once, more than once, or not at all.

106. A 32 year old man presents with headache, photophobia and sudden reduction in visual acuity. His fundi look pale.

107. A 34 year old woman has generalized headache described as a tight band, unrelieved by paracetamol. She has difficulty sleeping and says she has lost weight recently.

108. A 53 year old man has severe headache, worse on lying. You find bilateral papilloedema.

109. A 72 year old woman has a right-sided headache aggravated by brushing her hair. She says she has been generally unwell for a few months with aching muscles.

110. A 14 year old boy presents with drowsiness and generalized headache. He is recovering from a bilateral parotitis. His CT scan is normal.

Theme 24: Investigation of hoarseness

Options:

a. No investigation
b. Computed tomography (CT) scan of the neck
c. Sputum for Acid fast bacilli
d. Cervical spine X-ray
e. Laryngoscopy
f. Bronchoscopy
g. Bronchoalveolar lavage
h. Chest X-ray
i. Lymph node biopsy
j. Treponemal Haemagglutination assay

For each presentation below, choose the SINGLE most appropriate investigation from the above list of options. Each option may be used once, more than once, or not at all.

111. A 25 year old man complains of a two-day history of hoarseness of voice. He denies any history of weight but admits to 4-year history of smoking.

112. A 13 year old girl complains of a 2-day history of hoarseness of the voice associated with a dry cough. She feels feverish and on direct laryngoscopy her vocal cords are grossly oedematous.

113. A 34 year old woman had a partial thyroidectomy 3 hours ago. She complains of mild hoarseness of the voice. She had no history of phonation problems prior to surgery.

114. A 67 year old man with a history of weight loss complains of hoarseness of the voice. Computed tomography scan reveals an opacity in the right upper mediastinum. He denied any history of difficulty in breathing.

115. A 34 year old IV drug user has a 4 month history of a productive cough. He has lost 20 lbs in weight.

Theme 25: The treatment of infectious diseases

Options:

a. Metronidazole
b. Flucloxacillin
c. Gentamicin
d. Fluconazole
e. Ciprofloxacin
f. Niclosamide
g. Rifampicin
h. Benzylpenicillin (IV)
i. Dapsone
j. Clotrimazole
k. Griseofulvin
l. Co-trimoxazole
m. Hib Vaccine
n. Cefotaxime or any such drugs

For each presentation below, choose the SINGLE most appropriate current from the above list of options. Each option may be used once, more than once, or not at all.

116. Methicillin resistant staphylococcus aureus. (MRSA).
117. Giardiasis.
118. Amoebiasis.
119. Trichomonas vaginalis.
120. Bacterial vaginosis.
121. Pneumocystis carinii pneumonia.
122. Haemophilus meningitis.
123. Prophylaxis for children in contact in household with meningitis.

Theme 26: Causes of pneumonia

Options:

a. Staphylococcus aureus
b. Pneumocystis carinii
c. Mycoplasma pneumoniae
d. Bacteroides fragilis
e. Coxiella burnetii
f. Legionella pneumophila
g. Haemophilus influenzae
h. Mycobacterium avium
i. Streptococcus pneumoniae
j. Mixed growth of organisms
k. Escherichia coli
l. Mycobacterium tuberculosis

For each presentation below, choose the SINGLE most appropriate causative organism from the above list of options. Each option may be used once, more than once, or not at all.

124. A 23 year old haemophiliac presents with a 2 month history of a dry cough associated with exertional dyspnoea. He has lost 8 lbs of weight over this period. A chest X-ray shows a 'ground glass' appearance.

125. A 33 year old homosexual man presents with a 3 month history of a productive cough associated with fever and night sweats. He denied any history of haemoptysis, but says he has lost considerable weight.

126. A 33 year old previously healthy man presents with joint pains and a dry persistent cough. He'd been on holiday two weeks prior to presentation. His X-ray shows bilateral patchy consolidation and blood analysis shows an increased antibody titre.

127. A 31 year old woman has a one week history of general malaise, fever and productive cough. Her X-ray shows a left middle lobe consolidation with increased vocal resonance in the left middle zone on auscultation.

Theme 27: Diagnosis of a swollen knee

Options:

a. Rheumatoid arthritis
b. Gout
c. Osteoarthritis
d. Pseudogout
e. Ruptured baker's cyst
f. Septic arthritis
g. Trauma
h. Charcot's knee
i. Haemarthrosis
j. Tuberculous arthritis
k. Psoriatic arthritis
l. Bronchogenic carcinoma

For each presentation below, choose the SINGLE most appropriate condition from the above list of options. Each option may be used once, more than once, or not at all.

128. A 34 year old woman presents with a 2 month history of right knee joint pain. On examination she is found to have nodules on her elbows and, sausage shaped fingers.

129. A 33 year old rugby player presents with an acutely painful knee. He has a mild cough but has otherwise been well enough to compete in the national finals.

130. A 23 year old haemophiliac presents with a painful and swollen right knee. He attributes this to a fall he had in the bath.

131. A 12 year old girl with a 2 hour history of rigors, presents with a painful right knee. On examination the knee was found to be hot and swollen with a positive patellar tap sign.

132. A 67 year old man with a 4 month history of a productive cough and weight loss presents with a painful right knee. His chest X-ray shows numerous nodular opacities, involving both lung fields.

Theme 28: Diarrhoea and weight loss

Options:

a. Inflammatory bowel disease
b. Tuberculous enterocolitis
c. Cytomegalovirus infection
d. Coeliac sprue
e. Tropical sprue
f. Hyperthyroidism
g. Amyloidosis
h. Intestinal lymphoma
i. Whipple's disease
j. Chronic pancreatitis

For each presentation below, choose the SINGLE most appropriate diagnosis from the above list of options. Each option may be used once, more than once, or not at all.

133. A 48 year old man presents with watery stools 4 to 6 times a day, he also has abdominal cramps, flatulence and borborygmi. He has lost 20 pounds over the last 8 months. He is of Irish descent.

134. A thirty year old HIV positive man with a 3 week history of intermittent bloody diarrhoea, urgency, abdominal pain and malaise. Repeated stool examination is negative for ova and parasites including multiple stool cultures for enteric pathogens.

135. A 50 year old man presents with diarrhoea and migratory arthralgias for the last 6 months, he has lost 20 pounds in weight and relatives describe a decline in mental acuity.

136. A 28 year old man with diarrhoea and crampy abdominal pain of the right lower abdomen for the last 8 weeks, he also complains of fever, anorexia and weight loss. He has not responded to antitubercular therapy for the last 3 weeks.

137. A 63 year old woman with rheumatoid arthritis for the last 20 years presents with weight loss, foul smelling diarrhoea, easy bruising and peripheral oedema. On examination she has waxy skin plaques especially in the axillary folds.

Theme 29: Investigation of chest pain

Options:

a. ECG
b. Treadmill exercise test
c. CXR
d. V/Q scan
e. Abdominal USG
f. Thallium perfusion scan
g. CT scan–chest
h. Bronchoscopy
i. Coronary angiography
j. Sputum culture
k. Endoscopy
l. Arterial blood gases

For each presentation below, choose the SINGLE most appropriate investigation from the above list of options. Each option may be used once, more than once, or not at all.

138. A 50 year old male complains of intermittent chest pain radiating to the jaw and left shoulder relieved by rest. ECG is found to be normal.

139. A 40 year old smoker presents with 1 hour history of severe central chest pain radiating down the left arm. It is also associated with nausea and sweating.

140. A 25 year old woman who is on OCPs complains of sudden onset pleuritic chest pain and mild breathlessness. She has history of a swollen leg.

141. A 20 year old man complains of pleuritic chest pain and dyspnoea. He is 6 feet tall and smokes a lot.

142. A 45 year old obese woman complains of intermittent right lower chest pain. Her CXR is normal. She has tenderness in right hypochondrium.

Theme 30: Quadriparesis

Options:

a. Guillain Barré syndrome
b. Hypokalaemic paralysis (periodic)
c. Renal tubular acidosis
d. Brainstem infarction
e. Myasthenia gravis
f. Lambert Eaton syndrome
g. Polymyositis
h. Muscular dystrophies
i. Botulism
j. High cervical cord pathology

For each presentation below, choose the SINGLE most appropriate diagnosis from the above list of options. Each option may be used once, more than once, or not at all.

143. A 23 year old man with paraesthesia in both legs progressing to quadriparesis with dysphagia over the next 72 hours. He had history of a gastroenteritis two weeks ago.

144. An 8 year old boy presenting with weakness in all 4 limbs and hyperventilation. His lab reports show Na^+ 130 mmol/L, K^+ 2.0 mmol/L, HCO_3^- 11 mmol/L, chloride 113 mmol/L. X-ray abdomen shows nephrocalcinosis.

145. A 64 year old smoker with small cell carcinoma of the lung presents with weakness of the proximal limbs. The weakness improves with sustained contraction of the muscles.

146. A 60 year old widow presenting with double vision one day after eating home canned fruit. Within four hours of presentation, she has difficulty in speaking and limb weakness. Other symptoms include nausea, vomiting, dizziness, blurred vision and dry mouth. Patient is alert, oriented and afebrile.

147. A 65 year old woman with seropositive RA with a 6 week history of progressive gene-

ralized weakness and paraesthesias in all four limbs. Examination reveals depressed reflexes with upgoing plantars.

Theme 31: Wasting of the small muscles of the hand

Options:

a. Leprosy
b. Motor neurone disease
c. Ulnar nerve damage
d. Carpal tunnel syndrome
e. Syringomyelia
f. Cervical rib
g. Neurofibroma
h. Pancoast tumour
i. Metastatic carcinoma in deep cervical nodes
j. Peripheral neuropathy

For each presentation below, choose the SINGLE most appropriate diagnosis from the above list of options. Each option may be used once, more than once, or not at all.

148. A 66 year old woman with pain in the neck radiating into the left upper limb into the axilla and down the ulnar border of the arm. Oblique X-rays of the cervical spine demonstrate enlargement of the left C8/T1 intervertebral foramen.

149. A 34 year old male with deep aching pain in the right arm and hand. He also develops episodes of blanching and swelling of the fingers especially on turning his head towards the left shoulder.

150. A 36 year old woman 5 months pregnant with her third child with history of severe pain in both the hands especially in the thumb and index fingers. The pain is relieved on swinging the arm or flexing and extending the wrist.

151. A 38 year old male with progressive left foot drop. He has a history of severe cramps in the left leg. Examination reveals wasting of small muscles of the hands and left leg, widespread fasciculations, brisk reflexes and left extensor plantar response.

152. A 69 year old heavy cigarette smoker with

history of haemoptysis. He has severe pain in the right shoulder especially at night. Examination reveals wasting of the muscles of the right hand and drooping of the right eyelid.

Theme 32: Complications of cholecystectomy

Options:

a. Retained CBD stones
b. Reactionary haemorrhage
c. Subphrenic abscess
d. Atelectasis
e. Walter Waltman syndrome
f. Biliary stricture
g. Biliary fistula
h. Biliary cirrhosis
i. Air embolism
j. Faecal fistula

For each presentation below, choose the SINGLE most appropriate complication from the above list of options. Each option may be used once, more than once, or not at all.

153. A 34 year old female presents with jaundice at the end of 2 months after cholecystectomy. During surgery there was bleeding from the cystic artery.

154. A 36 year old male presents with jaundice 2 weeks after surgery. The intraoperative findings were multiple stones with a broad cystic duct. An intraoperative cholangiogram was not performed.

155. A 34 year old male presents on the 5th day after cholecystectomy with upper abdominal pain, hypotension and dyspnoea. The surgeon had not placed an intra-abdominal drain after surgery.

156. On the 4th day of cholecystectomy the patient develops dyspnoea. Air entry on the right side of chest is decreased.

157. A patient of cholecystectomy presents with slowly progressive jaundice of 3 years duration. On exploration the surgeon encounters vascular adhesions and has to abandon the procedure.

Theme 33: Anaesthesia

Options:

a. General anaesthesia
b. Spinal anaesthesia
c. Epidural anaesthesia
d. Pudendal block
e. Entonox
f. IM Morphine
g. IV Pethidine
h. NSAID
i. Paracetamol
j. Prochlorperazine
k. Transcutaneous nerve stimulation
l. Pressure massage
m. Acupuncture

For each presentation below, choose the SINGLE most appropriate type of anaesthesia required from the above list of options. Each option may be used once, more than once, or not at all.

158. A 32 year old primi is in labour. Her cervix is 8 cm dilated in 12 hours. She said that the contractions are more painful and she could no longer tolerate it.

159. A pregnant mother discusses about pain relief in the antenatal clinic. She insists upon her freedom of movement during her labour and she wants to walk during labour.

160. A 28 year old primi delivered a baby 30 minutes ago and she is still bleeding vaginally. The decision to remove the placenta manually was made.

161. A 32 year old gravida 2, complains of pain during uterine contractions. Cervix is 6 cm dilated. She has already received 2 injections of pethidine.

162. A 29 year old primi is in labour. Cervix is 9 cm dilated and the head is in occipito-posterior position.

Theme 34: Pelvic pain

Options:

a. Appendicitis
b. Chronic pelvic inflammatory disease
c. Endometrial cancer
d. Endometriosis
e. Fibroids
f. Irritable bowel syndrome
g. Ovarian cyst
h. Retroverted uterus

For each presentation below, choose the SINGLE most appropriate diagnosis from the above list of options. Each option may be used once, more than once, or not at all.

163. A 33 year old lady with no children who has been suffering worsening pelvic pain particularly prior to menstruation and is now complaining of deep dyspareunia.

164. A 55 year old lady on HRT who has been experiencing non specific pelvic pain and has occasional spotting of blood prior to her withdrawal bleed on HRT.

165. A 21 year-old lady on no form of contraception and sudden onset of colicky intermittent pain.

Theme 35: Pelvic inflammatory disease

Options:

a. Actinomyces israelii
b. Chlamydia trachomatis
c. Entamoeba histolytica
d. Escherichia coli
e. Gardnerella vaginalis
f. Herpes hominis
g. Mycobacterium tuberculosis
h. Neisseria gonorrhoea
i. Staphylococcus aureus

For each presentation below, choose the SINGLE most appropriate causative organism from the above list of options. Each option may be used once, more than once, or not at all.

166. A 24 year old sexually active girl has lower abdominal pain and pustules on hands.
167. A 42 year old presents with weight loss, night sweats, chronic abdominal pain and a tubo-ovarian mass.
168. A 30 year old lady presents with lower abdominal pain and has an intra-uterine device.
169. A teenage girl is admitted four months after menarche with a rash and septic shock.
170. A 25 year old lady has very mild lower abdominal pain . Laparoscopy reveals a severe inflammatory process.

Theme 36: Cause of shoulder pain

Options:

a. Rheumatoid arthritis
b. Osteoarthritis
c. Pyogenic arthritis
d. Trauma
e. PMR
f. Shoulder hand syndrome
g. Herpes zoster
h. Referred pain from neck
i. Painful arc syndrome

For each presentation below, choose the SINGLE most appropriate diagnosis .from the above list of options. Each option may be used once, more than once, or not at all.

171. A 55 year old man has shoulder pain which typically occurs only when he lifts his arm above a certain level. Deep tenderness is also present.
172. A 50 year old has shoulder pain which typically aggravates on turning his head to one side.
173. A 70 year old woman has morning stiffness and shoulder pain. She also complains of decreased appetite and fever. Her ESR is found to be 50 mm/hr.
174. A 50 year old woman has morning stiffness and shoulder pain. She has slowly developed stiffness of both of her wrist joints in the past few months. She remains afebrile.

175. A 35 year old gardener develops fever, cellulitis of his left leg and a red, hot, swollen right shoulder.

Theme 37: Causes of abdominal pain

Options:

a. Biliary colic
b. Peptic ulcer
c. Appendicitis
d. Renal colic
e. Pancreatitis
f. Diverticulitis
g. Peritonitis
h. Intussusception
i. Inflammatory bowel disease
j. Sigmoid volvulus

For each presentation below, choose the SINGLE most appropriate cause from the above list of options. Each option may be used once, more than once, or not at all.

176. A 45 year old woman complains of intermittent abdominal and right sided back pain. She has been vomiting. On examination there is tenderness in right lumbar region especially on the back side.

177. A 40 year old woman complains of pain abdomen and belching which wakes her up sometimes in the night. This has been intermittently present for the past 5 months.

178. A 50 year old chronic alcoholic describes sudden onset severe abdominal pain which appears to radiate into his back.

179. A 25 year old woman presents with upper abdominal pain radiating to the right scapula. She is afebrile but vomiting.

180. A 19 year old girl has a one day history of severe abdominal pain with episodes of vomiting. She is febrile. On examination there is tenderness in the right lower abdomen.

Theme 38: Diagnosis of dermatological conditions

Options:

a. Erythroplasia of querat
b. Malignant melanoma
c. Porokeratosis
d. Pyogenic granuloma
e. Seborrhoeic keratosis
f. Marjolin's ulcer
g. Lentigo maligna
h. Solar keratosis
i. Lupus vulgaris
j. Bowen's diseases
k. Pityriasis versicolor

For each presentation below, choose the SINGLE most appropriate diagnosis from the above list of options. Each option may be used once, more than once, or not at all.

181. A 45 year old male farmer with multiple marked brown lesions on the forehead and limbs.

182. A retired 60 year old who used to work in an Arsenic factory presents with flat scaly red crusted plaque on the right hand which is progressively increasing in size.

183. A 55 year old Australian male presents with cutaneous scaling of arms and forehead, which has no history of progression, induration or ulceration.

184. A 60 year old Hindu who is uncircumcised presents with scaly lesion on his penis. The dermatologist diagnoses it as Bowen's diseases.

185. A 45 year old male with multiple scaly lesions on upper trunk and back which seem to disappear and recur.

Theme 39: Cause of breathlessness

Options:

a. Aortic valve disease
b. Cardiac arrhythmia
c. HTN
d. MR
e. Pulmonary fibrosis
f. Viral myopericarditis
g. Alcoholic heart muscle disease
h. ASD
i. Dilated cardiomyopathy
j. Infective endocarditis
k. Pericardial effusion
l. Tuberculosis

For each presentation below, choose the SINGLE most appropriate cause of breathlessness from the above list of options. Each option may be used once, more than once, or not at all.

186. A 60 year old man develops shortness of breath over a few days. He is a known case of carcinoma of the lungs. His CXR shows a large cardiac silhouette but no pulmonary oedema.

187. A 20 year old female has felt unwell for the past 1 month. She also complains of chest pains which are worse if she lies flat. She has now become short of breath and is found to have acute pulmonary oedema.

188. A 25 year old Indian has come to work as a chef in UK. He has a 2 month history of cough, night sweats, weight loss and fever. He has been treated by his GP with a number of antibiotics, but remains unwell. His CXR shows a normal sized heart.

189. A 60 year old man had an attack of MI 1 month back. He has now become breathless. On cardiovascular examination he has a pan systolic murmur.

190. A 45 year old man admitted with complains of breathlessness and peripheral oedema.

On examination he has cardiomegaly but his liver function tests and CRP values are within normal limits.

Theme 40: Cause of cerebral lesions

Options:

a. AV malformation
b. Cerebral abscess
c. Extradural haematoma
d. Subdural haematoma
e. Carotid artery occlusion
f. Medulloblastoma
g. Berry aneurysm
h. Pituitary adenoma
i. Craniopharyngioma
j. Meningioma
k. Metastatic carcinoma

For each presentation below, choose the SINGLE most appropriate most likely cause from the above list of options. Each option may be used once, more than once, or not at all.

191. A 30 year old woman complains of worst headache of her life. She denies any history of head injury. She has no focal neurological signs.

192. A 65 year old male alcoholic has fluctuating levels of consciousness. His wife reports that he fell down the staircase 2 months ago. He has also developed focal neurological signs.

193. A 60 year old woman, treated with modified radical mastectomy 7 year ago, now presents with gradual onset of confusion and visual disturbances. CT head shows a cerebral mass.

194. A 60 year old woman, treated with total thyroidectomy for thyroid carcinoma, now presents with visual changes. On examination she has bitemporal hemianopsia. CT scan of the head shows a cystic lesion compressing the optic tracts.

195. A 30 year old motorcyclist is involved in road traffic accident. On examination he has dilated left pupil and is unconscious. Skull films show a left temporo-parietal fracture.

Theme 41: Treatment of acute breathlessness

Options:

a. IV adrenaline
b. Mechanical ventilation
c. Refer to psychiatrist
d. Rebreathe into paper bag
e. Heparin
f. Diuretics
g. Heimlich manoeuvre
h. Nebulized salbutamol
i. Chest drain
j. IM adrenaline
k. Forced alkaline diuresis
l. IV aminophylline

For each presentation below, choose the SINGLE most appropriate treatment from the above list of options. Each option may be used once, more than once, or not at all.

196. A 50 year old woman is admitted to the hospital with sudden onset breathlessness. On examination she has bilateral crepts in lower zones and her CXR reveals interstitial oedema.

197. A 25 year old has history of panic attacks and breathlessness. She is getting increasingly depressed because of this. She thinks she cannot cope up with this and is seriously contemplating suicide.

198. A 25 year old man comes to A & E, is too breathless to speak. He has tachycardia, respiratory rate > 25/min and PEF is 100 L/min. On examination he has bilateral wheeze with a normal CXR.

199. A 28 year old woman has just flown back to UK from holidays. She suddenly becomes breathless and cyanosed. She has tachycardia and her BP is 110/70. Her PEF is 300 L/min. CXR is normal.

200. A 60 year old man presents with acute breathlessness and cough with frothy pink sputum. He has orthopnoea. On examination he has bilateral crepts and wheeze.

ANSWERS

1. **(a)** Vasovagal syncope
2. **(d)** Cough induced
3. **(e)** Micturition
4. **(i)** Sick sinus syndrome
5. **(g)** Atrial myxoma
6. **(a)** Hypothyroidism
7. **(g)** Endometriosis
8. **(c)** DUB
9. **(l)** Ectopic pregnancy
10. **(i)** Polycystic ovarian syndrome
11. **(i)** Epiglotittis
12. **(e)** Cardiac failure
13. **(a)** Laryngomalacia
14. **(d)** Asthma
15. **(h)** Foreign body aspiration
16. **(i)** Leprosy
17. **(e)** Tuberculosis
18. **(b)** Hereditary haemorrhagic telangiectasia
19. **(d)** Pericarditis
20. **(a)** Parkinson's disease
21. **(k)** Sensory ataxia
22. **(h)** Peripheral neuropathy
23. **(d)** Vertebro basilar insufficiency
24. **(e)** Cerebellar ataxia
25. **(b)** Malabsorption
26. **(e)** Hyperthyroidism
27. **(d)** Depression
28. **(d)** Depression
29. **(d)** Infective arthritis
30. **(j)** Felty's syndrome
31. **(b)** Pseudogout
32. **(g)** Juvenile chronic arthritis
33. **(f)** Blood transfusion
34. **(g)** Oral analgesia
35. **(b)** Ruptured aorta
36. **(g)** Oral analgesia
37. **(b)** Ruptured aorta
38. **(h)** Observation
39. **(i)** Pralidoxime
40. **(b)** Desferrioxamine
41. **(d)** Ethanol
42. **(a)** Acetylcysteine
43. **(f)** Thyroid function tests
44. **(h)** Serum ACTH
45. **(l)** Plasma cortisol
46. **(g)** Galactose in urine
47. **(c)** Serum ADH
48. **(j)** 6 years
49. **(c)** 9 months
50. **(g)** 3 years
51. **(h)** 4 years
52. **(d)** 12 months
53. **(a)** Carcinoma
54. **(b)** Fibroadenoma
55. **(f)** Paget's disease
56. **(g)** Cystosarcoma phylloides
57. **(e)** Breast abscess
58. **(l)** Lithium
59. **(k)** Isotretinoin
60. **(j)** Alcohol
61. **(g)** Indomethacin
62. **(c)** Salbutamol
63. **(h)** Hyperthyroidism
64. **(f)** Hyperprolactinaemia
65. **(f)** Hyperprolactinaemia
66. **(b)** Endometriosis
67. **(g)** Venesection followed by hydroxyurea
68. **(l)** Secure haemostasis
69. **(n)** Tranexaemic acid
70. **(f)** Venesection
71. **(q)** SC Diamorphine with cyclizine
72. **(n)** Chronic pancreatitis

73. **(d)** Perforated peptic ulcer
74. **(l)** Hydatid disease
75. **(k)** Hepatocellular carcinoma
76. **(i)** Acute cholecystitis
77. **(a)** Paracetamol
78. **(d)** Dihydrocodiene
79. **(g)** Carbamazepine
80. **(f)** Oral glucose tolerance test
81. **(b)** GHRH/arginine test
82. **(d)** Insulin induced hypoglycaemia
83. **(h)** Short synacthen test
84. **(f)** Oral glucose tolerance test
85. **(h)** Phaeochromocytoma
86. **(h)** Phaeochromocytoma
87. **(k)** Cushing's disease
88. **(b)** Conn's syndrome
89. **(i)** Adrenogenital syndrome
90. **(e)** HCG
91. **(f)** NSE
92. **(a)** α fetoprotein
93. **(g)** PLAP
94. **(n)** 5-HIAA
95. **(d)** Insulin
96. **(c)** Methyldopa
97. **(i)** Heparin and aspirin
98. **(e)** Carbamazepine with 5 mg/day folate
99. **(b)** Paracetamol
100. **(d)** 5-7 months
101. **(a)** 1-2 months
102. **(i)** 7-10 months
103. **(h)** 18-22 months
104. **(f)** 2-3 years
105. **(g)** 14-16 months
106. **(i)** Carotid arteriography
107. **(a)** Mental state examination
108. **(h)** Computed tomography scan of the brain
109. **(f)** Erythrocyte sedimentation rate
110. **(c)** Lumbar puncture
111. **(a)** No investigation
112. **(a)** No investigation
113. **(a)** No investigation

114. **(e)** Laryngoscopy
115. **(c)** Sputum for Acid fast bacilli
116. **(a)** Metronidazole
117. **(a)** Metronidazole
118. **(a)** Metronidazole
119. **(a)** Metronidazole
120. **(a)** Metronidazole
121. **(l)** Co-trimoxazole
122. **(n)** Cefotaxime or any such drugs
123. **(g)** Rifampicin
124. **(b)** Pneumocystis carinii
125. **(l)** Mycobacterium tuberculosis
126. **(c)** Mycoplasma pneumoniae
127. **(i)** Streptococcus pneumoniae
128. **(a)** Rheumatoid arthritis
129. **(g)** Trauma
130. **(i)** Haemarthrosis
131. **(f)** Septic arthritis
132. **(j)** Tuberculous arthritis
133. **(d)** Coeliac sprue
134. **(c)** Cytomegalovirus infection
135. **(i)** Whipple's disease
136. **(a)** Inflammatory bowel disease
137. **(g)** Amyloidosis
138. **(b)** Treadmill exercise test
139. **(c)** CXR
140. **(d)** V/Q scan
141. **(c)** CXR
142. **(e)** Abdominal USG
143. **(a)** Guillain Barré syndrome
144. **(c)** Renal tubular acidosis
145. **(f)** Lambert Eaton syndrome
146. **(i)** Botulism
147. **(j)** High cervical cord pathology
148. **(g)** Neurofibroma
149. **(f)** Cervical rib
150. **(d)** Carpal tunnel syndrome
151. **(b)** Motor neurone disease
152. **(h)** Pancoast tumour
153. **(f)** Biliary stricture
154. **(a)** Retained CBD stones
155. **(e)** Walter Waltman syndrome

156. **(d)** Atelectasis
157. **(h)** Biliary cirrhosis
158. **(e)** Entonox
159. **(c)** Epidural anaesthesia
160. **(a)** General anaesthesia
161. **(c)** Epidural anaesthesia
162. **(c)** Epidural anaesthesia
163. **(d)** Endometriosis
164. **(c)** Endometrial cancer
165. **(g)** Ovarian cyst
166. **(h)** Neisseria gonorrhoea
167. **(g)** Mycobacterium tuberculosis
168. **(a)** Actinomyces israelii
169. **(i)** Staphylococcus aureus
170. **(b)** Chlamydia trachomatis
171. **(i)** Painful arc syndrome
172. **(h)** Referred pain from neck
173. **(e)** PMR
174. **(a)** Rheumatoid arthritis
175. **(c)** Pyogenic arthritis
176. **(d)** Renal colic
177. **(b)** Peptic ulcer
178. **(e)** Pancreatitis
179. **(a)** Biliary colic
180. **(c)** Appendicitis
181. **(h)** Solar keratosis
182. **(j)** Bowen's diseases
183. **(h)** Solar keratosis
184. **(a)** Erythroplasia of querat
185. **(k)** Ptiriasis versicolor
186. **(k)** Pericardial effusion
187. **(f)** Viral myopericarditis
188. **(l)** Tuberculosis
189. **(d)** MR
190. **(i)** Dilated cardiomyopathy
191. **(g)** Berry aneurysm
192. **(d)** Subdural haematoma
193. **(k)** Metastatic carcinoma
194. **(i)** Craniopharyngioma
195. **(c)** Extradural haematoma
196. **(f)** Diuretics
197. **(c)** Refer to psychiatrist
198. **(h)** Nebulized salbutamol
199. **(e)** Heparin
200. **(f)** Diuretics

Full Name

Test Centre/Date

- Use pencil only • Make heavy marks that fill the lozenge completely
- Write your candidate number in the top row of the box to the right **and** fill in the appropriate lozenge below each number
- Given **one** answer only for each question

0	0	0	0	0	0
1	1	1	1	1	1
2	2	2	2	2	2
3	3	3	3	3	3
4	4	4	4	4	4
5	5	5	5	5	5
6	6	6	6	6	6
7	7	7	7	7	7
8	8	8	8	8	8
9	9	9	9	9	9

Sample

Answer grid: Questions 1–50, each with answer options A, B, C, D, E, F, G, H, I, J, K, L, M, N, O, P, Q, R, S, T

Do not Write in this space

Five

Mock Test Paper

Theme 1: Investigation of chest pain

Options:

a. ECG
b. Treadmill exercise test
c. CXR
d. V/Q scan
e. Abdominal USG
f. Thallium perfusion scan
g. CT scan–chest
h. Bronchoscopy
i. Coronary angiography
j. Sputum culture
k. Endoscopy
l. Arterial blood gases

For each presentation below, choose the SINGLE most appropriate investigation from the above list of options. Each option may be used once, more than once, or not at all.

1. A 25 year old woman presents with 1 day history of cough, green coloured sputum, fever and breathlessness. She also complains of left sided chest pain which increases on deep inspiration.
3. A 60 year old man complains of daily episodes of central chest pain when he gets up in the morning. The pain lasts for 15–20 minutes and settles with rest. He is waiting to have a knee replacement surgery.
4. A 60 year old hypertensive man presents with sudden onset severe chest pain radiating to the back. The pulse in his left arm is weaker than his right arm.
5. A 50 year old male smoker complains of episodes of dull central chest pain on exertion or after heavy meals. The pain lasts 10–15 minutes and is relieved by rest.

Theme 2: Causes of dyspnoea

Options:

a. Anaemia
b. Bronchial asthma
c. Atypical pneumonia
d. Acute pulmonary oedema
e. Exacerbation of chronic bronchitis
f. Valvular disease
g. Atelectasis
h. Bronchial carcinoma
i. Metastatic carcinoma
j. Pulmonary embolus

For each presentation below, choose the SINGLE most appropriate cause of dyspnoea from the above list of options. Each option may be used once, more than once, or not at all.

6. A 65 year old man presents to A & E with shortness of breath and is slightly drowsy. He has history of chronic productive cough.

7. A 70 year old woman presents with dyspnoea to A & E. On examination she has decreased breath sounds in right lower lung fields. Her CXR reveals pleural effusion. She also has a firm mass in her left breast.

8. A 35 year old man presents with cough and breathlessness. CXR done shows diffuse consolidation of right lower lobe. His fever is persisting despite treatment with IV augmentin. CXR done shows hyper-expansion.

9. A 30 year old airhostess presents with 10 days history of fever, dry cough and is short of breath. On examination she has increased respiratory rate. Her lung fields are clear on auscultation.

10. A 50 year old male patient suffered an MI 1 week ago and was admitted. He wakes up in the night with dyspnoea and frothy sputum. On examination he is cyanosed and tachypnoeic. Auscultation of the lung reveals crepts.

Theme 3: Blood films

Options:

a. Iron deficiency anaemia
b. DIC
c. Megaloblastic anaemia
d. Multiple myeloma
e. Sickle cell disease

For each presentation below, choose the SINGLE most appropriate diagnosis from the above list of options. Each option may be used once, more than once, or not at all.

11. A 19 year old girl has menorrhagia and has microcytic, hypochromic RBCs.

12. A 20 year old boy has target cells, sickle cells and nucleated RBCs.

13. A 25 year old woman has macrocytes which are oval, tear drop cells with poikilocytosis and anisocytosis.

14. A 50 year old man with backache has abnormal plasma cells and stacking of RBCs into rouleaux.

15. A 25 year old woman presents with helmet cells, fragmented RBCs, polychromasia, spherocytosis and thrombocytopenia.

Theme 4: Adverse effects of medications

Options:

a. Enalapril
b. Bendrofluazide
c. Clonidine
d. Phenytoin
e. Hydralazine
f. Prednisolone
g. Lithium
h. Metformin
i. Simvastatin
j. Carbimazole
k. Amitriptyline
l. Bleomycin
m. Amiodarone
n. Nifedipine
o. Third generation cephalosporin

For each presentation below, choose the SINGLE most appropriate causative medication from the above list of options. Each option may be used once, more than once, or not at all.

16. A 40 year old man presents with coarse tremors. He is being treated for bipolar disorder.

17. A 55 year old man presents with sudden onset severe pain in one of his toes. On examination the joint is tender, swollen and hot. He is on treatment for essential hypertension.

18. A 45 year old man presents with sore throat. On examination he is found to be neutropenic.

19. A 70 year old man was found lying on the floor of his house. He is found to be pale and hypothermic. He has bradycardia. He has been diagnosed as a diabetic recently.

20. A 35 year old woman presents with a photosensitive rash over her face with joint pains and fever. She had been started on treatment for eclampsia.

Theme 5: Monitoring In anaesthesiology

Options:

a. Airway pressures
b. Disconnect alarm
c. End tidal carbon dioxide
d. Inspired oxygen concentration
e. Cardiac output
f. Pulmonary artery flotation catheter
g. Invasive arterial pressure
h. Central venous pressure
i. Hourly urine output
j. Peripheral nerve stimulator
k. Temperature

For each presentation below, choose the SINGLE most appropriate method of monitoring from the above list of options. Each option may be used once, more than once, or not at all.

21. An obese middle aged male is in the prone position having a 4 hour lumbar fusion under general anaesthesia. He has aortic stenosis, angina pectoris and long standing controlled hypertension.

22. During a general anaesthesia for a knee arthroscopy the surgeon notices that the knee feels stiff and that the muscle tone in the thigh has increased. The patient has been breathing isoflurane, nitrous oxide and oxygen spontaneously through an LMA for 30 mins. A nasopharyngeal temperature probe is inserted which reads 37.8° celcius.

23. A young female presents for elective tonsillectomy. Anaesthesia is induced and the patient intubated with some difficulty. No breath sounds are detected during auscultation of the chest. Shortly afterwards the patient starts to desaturate.

24. A patient undergoing laparoscopic nephrectomy has been on the operating table for over 3 hours during which 4 litres of intravenous normal saline has been given.

Saturation, pulse and blood pressure have all been normal, however only 30 ml of urine has been collected.

25. A 34 year old male with 25 % partial thickness burns to the legs is having his burns debrided under general anaesthesia. Pre-operative fluid resuscitation was less than adequate.

Theme 6: Diagnosis of infections

Options:

a. Pseudomonas aeruginosa
b. E. coli
c. Staphylococcus aureus
d. Proteus mirabilis
e. Streptococcus viridans
f. Chlamydia trachomatis
g. Chlamydia psittaci
h. Trichomonas vaginalis
i. Neisseria gonorrhoea
j. Neisseria meningitidis
k. Haemophilus influenzae

For each presentation below, choose the SINGLE most appropriate causative organism from the above list of options. Each option may be used once, more than once, or not at all.

26. A 25 year old man presents with a swelling in his right axilla. Aspiration yields yellowish-green pus.

27. A 32 year old man presents with a fever, dyspnoea and palpitations. On auscultatation, a pansystolic murmur is heard in the tricuspid area. He was previously healthy.

28. A 5 year old boy who has started school presents with a high fever, vomiting, headache and a stiff neck.

29. A 10 year old Nigerian boy presents with a 3 month history of a purulent eye discharge and increased lacrimation. His 16 year old brother has a similar condition.

30. A 20 year old woman presents with a subacute onset of lower abdominal pain associated with frequency and dysuria.

Theme 7: Diagnosis of arrhythmias

Options:

a. Atrial flutter
b. Atrial fibrillation
c. Ventricular tachycardia
d. Ventricular extrasystoles (ectopics)
e. Heart block
f. Sinus tachycardia
g. Sinus bradycardia
h. Supraventricular tachycardia
i. Blood loss
j. Wenckebach's phenomenon

For each presentation below, choose the SINGLE most appropriate diagnosis .from the above list of options. Each option may be used once, more than once, or not at all.

31. A 65 year old man, post myocardial infarction is found to have a regular pulse, with a rate of 50 beats/min.

32. A 50 year old man with palpitations is treated with a carotid massage. He now has no other complaints.

33. Following a road traffic accident, a 25 year old man is brought to the A & E. He is found to have pulse rate of 120 beats/min and blood pressure of 90/50 mmHg.

34. A 65 year old man is found to have an irregular pulse, with a rate of 110 beats/min.

35. A 23 year old footballer is examined by his GP and found to have a pulse rate of 50 beats/min. He is otherwise well.

36. A 50 year old man, post myocardial infarction in ITU is found to have a pounding heart beat which then disappeared spontaneously. The patient remains conscious.

Theme 8: Hypoglycaemia

Options:

a. Sulfonylurea ingestion
b. Exogenous insulin
c. Insulinoma
d. Gastrectomy
e. Hepatoma
f. Addison's disease
g. Ethanol ingestion
h. Uraemia
i. Reactive functional hypoglycaemia
j. Mesothelioma

For each presentation below, choose the SINGLE most appropriate cause of hypoglycaemia from the above list of options. Each option may be used once, more than once, or not at all.

37. A 55 year old woman has had increasingly recurrent episodes of confusion upon awakening in the morning over the last 2 months. She has also gained 15 pounds in the same period.

38. An 18 year old woman with anxiety neurosis and repeated episodes of sweating and palpitations 3 hours after meals.

39. A 35 year old IDDM with diabetes for the last 15 years presents with nocturia and frequent episodes of sweating and confusion.

40. A 28 year old HIV positive male with progressive asthenia and giddiness especially on suddenly standing up.

41. A chronic alcoholic with laenne's cirrhosis with recent onset increase in jaundice, ascites and abdominal pain.

Theme 9: Differential diagnosis of chest pain in children

Options:

a. Mitral insufficiency
b. Aortic stenosis
c. Pericarditis
d. Tricuspid incompetence
e. Costochondritic pain
f. Hiatus hernia
g. Pericardial tamponade
h. Reflux oesophagitis
i. Aortic insufficiency
j. Pleuritis

For each presentation below, choose the SINGLE most appropriate diagnosis.from the above list of options. Each option may be used once, more than once, or not at all.

42. A 4 year old boy wakes up frequently saying, "It hurts here" while pointing to his chest. He was born prematurely but has done well otherwise. On examination he has a 2/6 ejection systolic murmur between the left sternal border and the apex that radiates to the base and is accompanied by an apical S3.

43. A 7 year old girl who had chickenpox 4 weeks ago complains of shortness of breath and a squeezing tightness in her midchest. She is anxious and refuses to lie down. Her heart rate is 110 beats per minute and blood pressure 110/80. Her neck veins are distended.

44. A 14 year old boy scout complains of exercise induced sharp chest pain at the left lower sternal border that diminishes with resting and does not awaken him. He has never had anything like this before. Palpation along the sternal edge replicates the symptoms.

45. A 17 year old develops a tightening sensation in his mid sternum during exercise. On examination the pulse rate is 180/minute,

the respiratory rate is 38/minute, and the blood pressure is 120/90 mmHg. You hear a suprasternal notch thrill, an apical click, and a 3/6 ejection murmur at the right upper sternal border.

46. An 18 year old girl has dull retrosternal pain and shortness of breath. On examination she has a heaving apical pulse, an apical systolic thrill and a short mid-diastolic rumbling murmur.

Theme 10: Differential diagnosis of neuromuscular disease

Options:

a. Cerebrovascular accident
b. Guillain–Barré syndrome
c. Amyotrophic lateral sclerosis (ALS)
d. Neurosyphilis
e. Duchenne's muscular dystrophy
f. Friedreich's ataxia
g. Myasthenia gravis
h. Tranverse myelitis
i. Motor neurone disease
j. Syringomyelia

For each presentation below, choose the SINGLE most appropriate diagnosis .from the above list of options. Each option may be used once, more than once, or not at all.

47. A 39 year old white man presents to his GP because of progressive muscle weakness of 1 week's duration. His medical history is unremarkable, although he reports having had an influenza like episode 2 weeks ago. GP notes a marked decrease in reflexes and loss of light touch and vibration sensation in the distal extremities.

48. A 6 year old black boy is brought to GP by his mother. She is concerned that he can no longer keep up with his friends, and she notes that he is using his hands to pull himself up from the floor. GP notes that the boy's calf muscles appear enlarged and his muscle strength is extremely impaired.

49. A 55 year old man with no previous medical problems visits his GP because his arms have become progressively weaker over the past 2 months. The weakness and fatigue began first in one arm and developed later in the other. GP notices hyperreflexia, as well as generalized muscle weakness, in all four extremities. The man has no sensory dysfunction, and his gait is normal.

50. A 34 year old woman presents with muscular weakness of 3 month's duration and says that she tires easily when she's trying to work. After she rests for a while, some of her strength returns. GP notices bilateral fascial weakness and asymmetric distribution of proximal limb weakness. Tendon reflexes are normal.

Theme 11: Investigations in rheumatology

Options:

a. Full blood count
b. Kveim test
c. ANCA
d. ESR
e. Antibodies to double-stranded DNA
f. Skin biopsy
g. Skin biopsy for Ziehl– Nielsen staining for AFB
h. Fasting cholesterol and triglyceride levels
i. Anti–Ro antibodies
j. Serum pancreatic glucagon
k. Muscle biopsy
l. Serum glucose
m. Anti–La antibodies

For each presentation below, choose the SINGLE most appropriate investigation from the above list of options. Each option may be used once, more than once, or not at all.

51. A 38 year old man presents with malaise and arthragia. He is noted to have various skin lesions, including a purple bulbous nose and tender red raised nodules on his anterior shin.

52. A 70 year old woman presents with a mid–facial disfigurement. The nose appears to have been gnawed off by a condition. The cutaneous lesion shows granulomas with central caseations.

53. A 50 year old woman presents with fleshy coloured papules over her right distal interphalangeal joint of her thumb and with a brown waxy plaque over her right shin.

54. A 50 year old woman presents with weakness in her upper arms. She has difficulty combing her hair. On examination, she is noted to have ragged cuticles and nail fold capillary dilatation.

55. A 60 year old woman presents with crops of yellow papules on her elbows and knees. Her serum glucose is normal.

Theme 12: Investigations in upper GI bleeding

Options:

a. Barium swallow
b. Blood alchohol concentration
c. Blood glucose concentration
d. CVP monitoring and blood replacement
e. Coagulation screen
f. Diagnostic gastroscopy and biopsy
g. Full blood count the following morning
h. Immediate FBC
i. LFTs
j. Serum autoantibodies
k. Serum urea and electrolytes
l. Viral hepatic serology

For each presentation below, choose the SINGLE most appropriate investigation from the above list of options. Each option may be used once, more than once, or not at all.

56. A 30 year old man with known duodenal ulcer disease with profuse haematemesis and maelena. He has sinus tachycardia of 150 and blood pressure of 50/0 mm Hg.

57. A 50 year old man with a history of alcoholism, cirrhosis an a tense ascites with haematemesis and sudden onset of coma.

58. A 20 year old male student drank 10 pints of beer earlier in the evening. He presents now with a small fresh haematemesis. His initial Hb is 15 g/dl.

59. A 70 year old with a 3 month history of epigastric pain, anorexia and 15 kg weight loss presents with a small haematemesis. His Hb is 8 g/dl. Blood film suggests iron deficiency.

60. A 70 year old woman with atrial fibrillation on digoxin and warfarin, presents with haematemesis. The initial Hb is 11 g/dl.

Theme 13: Complications of total hip replacement (THR)

Options:

a. Anterior dislocation
b. Cellulitis
c. Chest infection
d. Deep infection
e. Deep vein thrombosis (DVT)
f. Haematoma
g. Posterior dislocation
h. Pulmonary embolism

For each presentation below, choose the SINGLE most appropriate complication from the above list of options. Each option may be used once, more than once, or not at all.

61. A 73 year old man complains of swelling and discoloration of the right leg seven days after a right THR. He has tenderness behind the right knee on palpation.

62. An 81 year old lady develops a pyrexia of 38 °C three weeks after her left THR. Her wound is oozing and her blood tests reveal a CRP of 150 mg/l and an ESR of 96 mm/hour.

63. A 67 year old lady develops swelling and bruising of the left thigh four days after her left THR. Blood tests are normal.

64. A 77 year old man develops sudden chest pain and breathlessness five days after his left THR. His pulse oximetry readings are 82% on air.

65. A 75 year old lady develops sudden severe pain in her right hip whilst sitting down three weeks after her right THR. She is unable to stand and her right leg is internally rotated, flexed and adducted at the hip.

Theme 14: Ethical practice of medicine in the United Kingdom

Options

a. Reversal of the circumcision.
b. Reversal of circumcision for catheter to be inserted and re-circumcising her.
c. Trial of labour
d. Termination
e. Refusal of termination since it's illegal after 24 weeks for social reasons.
f. Give her contraception
g. Withhold contraception
h. Call Police and then give her the contraception
i. Inform mother and Police immediately
j. Inform the General practitioner.(GP)

For each presentation below, choose the SINGLE most appropriate ethical practice from the above list of options. Each option may be used once, more than once, or not at all.

66. A 22 year Somalian primigravida who doesn't speak English presents in labour. On vaginal examination you notice a very small introitus, barely enough to admit your little finger. A CTG is done and it shows a baseline rate of 100 beats/min. Your team decides, she needs an emergency caesarean section but because of the small introitus you are unable to pass the catheter to proceed to theatre.

67. A 13 year old girl demands the morning after pill. She says the condom she used with her 13 year old boyfriend split in two, while having intercourse.

68. A tearful 19 year old girl at 27 weeks of pregnancy requests a termination, saying her boyfriend has just left her and that she would not want the baby to remind her of him. The boyfriend who is now in Jail is reported to have assaulted her during their stormy 2 year relationship.

Theme 15: Diagnosis of falls

Options:

a. Parkinson's disease
b. Impaired vision
c. Aortic stenosis
d. Vertebro-basilar insufficiency
e. Cerebellar ataxia
f. Postural hypotension
g. Drop attacks
h. Peripheral neuropathy
i. Acute labyrinthitis
j. Sick sinus syndrome
k. Sensory ataxia
l. Meniere's disease

For each presentation below, choose the SINGLE most appropriate diagnosis .from the above list of options. Each option may be used once, more than once, or not at all.

69. A 70 year old woman complains of giddiness on standing for long periods. She also gives history of frequent falls on getting up from the bed in morning.

70. A 65 year old man complains of frequent falls over the past 1 year. He says he has never lost consciousness and he falls without any prior warning symptoms.

71. A 72 year old woman is found lying outside her house. She has been walking recently with a stamping gait. On examination her Romberg test is positive.

72. A 60 year old man has had increasing number of falls in the last year. He has noticed a tremor of his hands and has cogwheel rigidity in both upper limbs.

73. A 68 year old man presents with several falls over last 1 year which are associated with dizziness. On examination he has a slow rising pulse with a low pulse pressure.

Theme 16: Diagnosis of weight loss

Options:

a. Anorexia nervosa
b. Carcinoid syndrome
c. Tuberculosis
d. Acute lymphobastic leukaemia
e. Hyperuricaemic gout
f. Peptic ulceration
g. Glucagonoma
h. Epstein Barr virus infection
i. Hypothyroidism
j. Cushing's syndrome
k. Addison's syndrome
l. Diabetes mellitus

For each presentation below, choose the SINGLE most appropriate diagnosis from the above list of options. Each option may be used once, more than once, or not at all.

74. A tall, active, lean, 29 year old single women is amenorrhoic and has had recent weight loss.

75. A 26 year old man has splenomegaly and nose bleeds. His serum uric acid levels are elevated.

76. A 35 year old women has headaches. Lymphocytosis and low glucose is noted on in her cerebrospinal fluid examination.

77. A 65 year old women complains of tiredness. She has developed dark spots inside her mouth. Hyperkalaemia is noted in her serum electrolyte profile.

78. A 67 year old man has hypoglycaemia that is very difficult to treat.

Theme 17: Drug overdose

Options:

a. Lithium overdose
b. Aspirin overdose
c. Ethanol overdose
d. Benzodiazepine overdose
e. Tricyclic antidepressant overdose
f. LSD overdose
g. Beta-blocker overdose
h. Paracetamol overdose
i. Methanol overdose
j. Amphetamine overdose
k. Digoxin overdose

For each presentation below, choose the SINGLE most appropriate overdosed drug from the above list of options. Each option may be used once, more than once, or not at all.

79. A 19 year old student was admitted to A & E with pyrexia and sweating. Pulse is 120/min, BP is 100/60. She has also complained of deafness and tinnitus.

80. A 34 year old man was admitted to A&E unconscious. His temperature was 37.7°C. Pulse is 130/min and BP is 90/65. Neurological examination showed bilateral extensor plantars. His pupils were dilated. ECG showed sinus tachycardia and occasional ventricular ectopics.

81. A 69 year old man presented with drowsiness and confusion. His pulse was 48/min and BP 98/68. ECG showed 1st degree heart block and widening of QRS complex.

82. A 77 year old woman presented with nausea, vomiting and diarrhoea. She also complained of blurring of vision and flashes of light. On examination she was slightly confused and her pulse was slow and irregular.

83. A 37 year old woman with long standing psychiatric illness was admitted with polyuria, diarrhoea, vomiting and coarse tremor involving both hands.

Theme 18: Gynaecomastia

Options:

a. Acromegaly
b. Anorexia nervosa
c. Congenital adrenal hyperplasia
d. Delayed puberty
e. Fragile X syndrome
f. Kallmann's syndrome
g. Klinefelter's syndrome
h. LH secreting pituitary tumour
i. Prolactinoma
j. Small cell cancer
k. Testicular carcinoma

For each presentation below, choose the SINGLE most appropriate diagnosis from the above list of options. Each option may be used once, more than once, or not at all.

84. A 30 year old male presents with reduced shaving frequency. He is tall, has absent pubic and axillary hair and has gynaecomastia.

85. A 16 year old male is referred with poor development. He is noted to be rather short and to have had a repair of a cleft palate. He has absent pubic and axillary hair, with delayed development of the genitalia.

86. A 16 year old male is seen in the clinic. His parents complain that he is prone to outbursts, has poor academic performance and he attends the remedial class in school. He has normal secondary sexual characterisitics and large testes.

87. A 25 year old male smoker complains of painful breasts. He is noted to have mild and tender gynaecomastia. He has a normal right testis but the left is not palpable.

88. A 15 year old male is referred with concerns regarding his development. He is thin with diffuse lanugo hair over the body, but absent secondary sexual character.

Theme 19: Respiratory diseases

Options:

a. Cystic fibrosis
b. ARDS
c. Tuberculosis
d. Cor pulmonale
e. Bronchial adenocarcinoma
f. Squamous cell carcinoma
g. Large cell carcinoma
h. Kartagner's syndrome
i. Hypertrophic pulmonary osteoarthropathy
j. Pulmonary oedema
k. Oat cell carcinoma

For each presentation below, choose the SINGLE most appropriate diagnosis from the above list of options. Each option may be used once, more than once, or not at all.

89. A 57 year old presents with weight loss and hyponatraemia. CXR has shown para-tracheal lymphadenopathy.

90. A 46 year old smoker presents with dull pain in wrist and ankles. He is cachexic and also complains of chest pain and dyspnoea.

91. A 45 year old smoker with weight loss and haemoptysis. He is clubbed and has reduced breath sounds in left upper zone of chest. CXR confirms left upper lobe collapse.

92. A 43 year old presents with long history of sinusitis, recurrent otitis media. He also has infertility and bronchiectasis.

93. A 35 year male brought to A&E after RTA. His pulse rate is 120/min and his respiratory rate is increased. On auscultation there are bilateral fine inspiratory crackles and CXR shows bilateral infiltrates.

Theme 20: Infectious disease investigations

Options:

a. Lyme disease serology
b. MRI hand
c. Hepatitis A serology
d. Hepatitis B serology
e. Viral antibodies
f. Blood film for malaria
g. Skin swab test
h. Skin prick test
i. Weil's disease serology
j. Blood culture

For each presentation below, choose the SINGLE most appropriate investigation from the above list of options. Each option may be used once, more than once, or not at all.

94. A police officer catches a heroine addict who bites him, now come in A&E with deep wound on the hand.

95. A girl comes with a rash on thigh with central clearing. She gives history of passing through thick forest.

96. A businessman comes from Zambia with a 10 day history of of rigors, fever and headache.

97. A fisherman 40 years of age presents in the A&E with fever, jaundice, headache and red conjunctivae. On examination he has mild neck rigidity and purpura.

Theme 21: Diagnosis of respiratory disorders

Options:

a. Acute Type I respiratory failure
b. Acute Type II respiratory failure
c. Chronic Type I respiratory failure
d. Chronic Type II respiratory failure
e. Metabolic acidosis
f. Metabolic alkalosis
g. Lactic acidosis
h. Hyperventilation syndrome
i. Mitochondrial myopathy
j. Normal finding

For each presentation below, choose the SINGLE most appropriate diagnosis from the above list of options. Each option may be used once, more than once, or not at all.

98. $PO_2 = 9$, $PCO_2 = 7$, pH = 7.4, $HCO_3 = 32$.
99. $PO_2 = 9$, $PCO_2 = 5$, pH = 7.4, $HCO_3 = 25$.
100. $PO_2 = 7.5$, $PCO_2 = 4.0$, pH = 7.6, $HCO_3 = 24$.
101. $PO_2 = 8$, $PCO_2 = 8$, pH = 7.2, $HCO_3 = 22$.
102. $PO_2 = 12$, $PCO_2 = 2$, pH = 7.8, $HCO_3 = 22$.

Note: Normal values are PO_2 = > 10.6 kPa, PCO_2 = 4.7–6.0 kPa, pH = 7.35-7.45, HCO_3 = 22–28 mmol/L

Theme 22: The diagnosis of acute vomiting in children

Options:

a. Acute appendicitis
b. Pancreatitis
c. Cyclical vomiting
d. Duodenal atresia
e. Overfeeding
f. Mesenteric adenitis
g. Meningitis
h. Meconium ileus
i. Gastroenteritis
j. Gastro-oesophageal reflux
k. Pyloric stenosis
l. Urinary tract infection
m. Psychogenic vomiting
n. Whooping cough

For each presentation below, choose the SINGLE most appropriate diagnosis from the above list of options. Each option may be used once, more than once, or not at all.

103. A two day old breast-fed male infant is vomiting after each feed. Abdominal X-ray demonstrated a "double bubble".

104. A six week old breast-fed boy has had projectile vomiting after each feed for the past two weeks. He is now lethargic, dehydrated and tachypnoeic.

105. A four month old baby who is thriving has persistent vomiting which is occasionally

blood stained and is associated with crying.

106. An eight year old girl shows signs of moderate dehydration. She has vomited all fluids for 24 hours and the vomit is not bile stained. Her abdomen is now soft and non-tender. She had two similar episodes in the past year.

107. A 12 week old thriving baby is vomiting after every feed. He is developmentally normal and is fed by the bottle at 260 ml/kg/day.

Theme 23: Prescribing for pain relief

Options:

a. A bolus of intravenous opiate
b. A subcutaneous opiate infusion
c. Acupuncture
d. Carbamazepine
e. Corticosteroids
f. Hypnotherapy
g. Intramuscular non-steroidal anti-inflammatory drugs
h. Oral non-steroidal anti-inflammatory drugs
i. Oral opiates
j. Proton pump inhibitor (eg. omeprazole)
k. Selective serotonin re-uptake inhibitor (e.g. fluoxetine)
l. Simple analgesics
m. Transcutaneous electrical nerve stimulation.
n. Tricyclic antidepressant

For each presentation below, choose the SINGLE most appropriate method from the above list of options. Each option may be used once, more than once, or not at all.

108. A 70 year old man presents with severe, retrosternal chest pain and sweating. An ECG shows acute myocardial infarction.

109. An 80 year old woman reports severe paroxysms of knife like or electric shock-like pain, lasting seconds, in the lower part of the right side of her face.

110. A 50 year old man with a known hiatus hernia, presents with recurrent, severe, burning retrosternal chest pain associated with acid regurgitation and increased belching.

111. A 30 year old woman has just been diagnosed as having rheumatoid arthritis and her rheumatologist has begun giving her gold injections. She continues to complain of joint pain and stiffness, particularly for the first two hours of each day.

112. A 70 year old man with inoperable gastric cancer causing obstruction and multiple liver metastases, is taking large doses of oral analgesia. Despite this, his pain is currently poorly controlled.

Theme 24: Differential diagnosis of palpitations

Options:

a. Ventricular ectopic
b. Ventricular fibrillation
c. Atrial fibrillation
d. Complete heart block
e. Wolff–Parkinson White syndrome
f. Phaeochromocytoma
g. Wenckebach phenomenon
h. Torsades de pointes
i. Diabetic neuropathy

For each presentation below, choose the SINGLE most appropriate diagnosis from the above list of options. Each option may be used once, more than once, or not at all.

113. A 56 year old man complains of palpitations. He reports 2 episodes of sudden loss of consciousness in the past 2 weeks. 24 hour ECG recording shows episodes of tachycardia with intervening periods showing a prolonged QT interval.

114. An obese 55 year old man with a 2-year history of palpitation is brought to the Accident and Emergency department unconscious. He is pulseless and his respiration is progressively becoming shallower. The ECG shows disorganised complexes.

115. A 45 year old man with a history of palpitations, complains of difficulty in breathing associated with chest pain. His ECG tracing shows a tachycardia of 100 beats/min and a wide QRS complex, which begins with a 'slur'.

116. A 33 year old woman with a history of weight loss despite an increased appetite complains of palpitations and diarrhoea.

Theme 25: The interpretation of common medical signs

Options:

a. Cardiomyopathy
b. Essential hypertension
c. Ischaemic heart disease.
d. Pulmonary hypertension
e. Osteoarthritis
f. Rheumatoid arthritis
g. Budd chiari malformation
h. Portal systemic shunting
i. Pulmonary fibrosis
j. Acute severe asthma
k. Reactive arthritis
l. Tuberculosis

For each presentation below, choose the SINGLE most appropriate cause of a raised JVP from the above list of options. Each option may be used once, more than once, or not at all.

117. A 67 year old man with a history of rheumatic heart disease complains of dyspnoea. On examination, his JVP is found to be raised with a large a wave. No cannon waves were visible.

118. A 43 year old man with a chronic history of cough and weight loss complains of dyspnoea. His JVP is raised with a pattern showing an abrupt X and Y descent . A 'pericardial knock' was clearly audible on auscultation.

119. A 54 year old woman with a 2 year history of symmetrical joint pains presents with a 3-month history of dyspnoea and cough. She is found to have a raised JVP.

Theme 26: Investigation of confusion

Options:

a. Serum and urine electrophoresis
b. Calcium and phosphate level
c. Stool microscopy and culture
d. Blood glucose
e. Blood culture
f. Thyroid function tests
g. Lipid profile
h. Mid stream urine specimen
i. Ultrasound of abdomen
j. Full blood count
k. Serum electrophoresis
l. ECG
m. Computed tomography (CT) scan of head
n. Chest X-ray
o. Urea and Electrolytes

For each presentation below, choose the SINGLE most appropriate answer from the above list of options. Each option may be used once, more than once, or not at all.

120. An 80 year old woman becomes suddenly confused. On examination, her blood pressure is 95/60 mmHg. Pulse rate is 55/min and is irregularly irregular.

121. An 83 year old woman in a nursing home has been constipated for a week. Over the past few days, she has become increasingly confused and incontinent.

122. An 80 year old woman presents with weakness on the left half of her body and a recent history of falls. Her daughter says that she has generally deteriorated over the past couple of weeks with periods of marked confusion.

123. An 81 year old woman is brought to the Accident and Emergency department confused. Over the past 3 months, she had been complaining of excessive passing of water and loss of weight.

124. An 81 year old man complains of general malaise and a chronic backache. She has a history of mild confusion with episodes of marked blurring of vision. An X-ray report shows a 'pepper pot' skull.

Theme 27: Diagnosis of constipation

Options:

a. Carcinoma of the colon
b. Parkinsonism
c. Anorexia nervosa
d. Myxoedema
e. Bulimia
f. Diverticulosis
g. Chronic pseudo-obstruction
h. Systemic sclerosis
i. Hypercalcaemia
j. Diabetic neuropathy
k. Irritable bowel syndrome
l. Multiple sclerosis

For each presentation below, choose the SINGLE most appropriate diagnosis from the above list of options. Each option may be used once, more than once, or not at all.

125. A 43 year old man complains of excessive thirst, polyuria, polydipsia and constipation. He admits to losing weight. His fasting blood glucose is 5.5 mmol/L.

126. A 23 year old woman being treated for myeloma is brought to the Accident and Emergency department, confused. This followed a hour history of severe abdominal pain, vomiting. Prior to this, the patient had complained of polyuria, polydipsia and constipation.

127. A 17 year old frail girl complains of constipation. Her body mass Index (BMI) is found to be 17. She is extremely afraid of eating and admits to sticking a finger down her throat to induce vomiting after meals. She is unusually sensitive to the cold.

128. A 65 year old man with a history of weight loss, complains of bleeding per rectum. He also reports a 2 month history of diarrhoea which seems to alternate with constipation. His Hb is 10 g/dl.

129. A 65 year old woman presents with constipation, and reports a 3 month history of difficulty in starting to walk and in stopping once started. She is found to have dysarthria and dribbling.

Theme 28: Types of bias in clinical trails

Options:

a. Recall bias
b. Chronologic bias
c. Lead-time bias
d. Publication bias
e. Selection bias
f. p–value bias
g. Randomisation bias
h. Commercial bias
i. Confounding bias
j. Observational bias

For each presentation below, choose the SINGLE most appropriate type of bias from the above list of options. Each option may be used once, more than once, or not at all.

130. A study was performed examining stroke rates when comparing people at work with people on long term sickness leave. Working people were found to have a lower stroke rate. It was concluded that work reduces your risk for stroke. The study suffers a bias.

131. A study aims to evaluate the impact of screening for colorectal cancer by means of faecal occult blood testing. It is found that patients detected by this method tend to survive longer than patients presenting with a complication of the tumour. It is concluded that faecal occult blood testing improves the chances of survival. The study suffers a bias.

132. Controversy surrounds the surgical treatment of Ebstein's anomaly. An author studies a population group undergoing surgery in early adulthood. He compares the results with those of a study performed twenty year previously in which surgery was performed in infancy. The study may result in a bias.

133. A study was performed in order to evaluate whether the age of first menstruation influenced the age of developing breast cancer. Patients first diagnosed with breast cancer were asked for the age of their first menstruation. The study may result in a bias.

134. A new type of antibiotic is gaining press attention. A certain journal informs authors that it would give preference to articles that are centered around this new antibiotic. Articles in the next edition of this journal are likely to suffer from a bias.

Theme 29: Vertigo

Options:

a. Benign positional vertigo
b. Vestibular neuronitis
c. Meniere's disease
d. Migraine
e. Multiple sclerosis
f. Alcohol
g. TIA (Vertebro-basilar)
h. Complex partial seizures
i. Posterior fossa tumours

For each presentation below, choose the SINGLE most appropriate cause of vertigo from the above list of options. Each option may be used once, more than once, or not at all.

135. A 50 year old woman with paroxysmal attacks of giddiness lasting 15-20 seconds. They occur on sitting up or lying down, looking up or looking down particularly with the head rotated to the left. The attacks persist for about 1 month and have occurred three times over the last 2 years.

136. A 14 year old boy with sudden vertigo and vomiting 3 days after contracting an upper respiratory infection. His hearing is normal.

137. A 60 year old woman with history of a bursting sensation in the head followed by a roaring noise in the right ear. She has episodes of intense vertigo which are reduced by lying still with the right ear uppermost.

138. A 54 year old hypertensive, diabetic with a history of sudden onset rotatory feelings accompanied by slurred speech and unsteadiness while walking. The episode lasted for 25 minutes.

Theme 30: Hyponatraemia

Options:

a. Addison's disease
b. Diuretics
c. Salt losing nephropathy
d. SIADH
e. Hypothyroidism
f. Cardiac failure
g. Cirrhosis
h. Nephrotic syndrome
i. Vomiting

For each presentation below, choose the SINGLE most appropriate diagnosis from the above list of options. Each option may be used once, more than once, or not at all.

139. A 12 year old boy presenting with periorbital puffiness and malaise. His serum cholesterol level is 300 mg/dl.

140. A 60 year old male chronic smoker presenting with anorexia, lethargy, confusion and cramps. Chest X-ray shows a hilar opacity.

141. A 25 year old male presenting with anorexia, weakness, weight loss and generalized pigmentation. The systolic BP falls by 15 mm on standing. He has a past history of pulmonary tuberculosis.

142. A 56 year old woman presents with progressive chest pain on exertion. Creatinine kinase 349 iu/L, LDH 334 iu/L, sodium 126 mmol/L. Examination reveals dry skin and periorbital oedema.

143. A 60 year old woman with progressive osteoarthritis. She has been consuming analgesics for the last 10 years.

Theme 31: Pain or swelling of joints

Options:

a. Rheumatoid arthritis
b. SLE
c. Systemic sclerosis
d. Polyarteritis nodosa
e. Ankylosing spondylitis
f. Reiter's syndrome
g. Behcet's disease
h. Mixed connective tissue disease
i. Henoch schönlein purpura
j. Sjögren's syndrome

For each presentation below, choose the SINGLE most appropriate diagnosis from the above list of options. Each option may be used once, more than once, or not at all.

144. A 43 year old man with 3 month history of fever, malaise, arthralgias, weight loss and abdominal pain. Two days ago he noticed a difficulty in extending the left wrist. Examination reveals a BP of 170/110 urinalysis shows 2 + proteinuria and polymorphonuclear leucocytosis with an ESR of 86 mm/hr.

145. A 29 year old male with history of asymmetric oligoarthritis for the last 3 years. He has history of painful lesions in the mouth for the last 8 years. He now presents with fever, headache, arthritis, abdominal pain and superficial thrombophlebitis of the left leg.

146. A 35 year old woman with Raynaud's phenomenon and week history of difficulty in climbing stairs. Examination reveals swollen fingers (sausage like), alopecia, red rash on the hands, facial telangiectasias and difficulty getting up from a squat. Her aldolase is 30 u/L with RA positive at 1:800. ANA 1:1600, speckled pattern with anti-RNP antibodies.

147. A 16 year old male with abdominal pain, nausea and vomiting for four days. He has

painful joints. Examination reveals a red rash over the buttocks and legs and stool is positive for occult blood.

148. A 50 year old woman with Raynaud's phenomenon for 10 years. For the last 6 months she has developed arthritis of the hands and feet with difficulty in swallowing. Also studies reveal positive ANA 1:160 with anticentromere antibodies.

Theme 32: Pathophysiology of breast cancer

Options:

a. Infiltration of ligaments of cooper
b. Infiltration of lactiferous ducts
c. Involvement of sweat glands
d. Bony metastases
e. Transcoelomic spread
f. Lymphatic spread
g. Extensive local dissemination
h. Spread to chest wall
i. Systemic spread to viscera
j. Nonmetastatic systemic manifestation

For each presentation below, choose the SINGLE most appropriate pathology from the above list of options. Each option may be used once, more than once, or not at all.

149. A 34 year old female presents with a lump in the breast and nipple retraction.

150. A 38 year old female presents with dimpling of the skin when she lifts her hands above the head for examination.

151. A 45 year old female presents with sudden onset paraplegia. She had undergone surgery forcarcinoma breast 2 years back.

152. A 37 year old female presents with a lump in the breast. The affected breast does not fall freely from the chest wall on bending forward.

153. A 43 year old female presents with ascites with bilateral ovarian masses. The histopathology shows signet ring cells. There is an associated breast lump.

Theme 33: Teratogenicity

Options:

a. Betamethasone
b. Norethisterone
c. Salbutamol
d. Ergometrine
e. Oxytocin
f. Prostaglandin F_2 alpha
g. Indomethacin
h. Oxytetracycline
i. Amoxicillin
j. Alcohol
k. Isotretinoin
l. Lithium
m. Valproic acid
n. Dilantin
o. Streptomycin
p. Thalidomide

For each pathology below, choose the SINGLE most appropriate involved drug from the above list of options. Each option may be used once, more than once, or not at all.

154. Virilization of a female fetus.
155. Premature closure of ductus arteriosus.
156. Defective dentition of the fetus after 4th month.
157. Fetal hydantoin syndrome.
158. Neural tube defects.

Theme 34: Diagnosis of gastrointestinal conditions

Options:

a. Hepatoma
b. Oesophageal varices
c. Mallory-Weiss tear
d. Perforated peptic ulcer
e. Fractured rib
f. Haematoma of the rectus sheath
g. Umblical hernia
h. Sigmoid volvulus
i. Splenic rupture
j. Pancreatic pseudocyst
k. Divarication of the recti
l. Acute pancreatitis

For each presentation below, choose the SINGLE most appropriate diagnosis from the above list of options. Each option may be used once, more than once, or not at all.

159. A 50 year old alcoholic man prsents with nausea, vomiting, and epigastric pain. On examination, he has a palpable epigastric mass and a raised amylase. CT scan of the abdomen shows a round well circumscribed mass in the epigastrium.

160. A 40 year old multiparous woman presents with a midline abdominal mass. The mass is nontender and appears when she is straining. On examination, the midline mass is visible when she raises head off the examining bed.

161. A 19 year old man presents with sudden severe upper abdominal pain after being tackled during rugby practice. He was recently diagnosed with gladular fever.

162. A 7 year old girl presents with spontaneous massive haematemesis.

163. A 55 year old male alcoholic presents after vomiting 800 ml of blood. His blood pressure is 80/50 with a pulse rate of 120. He also has ascites.

Theme 35: Treatment of drug and alcohol abuse

Options:

a. Alcoholics anonymous
b. Antipsychotic medication
c. Aversion treatment
d. Controlled drinking
e. Disulfiram
f. Inpatient detoxification with chlordiazepoxide
g. Methadone maintenance treatment
h. Motivational interviewing
i. Simple advice
j. Token economy
k. Treatment under Section 3, Mental Health Act 1984

For each presentation below, choose the SINGLE most appropriate treatment from the above list of options. Each option may be used once, more than once, or not at all.

164. A 32 year old man with a 10 year history of heroin addiction has a string of convictions for theft. He is at risk of HIV and other transmissible diseases due to needle sharing. He wants to stabilise his lifestyle, but does not feel ready to give up opiates.

165. A 43 year old businessman, who has a history of alcohol dependence, has managed to stop drinking. He is afraid of relapsing during a forthcoming business trip and wants help to remain abstinent from alcohol.

166. A 25 year old male student drinks about 4 pints of beer a day every day. He has no symptoms of alcohol dependency or physical problems. He is concerned his level of drinking may be harmful.

167. A 33 year old homeless man drinks a bottle of whisky per day. He has begun to have episodes of amnesia. He wants to stop drinking. When he last tried to give up drinking, he suffered a grand mal convulsion.

168. A 45 year old man would like to have support to give up drinking.

Theme 36: Causes of numbness and paraesthesia in upper limbs

Options:

a. Carpal tunnel syndrome
b. Ulnar nerve lesion
c. Peripheral neuropathy
d. Cervical spondylosis
e. Multiple sclerosis
f. Syringomyelia
g. Cortical lesions
h. Radial nerve lesion

For each presentation below, choose the SINGLE most appropriate cause from the above list of options. Each option may be used once, more than once, or not at all.

169. A 45 year old lady who is an author of many books complains of tingling sensation in one of her hands. She complains that the problem lies mainly in her index and middle finger and it gets worse in the night.

170. A 50 year old bricklayer complains of tingling sensation in one of his arms and hand. Some degree of neck stiffness is also present.

171. A 40 year old lady complains of tight band like sensation around her arms and ribs. She also complains of 'electric shock' like pains which increase on flexing the neck.

172. A 45 year male teacher complains of tingling in his left little finger. On examination slight wasting of the small muscles of the affected hand are noted.

173. A 40 year old bricklayer injured his left index finger but did not feel the pain. On examination it was found that he had lost pain and temperature sensation in his left hand and arm with some degree of weakness.

Themes 37: Diagnosis of bowel disease

Options:

a. Irritable bowel syndrome
b. Diverticular disease
c. Crohns disease
d. Ulcerative colitis
e. Ischaemic colitis
f. Intususseption
g. Small bowel obstruction
h. Large bowel obstruction

For each presentation below, choose the SINGLE most appropriate diagnosis from the above list of options. Each option may be used once, more than once, or not at all.

174. A 30 year old man presents with painless bloody diarrhoea. He also complains of passing mucus in the stool. On examination there is no abdominal tenderness or mass palpable per abdomen.

175. A 50 year old clerk complains of pain abdomen with alternating diarrhoea and constipation. On examination left iliac fossa was found to be tender.

176. A 45 year old man complains of pain abdomen and diarrhoea. On examination there is abdominal tenderness and anal tags.

177. A 30 year old woman complains of pain abdomen which is relieved by defecation. She also complains of wind and loose motions after meals. On examination tenderness was present in left lower abdomen.

178. A 60 year old woman complains of pain abdomen and bloody diarrhoea. She has history of CAD. On examination generalized tenderness noted in abdomen.

Theme 38: Diagnosis of renal conditions

Options:

a. Dilatation of the ureter
b. Medullary sponge kidney
c. Renal papillary necrosis
d. Ectopic kidney
e. Posterior urethral valves
f. Horse shoe kidney
g. Renal tuberculosis
h. VUR
i. Pelvi-ureteric obstruction
j. Duplex kidney

For each presentation below, choose the SINGLE most appropriate diagnosis from the above list of options. Each option may be used once, more than once, or not at all.

179. A 13 year old with recurrent UTI and haematuria undergoes cystoscopy. A shallow diverticulum is seen just above and lateral to the ureteric orifice.

180. A 25 year old male has acute left loin pain radiating to the left groin. Urine analysis shows pyuria. He undergoes an IVU which reveals collections of contrast medium in dilated papillary collecting ducts of both right and left kidneys. Both kidneys are enlarged.

181. A 25 year old woman in the 3rd month of her 1st pregnancy developed asymptomatic pyuria.

182. A 65 year old man has a deteriorating renal function. He is a diabetic and an IVU reveals filling defects within dilated calyces and ring shadows.

183. 25 year old male presents with increased frequency of micturition and left loin pain. Urine analysis demonstrates an acidic pH and low specific gravity.

72. **(a)** Parkinson's disease
73. **(c)** Aortic stenosis
74. **(a)** Anorexia nervosa
75. **(d)** Acute lymphobastic leukaemia
76. **(c)** Tuberculosis
77. **(k)** Addisons syndrome
78. **(g)** Glucagonoma
79. **(b)** Aspirin overdose
80. **(e)** Tricyclic antidepressant overdose
81. **(g)** Beta-blocker overdose
82. **(k)** Digoxin overdose
83. **(a)** Lithium overdose
84. **(g)** Klinefelter's syndrome
85. **(f)** Kallmann's syndrome
86. **(e)** Fragile X syndrome
87. **(k)** Testicular carcinoma
88. **(b)** Anorexia nervosa
89. **(k)** Oat cell carcinoma
90. **(i)** Hypertrophic pulmonary osteoarthropathy
91. **(f)** Squamous cell carcinoma
92. **(h)** Kartagner's syndrome
93. **(b)** ARDS
94. **(d)** Hepatitis B serology
95. **(a)** Lyme disease serology
96. **(f)** Blood film for malaria
97. **(i)** Weil's disease serology
98. **(d)** Chronic Type II respiratory failure
99. **(c)** Chronic Type I respiratory failure
100. **(a)** Acute Type I respiratory failure
101. **(b)** Acute Type II respiratory failure
102. **(h)** Hyperventilation syndrome
103. **(d)** Duodenal atresia
104. **(k)** Pyloric stenosis
105. **(j)** Gastro-oesophageal reflux
106. **(c)** Cyclical vomiting
107. **(e)** Overfeeding
108. **(a)** A bolus of intravenous opiate
109. **(d)** Carbamazepine
110. **(j)** Proton pump inhibitor (eg. omeprazole)
111. **(h)** Oral non-steroidal anti-inflammatory drugs
112. **(b)** A subcutaneous opiate infusion
113. **(h)** Torsades de pointes
114. **(b)** Ventricular fibrillation
115. **(e)** Wolf-Parkinson White syndrome
116. **(f)** Phaeochromocytoma
117. **(d)** Pulmonary hypertension
118. **(l)** Tuberculosis
119. **(f)** Rheumatoid arthritis
120. **(l)** ECG
121. **(h)** Mid stream urine specimen
122. **(m)** Computed tomography (CT) scan of head
123. **(d)** Blood glucose
124. **(a)** Serum and urine electrophoresis
125. **(j)** Diabetic neuropathy
126. **(i)** Hypercalcaemia
127. **(c)** Anorexia nervosa
128. **(a)** Carcinoma of the colon
129. **(b)** Parkinsonism
130. **(e)** Selection bias
131. **(c)** Lead-time bias
132. **(b)** Chronologic Bias
133. **(a)** Recall bias
134. **(d)** Publication bias
135. **(a)** Benign positional vertigo
136. **(b)** Vestibular neuronitis
137. **(c)** Meniere's disease
138. **(g)** TIA (Vertebrobasilar)
139. **(h)** Nephrotic syndrome
140. **(d)** SIADH
141. **(a)** Addison's disease
142. **(e)** Hypothyroidism
143. **(c)** Salt losing nephropathy
144. **(d)** Polyarteritis nodosa
145. **(g)** Behcet's disease
146. **(h)** Mixed connective tissue disease
147. **(i)** Henoch schönlein purpura
148. **(c)** Systemic sclerosis
149. **(b)** Infiltration of lactiferous ducts
150. **(a)** Infiltration of ligaments of cooper

151. **(d)** Bony metastases
152. **(h)** Spread to chest wall
153. **(e)** Transcoelomic spread
154. **(b)** Norethisterone
155. **(g)** Indomethacin
156. **(h)** Oxytetracycline
157. **(n)** Dilantin
158. **(m)** Valproic acid
159. **(j)** Pancreatic pseudocyst
160. **(k)** Divarication of the recti
161. **(i)** Splenic rupture
162. **(b)** Oesophageal varices
163. **(b)** Oesophageal varices
164. **(g)** Methadone maintenance treatment
165. **(e)** Disulfiram
166. **(i)** Simple advice
167. **(f)** Inpatient detoxification with chlordiazepoxide
168. **(a)** Alcoholics anonymous
169. **(a)** Carpal tunnel syndrome
170. **(d)** Cervical spondylosis
171. **(e)** Multiple sclerosis
172. **(b)** Ulnar nerve lesion
173. **(f)** Syringomyelia
174. **(d)** Ulcerative colitis
175. **(b)** Diverticular disease

176. **(c)** Crohns disease
177. **(a)** Irritable bowel syndrome
178. **(e)** Ischaemic colitis
179. **(h)** VUR
180. **(b)** Medullary sponge kidney.
181. **(a)** Dilatation of the ureter
182. **(c)** Renal papillary necrosis
183. **(g)** Renal tuberculosis
184. **(j)** Von Willebrand's disease
185. **(k)** Vaginal carcinoma
186. **(c)** DUB
187. **(b)** Endometrial carcinoma
188. **(a)** Fibroid
189. **(g)** One and half year
190. **(h)** Two year
191. **(i)** Three year
192. **(a)** Two months
193. **(j)** Four year
194. **(d)** Eleven months
195. **(h)** Two year
196. **(d)** Eleven months
197. **(f)** One year
198. **(k)** Five year
199. **(e)** Five months
200. **(b)** Six months

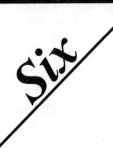

Mock Test Paper

Theme 1: Choice of contraception

Options:

a. POP
b. Condoms
c. IUCD
d. Condoms + OCPs
e. COCPs
f. Mirena coil
g. Depot progestagen injection
h. Natural method
i. Diaphragm
j. Spermicidal jellies
k. Vasectomy
l. Fallopian tube ligation

For each presentation below, choose the SINGLE most appropriate method of contraception from the above list of options. Each option may be used once, more than once, or not at all.

1. A 45 year old married woman is in a stable relationship. She smokes a pack of cigarettes everyday.
2. A 35 year old woman recently underwent her sterilization surgery. She wants an immediate contraceptive cover.
3. A 20 year old student wants a contraception 4 days after unprotected intercourse with her boyfriend.
4. A 20 year old woman who has multiple partners wants contraception.
5. A 25 year old who has history of ectopic pregnancy wants a suitable contraception.

Theme 2: Causes of haematuria

Options:

a. Bladder carcinoma
b. Renal cell carcinoma
c. Renal tract calculi
d. Alport's syndrome
e. SLE
f. Polycystic kidney disease
g. Goodpasture's syndrome
h. Cystitis
i. Nephroblastoma
j. Wegener's granulomatosis
k. Glomerulophritis

For each presentation below, choose the SINGLE most appropriate cause of haematuria from the above list of options. Each option may be used once, more than once, or not at all.

6. A 4 year old child with gross abdominal distension. On examination he has a mass palpable in right flank. His family history is insignificant.

7. A 60 year old woman presents with haematuria and right sided loin pain. On examination she has a mass palpable in right loin. She is anaemic and has lost some weight in last 2 months.

8. A 13 year old girl presents with recurrent episodes of haematuria. She has a history of URTI. On examination no abnormality was found.

9. A 10 year old boy presents with haematuria and sensorineural deafness which is hereditary.

10. A 20 year old woman presents with a non-specific rash after sun bath. She also has aprthous ulcers and haematuria.

Theme 3: Choice of antibiotics

Options:

a. Zidovudine
b. Amoxicillin and gentamycin
c. Clindamycin
d. IV ampicillin
e. Rifampicin
f. Penicillin V
g. Benzylpenicillin
h. Trimethoprim
i. Metronidazole
j. Ciprofloxacin
k. Mefloquine
l. Chloroquine and proguanil
m. Amoxicillin

For each presentation below, choose the SINGLE most appropriate antibiotic from the above list of options. Each option may be used once, more than once, or not at all.

11. A 35 year old man develops bloody diarrhoea. He had attended a party last night. Many guests which attended the party also complain of same problem.

12. A 60 year old woman with a prosthetic heart valve is due for gynaecological procedure.

13. A 7 year old boy presents with a painful right ear. On examination the boy is found to be febrile with a bulging red tympanic membrane.

14. A 40 year old obese woman due to undergo cholecystectomy.

15. An 18 year old boy complains of headache, neck stiffness, fever has and a purpuric rash.

Theme 4: Diagnosis of urological conditions

Options:

a. Carcinoma of bladder
b. Carcinoma prostate
c. Carcinoma kidney
d. Testitular tumour
e. Testicular torsion
f. Acute epididymo-orchitis
g. Hydrocele
h. Acute pyelonephritis
i. Inflamed hydatid de Morgani
j. ATN
k. CRF
l. Ureteric colic

For each presentation below, choose the SINGLE most appropriate diagnosis of from the above list of options. Each option may be used once, more than once, or not at all.

16. 12 year old boy presents to A and E with red, painful swollen scrotum. His midstream urine investigation is normal.

17. A 7 year old boy presents with scrotal oedema of 2 days duration and painless haematuria. His urine examination reveals granular casts.

18. A 25 year old man presents with a painless lump in one of his testes of 2 months duration. He is found to have no inguinal lymphadenopathy. He has an elevated serum alpha–fetoprotein.

19. A 65 year old man presents with poor stream and nocturia. On examination he has lemon tinge to his skin, ascites and a palpable bladder. He also has an enlarged prostate and his B.P. is found to be 170/94.

20. An 80 year old man presents with increased micturition and backache. On examination he has a palpable bladder and an enlarged prostate. His serum alkaline phosphatase and serum acid phosphatase are both elevated.

Theme 5: Disorders affecting the mouth

Options:

a. Candidiasis
b. Squamous cell carcinoma
c. Stevens–Johnson syndrome
d. Lichen planus
e. Iatrogenic gingivitis
f. Psoriasis
g. Leukoplakia
h. Folate deficiency
i. Behcet's disease
j. Peutz–Jegher's syndrome
k. Addison's disease
l. Iron deficiency

For each presentation below, choose the SINGLE most appropriate diagnosis .from the above list of options. Each option may be used once, more than once, or not at all.

21. A 75 year old man complains of soreness the corners of his mouth. He has poorly fitting dentures. On examination he has marked angular stomatitis.

22. A 65 year old male complains of large mouth ulcer which was initially painful but is painless now. He has been a chronic smoker for the past 30 year. On examination he has a 2 cm ulcer on the inside of his cheek with rolled out edges.

23. A 30 year old woman complains of multiple painful blisters affecting her skin and mouth. She has been on amoxicillin for a chest infection.

24. A 50 year old male presents which painful white web–like lesions on his tongue. He also complains of purplish paules around his wrist which are intensely itchy.

25. A 50 year old man who is on treatment for his epilepsy presents with painful swollen gums.

Theme 6: Hormonal disease

Options:

a. Cortisol
b. Adrenocorticotrophic hormone (ACTH)
c. Growth hormone
d. Calcitonin
e. Somatostatin
f. Thyroxine
g. Parathyroid hormone
h. Insulin
i. Adrenaline
j. Thyroid stimulating hormone (TSH)
k. Serotonin
l. Glucagon
m. Aldosterone

For each presentation below, choose the SINGLE most appropriate involved hormone from the above list of options. Each option may be used once, more than once, or not at all.

26. A 20 year old known diabetic is brought to A & E unconscious. He has up-going plantar reflexes.

27. A 38 year old man with an enlarged right adrenal gland and normal left gland presents with weakness. His Na^+ is 140 mmol/L and K^+ is 2.5 mmol/L.

28. A 35 year old man complains of polyuria, excessive drinking of water, associated with excessive thirst.

29. A 35 year old woman with polyuria presents with a one month history of palpitations and diarrhoea.

30. An obese 34 year old woman is found to have a 'moon face', a blood pressure of 145/95 mmHg and raised blood glucose.

Theme 7: Immediate investigation of the unconscious patient

Options:

a. Arterial blood gases
b. Blood carbondioxide
c. Blood culture
d. Blood glucose
e. Blood paracetamol
f. Blood salicyclate level
g. Chest X-ray
h. Computed tomography scan
i. Electrocardiogram (ECG)
j. Lumbar puncture
k. Serum osmolality
l. Skull X-ray
m. Temperature

For each presentation below, choose the SINGLE most appropriate investigation from the above list of options. Each option may be used once, more than once, or not at all.

31. A 28 year old woman is brought to A & E unconscious (GCS=7). On initial examination, her pulse rate is 110 beats/min, SaO_2 95% on air and BM (glucose) 4.5 mmol/L. A purpuric rash is noted on both her arms.

32. A 47 year old female is brought to the A & E unconscious (GCS=7). On initial examination her pulse rate is 110 beats/min. SaO_2 100% on air and BM (glucose) 4.3 mmol/L.

33. A 45 year old man is brought to the A & E unconscious (GCS=7). On initial examination his pulse rate is 90 beats/min, BM (glucose) 5.3 mmol/L and SaO_2 97% on air. He smells of alcohol and there are no external signs of injury.

34. A 45 year old woman is brought to the A & E unconscious (GCS=7). On initial examination, her pulse rate is 80 beats/min, she is sweating and has a SaO_2 of 98% on air.

35. A 45 year old woman is brought to the A & E unconscious (GCS=7). On examination

her pulse rate is 110 beats/min, temperature normal and BM (glucose) 4.6 mmol/L. She was found with an empty bottle of antidepressant (Dothiepin).

Theme 8: Treatment of intestinal obstruction

Options:

a. Anterior resection
b. Sigmoid colectomy
c. Subtotal colectomy and ileorectal anastomosis.
d. Transverse colectomy
e. Right hemicolectomy
f. Exploratomy laparotomy and Hartmann's procedure
g. Abdominoperineal resection with end colostomy
h. Urgent herniorraphy

For each presentation below, choose the SINGLE most appropriate treatment from the above list of options. Each option may be used once, more than once, or not at all.

36. An 86 year old man presents with abdominal distension and pain. Sigmoidoscopy and barium enema confirm a obstructing carcinoma of rectosigmoid.

37. A 60 year old male presents with abdominal pain in RIF with distension. X-ray shows a dilated loop bowel 12 cm in diameter with convexity towards left hemidiaphragm.

38. An elderly male with high grade fever, vomiting and intense pain in RIF. On examination hard rigid distended mass seen on abdomen with rebound tenderness on the left. X-ray shows free air under the diaphragm.

39. A 46 year old man presents with bowel obstruction and pain in rectum. Rectal examination and X-rays confirm obstruction and carcinoma rectum.

40. Middle aged man complains of constant groin pain along with nausea and vomiting. On examination he has positive cough impulse. A tender lump is also palpated which is not reducible.

Theme 9: Localisation of neurological disorder

Options:

a. Non–dominant frontal lobe
b. Dominant frontal lobe
c. Non–dominant temporal lobe
d. Dominant temporal lobe
e. Non–dominant parietal lobe
f. Dominant parietal lobe
g. Occipital lobes
h. Temporo–occipito–parietal junction

For each presentation below, choose the SINGLE most appropriate affected cerebral area from the above list of options. Each option may be used once, more than once, or not at all.

41. A 45 year old stroke patient can clearly understand what someone says to him but he is unable to respond verbally to that person.

42. Although he can repeat phrases, the speech of a 52 year old stroke patient is impaired and has difficulty understanding what someone says to him.

43. A well educated stroke patient cannot add a column of four single digit numbers .

44. A 58 year old stroke patient is unable to copy completely; a simple drawing of a clock face.

Theme 10: Tumour risk factors

Options:

a. Pernicious anaemia
b. Dye and printing chemicals
c. Asbestos
d. Ulcerative colitis
e. Epstein–Barr virus
f. Nickel
g. Smoking
h. CMV
i. Excessive sunlight and UV exposure
j. Human papilloma virus

For each presentation below, choose the SINGLE most appropriate association from the above list of options. Each option may be used once, more than once, or not at all.

45. Burkitt's lymphoma.
46. Bladder carcinoma.
47. Gastric carcinoma.
48. Colorectal carcinoma.
49. Lung carcinoma.
50. Nasopharyngeal carcinoma.

Theme 11: Causative organisms in infection

Options:

a. Bacillus anthracis
b. Clostridium difficile
c. Campylobacter jejuni
d. Clostridium perfringens
e. Clostridium welchii
f. Haemophilus influenzae
g. Mycobacterium kansasii
h. Neisseria gonorrhoea
i. Neisseria meningitidis
j. Treponema pallidum

For each presentation below, choose the SINGLE most appropriate causative organism from the above list of options. Each option may be used once, more than once, or not at all.

51. A 10 year old boy rushed to hospital with a days' history of fever, a blotchy rash and confusion.
52. A 14 day old neonate presenting with a purulent eye discharge.
53. A 37 year old man, previously fit and well, presenting with a 2 day history of bloody diarrhoea, abdominal pain and vomiting.
54. A 3 year old boy who has gone of his food, presenting with fever and left ear pain.
55. An 80 year old nursing home resident admitted to hospital with profuse diarrhoea, one week after completing a course of augmentin for a urinary tract infection.

Theme 12: Decision making in terminal care

Options:

a. Administer enema
b. Gastric intubation
c. High fibre diet
d. Increase opiate analgesia
e. IV fluids
f. Nutritional supplements
g. Palliative radiotherapy
h. Prescribe a corticosteroid
i. Laxative
j. Amitriptyline
k. ABGs
l. Biphosphonate
m. Methotrimeprasin
n. Reduce opiate analgesia
o. Set up syringe drive

For each presentation below, choose the SINGLE most appropriate management from the above list of options. Each option may be used once, more than once, or not at all.

56. An 80 year old man with metastatic carcinoma becomes confused with abdominal distention and faecal incontinence. He is on high opiate doses.
57. A 55 year old woman with known spinal metastases from breast cancer becames nauseated and confused. Serum creatinine is 120 umol/L, blood glucose is 5.4 mmol/L, serum calcium 3.2. She is receiving IV fluids.
58. A 45 year old man is dying of AIDS. He is in considerable pain despite morphine sulfate, slow release, 20 mg daily, amount 100 mg at night and naproxen 500 mg twice a day.
59. A 65 year old man with prostate carcinoma has extensive pelvic spread of disease with pain not adequately controlled by full dosage of analgesia.

60. An 82 year old man with bronchial carcinoma with known cerebral metastases develops weakness of his right arm but is in no pain.

Theme 13: Amputations in orthopaedic practice

Options:

a. Below knee amputation
b. Transmetatarsal amputation.
c. Syme's amputation
d. Ray amputation with "racket incision"
e. Supracondylar amputation
f. Tarsal amputation
g. Hindquarter amputation
h. Chopart's amputation
i. Above knee amputation

For each presentation below, choose the SINGLE most appropriate amputation from the above list of options. Each option may be used once, more than once, or not at all.

61. An 85 year old man with pain and deformity of the left knee due to congenital malformation. He was able to walk up to the last 5 year when the pain became unbearable.

62. Ischaemic gangrene of the lower leg with ulceration over the medial malleolus and spreading infection proximally.

63. A 90 year old lady who is immobile due to severe osteoartritis in the hips and knees. She has developed marked arterial ulceration in the right lower limb. She requires full nursing care.

64. A gangrenous toe due to peripheral vascular disease with superimposed infection in a 70 year old diabetic.

65. A 64 year old man with a tumour of the upper femur.

Theme 14: Investigation of hoarseness

Options:

a. No investigation
b. Computed tomography (CT) scan of the neck
c. Sputum for Acid fast bacilli
d. Cervical spine X-ray
e. Laryngoscopy
f. Bronchoscopy
g. Bronchoalveolar lavage
h. Chest X-ray
i. Lymph node biopsy
j. Treponemal haemagglutination assay

For each presentation below, choose the SINGLE most appropriate investigation from the above list of options. Each option may be used once, more than once, or not at all.

66. A 25 year old man complains of a two day history of hoarseness of the voice. He denies any history of loss of weight but admits to 4 year history of smoking.

67. A 13 year old girl complains of a 2 day history of hoarseness of the voice associated with a dry cough. She feels feverish and on direct laryngoscopy her vocal cords are grossly oedematous.

68. A 34 year old woman had a partial thyroidectomy 3 hours ago complains of mild hoarseness of the voice. She had no history of phonation problems prior to surgery.

69. A 67 year old man with a history of weight loss complains of hoarseness of the voice. Computed tomography scan reveals an opacity in the right upper mediastinum. He denied any history of difficulty in breathing.

70. A 34 year old IV drug user complains of a 4 month history of a productive cough. He has lost 20 lb in weight.

Theme 15: Treatment in eye conditions

Options:

a. Pilocarpine drops
b. Tetracycline ointment + sulfadimethoxine
c. Peripheral iridectomy
d. Pressure on the eyeball
e. ECCE
f. ICCE
g. Tetracycline ointment + ciprofloxacin
h. Scleral buckling
i. 1% tropicamide
j. 1% cyclopentolate
k. Corticosteroids

For each presentation below, choose the SINGLE most appropriate treatment from the above list of options. Each option may be used once, more than once, or not at all.

71. A 54 yearr old myopic develops flashes of light and then sudden loss of vision.

72. A 54 year hypertensive presents with sudden loss of vision and on fundoscopy there is pale retina with cherry red spot at fovea.

73. A 29 year old man presents with meiosis and photophobia. The ophthalmologist prescribes a drug so that he may not develop synechiae as a sequel to this presentation.

74. An 8 year old African boy with complaints of grittiness and lacrimation in eyes. His siblings also have this problem.

75. A 47 year old male with mild headache. He has changed his spectacles thrice in one year. There is mild cupping and sickle shaped scotoma in both eyes.

Theme 16: The diagnosis of abnormal chest X-rays

Options:

a. Sarcoidosis
b. Histiocytosis
c. Aspergillus fumigatus
d. Idiopathic thrombocytopenia
e. Polyarteritis nodosa
f. Hyperparathyroidism
g. Silent infarction
h. Asthma
i. Emphysema
j. Lung fibrosis
k. Pleurisy
l. Lung collapse
m. Tuberculosis

For each presentation below, choose the SINGLE most appropriate diagnosis from the above list of options. Each option may be used once, more than once, or not at all.

76. A young woman complains of sore eyes, a dull chest pain, malaise and a low grade fever. She has had recurrent low grade fever for 4 months. A CXR shows bilateral hilar enlargement.

77. A middle aged pharmaceutical engineer presents with increasing breathlessness and cough. He is a non smoker. CXR shows diffuse bilateral mottling and multiple small cystic lesions. 6 months ago he had pneumothorax.

78. For the past 3 years, a young man has complained of recurrent bouts of pneumonia with wheeziness, cough, fever and malaise. His sputum is tenacious. Peripheral blood shows very high ESR and IgE.

79. A 30 year old computer engineer with a long history of asthma and rhinitis presents with wheezing, cough and fever. CXR shows patchy consolidation. Physical examination shows multiple tender subcutaneous nodules and purpura.

80. A 43 year old man presents with chest pain and a cough. He complains of fullness and pressure in the chest and a sharp pain affecting 2 or 3 ribs on the right side. A CXR shows right sided hilar enlargement.

Theme 17: Tumour markers

Options:

a. Alpha fetoprotein
b. Carcinoembryonic antigen
c. HCG
d. Placental alkaline phosphatase
e. Oestrogen receptors
f. TdT
g. Squamous cell carcinoma Ag
h. CA 19-9 RIA
i. Calcitonin
j. CA-125
k. Neuron specific enolase
l. CA-153

For each malignancy below, choose the SINGLE most appropriate tumour marker from the above list of options. Each option may be used once, more than once, or not at all.

81. Hepatocellular carcinoma.
82. Mucinous cystadenoma of ovary.
83. Epithelial tumours of ovary.
84. Functional germ cell tumours.
85. Medullary carcinoma thyroid.
86. Bronchial carcinoma.
87. Colorectal carcinoma.
88. Seminoma.

Theme 18: Adverse effects of anti-cancer drugs

Options:

a. Haemorrhagic cystitis
b. Seizures
c. Pancreatitis
d. Pulmonary fibrosis
e. Visceral fibrosis
f. GI ulceration
g. Peripheral neuropathy
h. Bone marrow suppression
i. Cardiotoxicity
j. Hepatotoxicity
k. Vomiting

For each drug below, choose the SINGLE most appropriate adverse effect from the above list of options. Each option may be used once, more than once, or not at all.

89. Vinblastine.
90. Vincristine.
91. Cyclophosphamide.
92. Actinomycin D.
93. L-asparaginase.
94. Melphalan.

Theme 19: Investigations in vaginal pathology

Options:

a. Plain abdominal X-rays
b. Bimanual pelvic examination
c. Micturating cystourethrogram
d. Smear
e. Biopsy
f. Wide excision
g. High vaginal swab
h. Urethral swab
i. Oestrogen pessary
j. Nystatin pessary
k. Metronidazole pessary
l. Serology
m. Skin scrapings
n. Dilatation and curettage

For each presentation below, choose the SINGLE most appropriate investigation from the above list of options. Each option may be used once, more than once, or not at all.

95. A recently married 29 year old woman presents to you with vaginal soreness, especially after intercourse. On physical examination, the vaginal walls are found to be inflamed with adherent patches of white exudates.

96. A 33 year old sexually active woman presents with history of profuse, frothy and offensive discharge. She says that urination is very painful and burning.

97. A young outgoing woman complains of painful vaginal lesions. On examination you find numerous erythematous shallow ulcers on the inner vulva. The ulcers are 2 cm in diameter and recur at regular intervals.

98. A 35 year old New Zealander visiting UK just arrives after spending a three month holiday in the Carribean. She is worried about a painless black lesion on her vulva. She says it may have been a freckle.

99. A 75 year old woman has had very painful micturition for over 6 months. She has had been taking antibiotics but they helped her only intermittently. On examination the vaginal epithelium is found to be white, thickened and granular.

Theme 20: Differential diagnosis of rectal bleeding

a. Piles
b. Fissure in ano
c. Colorectal carcinoma
d. Diverticular disease
e. Ulcerative colitis
f. Irritable bowel disease
g. Coeliac disease
h. Hirschprung's disease
i. Fistula in ano
j. Sigmoid carcinoma

For each presentation below, choose the SINGLE most appropriate diagnosis from the above list of options. Each option may be used once, more than once, or not at all.

100. A patient presents with large volumes of blood in pan.
101. A patient presents with blood and mucus mixed with stools.
102. A patient presents with painful bright red bleed, blood on paper and outside the stool.
103. A patient presents with painless bright red bleed, blood on paper and in pan.
104. Painless bleeding, blood often mixed with stool in an elderly with 6 month history weight loss.

Theme 21: Auto-antibodies in rheumatology

Options:

a. Anti-centromere antibodies
b. Anti-Ro antibodies
c. Anti-La antibodies
d. Anti-Jo-1 antibodies
e. Anti-dsDNA antibodies
f. Anti-topoisomerase
g. cANCA
h. pANCA
i. Anti-histone H1, H3, H4
j. Anti-histone H2a, H2b
k. Anti-mitochondrial antibodies

For each presentation below, choose the SINGLE most appropriate antibody from the above list of options. Each option may be used once, more than once, or not at all.

105. A 75 year old man presents with Bell's palsy. His past medical history is significant for late onset asthma and heart failure. He also reports to have consulted his GP for a generalized rash sometime back. His CXR shows multiple soft shadows and FBC shows an eosinophilia.
106. A 75 year old man presents in ARF. He has been troubled by recurrent epistaxis but over the last three weeks he reports to have coughed up blood too. His CXR shows multiple nodules.
107. A 65 year old woman complains of symptoms suggestive of Raynaud's phenomenon and difficulty in swallowing. On examination she has painful lesions on her finger tips and facial telangiectasia.
108. A 50 year old woman complains of several months history of weakness and difficulty climbing stairs. On examination she has fissuring of the skin of her hands and her CXR shows pulmonary fibrosis.
109. A 50 year old woman complains of dry eyes and a dry mouth. Schirmer's tear test reveals reduced lacrimation secretion.

Theme 22: Differential diagnosis of ectopic pregnancy

Options:

a. Renal colic
b. Pelvic inflammatory disease
c. Normal pregnancy
d. Missed abortion
e. Septic abortion
f. Threatened miscarriage
g. Torsion of ovarian mass
h. Irritable bowel syndrome
i. Inevitable miscarriage
j. Endometriosis
k. Ectopic pregnancy
l. Crohn's disease
m. Bacterial vaginosis
n. Ulcerative colitis
o. Appendicitis

For each presentation below, choose the SINGLE most appropriate diagnosis from the above list of options. Each option may be used once, more than once, or not at all.

110. A 21 year old woman presents as an emergency with a four-hour history of a lower abdominal pain and bright red vaginal blood loss. She had not had menstrual period for nine weeks and has a positive home pregnancy test one week ago. On vaginal examination, the uterus is tender and bulky. The cervical os is open.

111. A 16 year old woman presents with a sudden onset of severe right iliac fossa pain. On vaginal ultrasound examination a 6 cm diameter echogenic cystic mass is seen in the right fornix.

112. An 18 year old student, due to take her examinations, reports that she missed her last period and that a pregnancy test is negative. She has worsening abdominal pain, which has been troublesome for three months. She is otherwise well.

113. A 22 year old lady who has had two terminations of pregnancy, reports that she is pregnant again. She has noted a small amount of watery brown vaginal discharge and tenderness in the right iliac fossa.

114. A 27 year old, who conscientiously uses the oral contraceptive pill, has experienced intermittent vaginal bleeding and malodorous discharge for several weeks. When examined she has pain over the lower abdomen, worse on the left. Her temperature is 39°C and her white cell count is elevated.

Theme 23: The management of chronic joint pain

Options:

a. Paracetamol

b. Sulphasalazine

c. Joint aspiration and blood culture

d. Oral non-steroidal anti-inflammatory drugs with gastric protection

e. Oral non-steroidal anti-inflammatory drugs

f. Methotrexate

g. Gold

h. Allopurinol

i. Joint replacement surgery

j. Colchicine

k. Antidepressant

l. Cognitive behavioural therapy

For each presentation below, choose the SINGLE most appropriate initial management from the above list of options. Each option may be used once, more than once, or not at all.

115. An elderly woman with severe ischaemic heart disease complains of stiff, painful hands, neck, knees and feet. Examination of the hands reveals Heberden's nodes.

116. A 22 year old bricklayer with ankylosing spondylitis has increasing early morning back pain and stiffness. He is on medication at present.

117. A 54 year old obese asthmatic businessman, who drinks 40 units of alcohol a week, presents with a fifth episode of a red hot ankle. Aspiration of the joint has revealed uric acid crystals.

118. A 40 year old woman with long standing rheumatoid arthritis presents with a red, swollen and inflamed right knee. She has swinging pyrexia.

119. A healthy 75 year old independent woman complains of increasing pain in her left knee and episodes of the joint "giving way". She is no longer able to climb her stairs. On examination, she is found to have marked valgus deformity with obvious instability.

Theme 24: The management of suicide

Options:

a. Imipramine
b. Cognitive therapy
c. Coagulation profile
d. Detain under section II of the mental health act
e. Fluoxetine
f. Carbamazepine
g. Detain under section I of the mental health
h. Admit and observe
i. Intensive psychiatric care
j. Electroconvulsive therapy
k. Psycho-surgery
l. Diazepam
m. Detain under section IV of the mental health act
n. No action

For each presentation below, choose the SINGLE most appropriate management from the above list of options. Each option may be used once, more than once, or not at all.

120. A 34 year old man starts punching people at the local tube station with no provocation. He is arrested by Police and asked to go for a mental health review. He disagrees strongly.

121. A known Schizophrenic goes missing from the local hospital. He is arrested by the police, but refuses to go back to hospital, despite the fact that he hasn't finished the course of anti-psychotic medication prescribed by his doctor.

122. A 16 year old boy refuses to go to church despite the constant insistence of his deeply religious mother. He had previously been a regular church-goer.

123. A 23 year old woman complains of tearfulness and feeling low but denies any suicidal thoughts. She had her first child 3 days ago.

124. A 45 year old man has been on anti-depressant therapy for 6 months. He continues to deteriorate and has had 4 serious suicidal attempts in the last 10 days.

Theme 25: Diagnosis of abdominal pain in children

Options:

a. Crohn's disease
b. Ulcerative colitis
c. Mesenteric adenitis
d. Appendicitis
e. Henoch schönlein purpura
f. Wilms tumour
g. Nephroblastoma
h. Sickle cell crisis
i. Acute gastroenteritis
j. Juvenile rheumatoid arthritis
k. Salpingitis
l. Testicular torsion
m. Diabetes mellitus
n. Acute gastritis
o. Anorexia nervosa
p. Bulimia

For each presentation below, choose the SINGLE most appropriate diagnosis from the above list of options. Each option may be used once, more than once, or not at all.

125. A 12 year old boy with a 3 week history of coryza is brought to the Accident and Emergency department complaining of severe abdominal pain. He is found to have nodules, which don't disappear on pressure on the buttocks.

126. A 12 year old Jamaican boy is brought to the Accident and Emergency department complaining of severe abdominal pain. On examination, he is found to have a prominent forehead.

127. A 12 year old girl has just returned with her parents from Thailand. She is brought to the Accident and Emergency department with a 5-hour history of diarrhoea associated with abdominal pain. Her mother, a known diabetic, has similar symptoms.

128. A 12 year old girl with a 3 month history of weight loss and increased appetite for food and drink is brought to the Accident and Emergency Department complaining of severe abdominal pain. She denied any history of vomiting or excessive exercise but her mother says she has been wetting the bed at night for the past 6 months.

129. A 10 year old Italian girl is brought to the Accident and Emergency department complaining of severe abdominal pain. On examination she is found to have yellow sclerae and tender fingers.

130. An 11 year old boy with a history of anorexia and polyuria is brought to the Accident and Emergency department complaining of severe abdominal pain. On examination she is found to be tender posteriorly on a per rectal examination. Blood sugar is 5 mmol/L. Temperature is 38°C.

Theme 26: The management of joint pain

Options:

a. Weight loss
b. Colchicine
c. Allopurinol
d. Naproxen
e. Blood culture and sensitivity testing.
f. Paracetamol
g. Gold
h. Laparoscopic surgery
i. Radiotherapy
j. Flucloxacillin before any investigation
k. Probenecid
l. Aspirin

For each presentation below, choose the SINGLE most appropriate treatment from the above list of options. Each option may be used once, more than once, or not at all.

131. A 33 year old man presents with a 2 year history of knee joint stiffness and pain which typically becomes better during the day.

132. A 32 year old man presents with a 10 day history of a painful and swollen left knee. On examination he is found to have conjunctivitis. Two weeks prior to presentation he had complained of diarrhoea.

133. An elderly woman with heart failure is being treated with chlorthalidone. She develops an acutely painful and red right toe.

134. A 45 year old man has been treated for acute gouty arthritis on multiple occasions. Investigations show hyperuricaemia.

135. A 67 year old labourer presents with pain on weight bearing and restricted movements of the left knee, especially worse at the end of the day.

136. An 34 year old man with a Body Mass Index (BMI) of 32 presents with a red, hot, swollen distal interphalangeal joint.

Theme 27: The diagnosis of infertility

Options:

a. Polycystic ovary disease
b. Endometriosis
c. Adenomyosis
d. Chronic salpingitis
e. Diabetes mellitus
f. Hyperprolactinaemia
g. Hypopituitarism
h. Hyperthyroidism
i. Hypothyroidism
j. Pulmonary tuberculosis
k. Possible malignancy

For each presentation below, choose the SINGLE most appropriate diagnosis from the above list of options. Each option may be used once, more than once, or not at all.

137. A 42 year old woman complains of being unable to conceive for 2 years despite have regular unprotected sex. She complains of excessive sweating, frequent stools and says this explains her loss in weight over recent weeks. She denied starving herself and says she a very good appetite. Glycosylated Hb (HbA$_{1c}$) is 5 %.

138. A 28 year old woman complains of infertility and is otherwise well. She had been on haloperidol to treat a schizophreniform illness she had for six year. She has a healthy 3 year old daughter.

139. A 26 year old woman complains of infertility for 3 year. She has a low libido, and has put on a lot of weight over the last couple of year. Her breasts were found to be discharging on examination.

140. A 31 year old woman complains of abdominal pain which seems to increase during her periods.Over the last year,she has noticed difficulty in breathing and chest pain associated with occasional haemoptysis, following her periods.She has been unable to conceive. On examination she is found to have an enlarged and tender uterus. Her BMI is 20.

Theme 28: Lower abdominal pain

Options:

a. Acute appendicitis
b. Ureteral calculus
c. Ectopic pregnancy
d. Pelvic inflammatory disease
e. Meckel's diverticulitis
f. Ovarian cyst
g. Muscle strain
h. Psoas haematoma
i. Diverticulitis
j. Inflammatory bowel disease

For each presentation below, choose the SINGLE most appropriate diagnosis from the above list of options. Each option may be used once, more than once, or not at all.

141. A 38 year old woman with severe crampy right lower abdominal pain for the last 12 days. She has 4 to 6 loose stools daily. Examination reveals a temperature of 38.8 °C, tender right lower quadrant and anal fistulae.

142. A 48 year old woman presents with severe left lower quadrant pain for 2 days. Pain is constant. There is marked tenderness, with temperature of 38.3°C, WBC count is 18,500 per mm with 86% polymorphonuclear leucocytes.

143. A 12 year old boy with crampy umbilical pain for the last 4 days. The pain is now in both lower quadrants, right greater than left, with a sharp steady character. He has anorexia, nausea, fever and has not passed a bowel movement in 24 hours.

144. A 14 year old haemophiliac presents with sudden onset left lower abdominal pain. Examination reveals a flexion deformity of the left hip. Attempts to straighten the leg result in excruciating pain.

145. A 22 year old unmarried physiotherapist presents with sudden onset pain in the right lower quadrant. She has a history of amenorrhoea for 1 month.

Theme 29: Confusion

Options:

a. Hyponatraemia
b. Hypoglycaemia
c. Hypothyroidism
d. Hyperthyroidism
e. Hypercapneic encephalopathy
f. Hepatic encephalopathy
g. Uraemic encephalopathy
h. Subacute combined degeneration
i. Wernicke's encephalopathy
j. Hypertensive encephalopathy
k. Herpes simplex encephalitis

For each presentation below, choose the SINGLE most appropriate cause of confusion from the above list of options. Each option may be used once, more than once, or not at all.

146. A 72 year old man on chlorpropamide for diabetes mellitus presents with confusion, after a attack of gastroenteritis.

147. A 68 year old vegan presenting with confusion, disorientation and ataxia. Examination reveals pallor and a tinge of icterus.

148. A 48 year old widower with history of peptic ulcer disease with vomiting after meals for the past 2 weeks. He is found in a drowsy inebriated state in his flat by the neighbour. Examination reveals an ataxic gait with dysconjugate eye movements and gaze evoked nystagmus in all directions.

149. A 40 year old man admitted with history of confusion for one day. His wife says that he has had fever for the past 48 hours. Examination reveals a temperature of 39°C. No neck stiffness but very poor recent memory. CSF reveals $50000/mm^3$ cells with 90% lymphocytes and 20 $RBCs/mm^3$. CSF protein is 80 mg/dl and glucose 90 mg/dl with a RBS of 130 mg/dl.

150. A 56 year old chronic smoker presenting with progessive dyspnoea, anasarca and confusion. Examination reveals bounding pulses, papilloedema and asterixis.

Theme 30: Low backache

Options:

a. Prolapsed intervertebral disc
b. Osteoarthritis
c. Spondylolisthesis
d. Spinal stenosis
e. Ankylosing spondylitis
f. Osteomyelitis
g. Metastatic carcinoma
h. Myeloma
i. Aortic aneurysm
j. Paget's disease

For each presentation below, choose the SINGLE most appropriate cause of backache from the above list of options. Each option may be used once, more than once, or not at all.

151. A 58 year old woman with history of breast surgery 2 years ago presents with pain in the low back since the last 2 months. The pain is constant, progressive and often awakens her at night.

152. A 22 year old male has had low back pain for the last 4 weeks. It is accompanied by morning stiffness and for the last 3 days he has noticed swelling of the left ankle.

153. A 26 year old weight lifter develops sudden severe back pain after a workout in the gym. The pain radiates down the right lower limb all the way to the sole of the foot.

154. A 63 year old female with known osteoarthritis develops low back pain and a discomfort in the buttock and thigh. This discomfort is brought on by walking and also by prolonged standing. Bending over to touch her toes relieves the pain.

155. An 80 year old man presents with progressive low back pain. He complains of an increase in his hat size. Urinary examination reveals increased hydroxyproline.

Theme 31: Causes of coma

Options:

a. Cinchonism
b. Alcohol poisoning
c. Phaeochromocytoma
d. Renal failure
e. Status epilepticus
f. Hysteria
g. Typhoid
h. Porphyria
i. Barbiturate poisoning
j. Meningococcal meningitis
k. TTP
l. Antidepressant poisoning
m. Narcotic overdose

For each presentation below, choose the SINGLE most appropriate diagnosis from the above list of options. Each option may be used once, more than once, or not at all.

156. A 33 year old male is found unconscious, with shallow and slow breathing, pin-point pupils.
157. A 16 year old girl develops high fever and is unconscious. Her BP is 84 mmHg systolic and she has a purpuric rash.
158. A middle aged woman is confused and dypnoeic. Her blood pressure is 160/110 mm Hg. She is pale and has basal crepitations. She also has evidence of peripheral neuropathy.
159. A tourist recently returned from Pakistan and brought to the emergency room, unconscious with a faint rash on the abdomen. His temperature is 38.4°C and blood pressure is 90/60 mmHg.
160. A young man is brought in the Accident and emergency room, unconcious. He has soiled his clothes. His pulse is 46/minute and BP of 210/110 mm Hg. On examination of the retina, you notice a congested fundus.

Theme 32: Cardiac pathology

Options:

a. Papillary muscle rupture
b. Ventricular septal defect
c. Valvular aortic stenosis
d. Supravalvular aortic stenosis
e. Subvalvular aortic stenosis
f. Atrial septal defect
g. Mitral regurgitiation
h. Pulmonary valve stenosis
i. Acute pericarditis
j. Tricuspid regurgitation

For each presentation below, choose the SINGLE most appropriate cardiac pathology from the above list of options. Each option may be used once, more than once, or not at all.

161. Coxsackie virus group B is a common cause of this condition.
162. Aschoff nodules are most likely to be associated with this condition.
163. A 50 year old patient has an asymptomatic apical midsystolic murmur.
164. The left fourth intercostal space adjacent to the sternum is the preferred location for ausculatation of this condition.
165. Ischaemia of the papillary muscles are likely to cause this pathology.

Theme 33: Skin rashes

Options:

a. Bullous impetigo
b. Bullous pemphigoid
c. Anaphylaxis
d. Chicken pox
e. Dermatitis herpetiformis
f. Epidermolysis bullosa
g. Erythema multiforme
h. Erythema ab igne
i. Hand, foot and mouth disease
j. Meningococcal meningitis
k. Pemphigus

For each presentation below, choose the SINGLE most appropriate diagnosis from the above list of options. Each option may be used once, more than once, or not at all.

166. A week old baby presents with fragile skin that blisters on contact.

167. A 6 year old presents with a 5 day history of flu-like symptoms with an irritating cough. Her parents have noticed a widespread erythematous, pruritic rash.

168. A 70 year old female presents with large, tense blisters on the legs. The blisters have an erythematous base and some are blood-filled.

169. A 60 year old female has flat, fragile blisters and erosions on the trunk . She also has similar lesions on the inside of the mouth.

170. An 18 year old male presents with an intensely pruritic vesicular rash on the buttocks, elbows, knees and shins. Over the last 6 months he has been aware of a 12 1b unintentional weight loss and loose motions.

Theme 34: Neuro-pharmacology

Options:

a. Baclofen
b. Carbamazepine
c. Donepezil
d. Gabapentin
e. Haloperidol
f. Interferon
g. Levodopa
h. Propranolol
i. Riluzole
j. Sodium valproate

For each condition below, choose the SINGLE most appropriate drug from the above list of options. Each option may be used once, more than once, or not at all.

171. The drug used to treat cognitive impairment in Alzheimer's disease.

172. The drug used in the treatment of Parkinson's disease.

173. The drug used with limited success to delay motor progression in motor neurone disease.

174. The drug used to treat spasticity.

175. The drug used to treat essential tremor.

Theme 35: Cause of visual loss

Options:

a. Migraine
b. CRVO.
c. Senile macular degeneration
d. Optic neuritis
e. RD
f. Vitreous haemorrhage
g. CRAO
h. Glaucoma

For each presentation below, choose the SINGLE most appropriate cause of visual loss from the above list of options. Each option may be used once, more than once, or not at all.

176. A 30 year old woman develops gradual loss of vision which recovers. The loss never involves the peripheral field and is always accompanied by pain in her temporal region.

177. A 40 year old woman has a sudden loss of vision which recovers. She complains of visual distortion and headache before the episode began and complains of nausea during the attack.

178. An 80 year old man develops progressive loss of vision with difficulty in reading. The loss does not involve the peripheral vision.

179. A 60 year old woman wakes up in the morning with blurred vision which progresses to visual loss in few hours. On examination extensive retinal haemorrhages are seen.

180. A 45 year old teacher, who is very myopic develops rapidly progressive loss of vision. She describes the loss as 'curtain falling down'.

Theme 36: Causes of chest pain

Options:

a. Pulmonary embolism
b. MI
c. Pericarditis
d. Pneumothorax
e. Oesophageal reflux
f. Spinal cord lesion.
g. Aortic aneurysm
h. Cardiac neurosis
i. Herpes zoster
j. Fractured ribs
k. Pleurisy

For each presentation below, choose the SINGLE most appropriate cause of chest pain from the above list of options. Each option may be used once, more than once, or not at all.

181. A 45 year old complains of pain under his right nipple. He cannot take a deep breath due to pain and is tender in the precordial region.

182. A 65 year old lady complains of severe chest pain which has been present since last ½ hr. She is pale and sweating and has difficulty breathing. She also complains of pain in her left arm.

183. A 70 year old hypertensive man complains of dull ache which suddenly becomes tearing in nature. He also complains that the pain radiates in between the scapulae. He is found to be cold and clammy.

184. A 25 year old tall man who is a chronic smoker becomes short of breath all of a sudden and complains of tight chest pain.

185. A 45 year old obese lady complains of repeated burning sensation in the centre of her chest especially on bending and taking heavy meals.

Theme 37: Management after renal investigations

Options:

a. Dialysis
b. IV methylprednisolone
c. Oral azathioprine
d. Adequate IV fluids
e. IV glucose and insulin
f. Urinary catheter
g. ACE inhibitor
h. IV pamidronate

For each presentation below, choose the SINGLE most appropriate management from the above list of options. Each option may be used once, more than once, or not at all.

186. An elderly male of age 62 year has features of urinary tract obstruction. His blood urea, serum creatinine and potassium levels are raised.

187. A patient is a known case of multiple myeloma. He has the following reports with him–urea 18 mmol/L, S. creatinine 350 μmol/L, Na 143 mmol/L, K 3.7 mmol/L, carcinoma 3.4 mmol/L.

188. A patient with rhabdomyolysis has the following investigations done: B. urea 19 mmol/L, S. creatinine 350 μmol/L, CPK 2500 IU, K 5.3 mmol/L.

189. A known diabetic presents with mild renal impairment. His B. urea 18 mmol/L, S. creatinine 340 μmol/L, Na 138 mmol/L, carcinoma 2.4 mmol/L, K 7.2 mmol/L.

190. A patient with SLE has B. urea 18 mmol/L, S. creatinine 350 μmol/L. Urine microscopy contains red cell casts.

Theme 38: Cause of hypercalcaemia

Options:

a. Bronchial carcinoma
b. William's syndrome
c. Primary hyperparathyroidism
d. Excess intake of vitamin D
e. Tertiary hyperparathyroidism
f. Breast metastasis
g. Sarcoidosis
h. Multiple myeloma
i. Excess intake of milk
j. Phosphate depletion

For each presentation below, choose the SINGLE most appropriate cause of hypercalcaemia from the above list of options. Each option may be used once, more than once, or not at all.

191. A 25 year old farmer complains of persistent dry coughs and vague abdominal pain. A CXR reveals bilateral hilar adenopathy. Abdominal X-rays reveals bilateral renal calcification. Investigations reveal mild anaemia, hypercalcaemia, a low PTH and low urinary cAMP and high levels of 1, 25 $(OH)_2D$.

192. A 70 year old man presents with weight loss and general deterioration. He also complains of bone pain. Investigations reveal hypercalcaemia.

193. A 2 weeks old premature neonate is having hypercalcaemia.

194. A 60 year old man with long standing chronic renal disease requires renal transplantation. His renal failure persists despite a successful renal transplantation and he is found to be having hypercalcaemia.

195. A 40 year old man complains of progressively worsening muscular pains. His S. calcium is 3.0 mmol/L and parathormone assay level is 10 pmol/L. His S. albumin, protein, magnesium and chloride are within normal limits.

Theme 39: Adverse effects of medications

Options:

a. Enalapril
b. Bendrofluazide
c. Clonidine
d. Phenytoin
e. Hydralazine
f. Prednisolone
g. Lithium
h. Metformin
i. Simvastatin
j. Carbimazole
k. Amitriptyline
l. Bleomycin
m. Amiodarone
n. Nifedipine
o. Third generation cephalosporin

For each presentation below, choose the SINGLE most appropriate causative medication from the above list of options. Each option may be used once, more than once, or not at all.

196. A 40 year old woman presents with a fracture. She has recently noticed weight gain, thirst and mood swings.

197. A 60 year old woman presents with dry cough. She has recently been started on a different antihypertensive.

198. A 40 year old man presents with nystagmus. He also complains of ataxia and blurring of vision. He has been on treatment for his seizures for quite some time now.

199. A 40 year old man presents with painful and tender shoulder and thigh muscles. His creatine kinase levels are found to be increased.

200. A 50 year old man presents with a TIA. His BP was found to be 180/110. He has been on some antihypertensive for the past 6 months but missed his medication in the last 2 days.

ANSWERS

1. **(a)** POP
2. **(b)** Condoms
3. **(c)** IUCD
4. **(b)** Condoms
5. **(e)** COCPs
6. **(i)** Nephroblastoma
7. **(b)** Renal cell carcinoma
8. **(k)** Glomerulophritis
9. **(d)** Alport's syndrome
10. **(e)** SLE
11. **(j)** Ciprofloxacin
12. **(b)** Amoxicillin and gentamycin
13. **(m)** Amoxicillin
14. **(d)** IV ampicillin
15. **(g)** Benzylpenicillin
16. **(e)** Testicular torsion
17. **(j)** ATN
18. **(d)** Testitular tumour
19. **(k)** CRF
20. **(b)** Carcinoma prostate
21. **(h)** Folate deficiency
22. **(b)** Squamous cell carcinoma
23. **(c)** Stevens–Johnson syndrome
24. **(d)** Lichen planus
25. **(e)** Iatrogenic gingivitis
26. **(h)** Insulin
27. **(m)** Aldosterone
28. **(g)** Parathyroid hormone
29. **(f)** Thyroxine
30. **(a)** Cortisol
31. **(j)** Lumbar puncture
32. **(c)** Blood culture
33. **(h)** Computed tomography scan
34. **(d)** Blood glucose
35. **(i)** Electrocardiogram (ECG)
36. **(g)** Abdominoperineal resection with end colostomy
37. **(b)** Sigmoid colectomy
38. **(f)** Exploratomy laparotomy and Hartmann's procedure
39. **(a)** Anterior resection
40. **(h)** Urgent herniorraphy
41. **(b)** Dominant frontal lobe
42. **(h)** Temporo–occipito–parietal junction
43. **(f)** Dominant parietal lobe
44. **(e)** Non–dominant parietal lobe
45. **(e)** Epstein–Barr virus
46. **(b)** Dye and printing chemicals
47. **(a)** Pernicious anaemia
48. **(d)** Ulcerative colitis
49. **(c)** Asbestos
50. **(e)** Epstein–Barr virus
51. **(i)** Neisseria meningitidis
52. **(h)** Neisseria gonorrhoea
53. **(c)** Campylobacter jejuni
54. **(f)** Haemophilus influenzae
55. **(b)** Clostridium difficile
56. **(i)** Laxative
57. **(l)** Biphosphonate
58. **(d)** Increase opiate analgesia
59. **(g)** Palliative radiotherapy
60. **(h)** Prescribe a corticosteroid
61. **(i)** Above knee amputation
62. **(a)** Below knee amputation
63. **(i)** Above knee amputation
64. **(d)** Ray amputation with "racket incision"
65. **(g)** Hindquarter amputation
66. **(a)** No investigation
67. **(a)** No investigation
68. **(a)** No investigation
69. **(e)** Laryngoscopy
70. **(c)** Sputum for Acid fast bacilli
71. **(h)** Scleral buckling

72. **(d)** Pressure on the eyeball
73. **(j)** 1% cyclopentolate
74. **(b)** Tetracycline ointment +
          sulfadimethoxine
75. **(a)** Pilocarpine drops
76. **(a)** Sarcoidosis
77. **(b)** Histiocytosis
78. **(c)** Aspergillus fumigatus
79. **(e)** Polyarteritis nodosa
80. **(j)** Lung fibrosis
81. **(a)** Alpha fetoprotein
82. **(b)** Carcinoembryonic antigen
83. **(j)** CA-125
84. **(c)** HCG
85. **(i)** Calcitonin
86. **(k)** Neuron specific enolase
87. **(h)** CA 19-9 RIA
88. **(d)** Placental alkaline phosphatase
89. **(h)** Bone marrow suppression
90. **(g)** Peripheral neuropathy
91. **(a)** Haemorrhagic cystitis
92. **(k)** Vomiting
93. **(j)** Hepatotoxicity
94. **(d)** Pulmonary fibrosis
95. **(j)** Nystatin pessary
96. **(g)** High vaginal swab
97. **(l)** Serology
98. **(f)** Wide excision
99. **(e)** Biopsy
100. **(d)** Diverticular disease
101. **(e)** Ulcerative colitis
102. **(b)** Fissure in ano
103. **(a)** Piles
104. **(c)** Colorectal carcinoma
105. **(h)** pANCA
106. **(g)** cANCA
107. **(a)** Anti-centromere antibodies
108. **(d)** Anti-Jo-1 antibodies
109. **(c)** Anti-La antibodies
110. **(i)** Inevitable miscarriage
111. **(g)** Torsion of ovarian mass
112. **(h)** Irritable bowel syndrome

113. **(k)** Ectopic pregnancy
114. **(e)** Septic abortion
115. **(a)** Paracetamol
116. **(d)** Oral non-steroidal anti-inflammatory
          drugs with gastric protection
117. **(j)** Colchicine
118. **(c)** Joint aspiration and blood culture
119. **(i)** Joint replacement surgery
120. **(h)** Admit and observe
121. **(h)** Admit and observe
122. **(n)** No action
123. **(b)** Cognitive therapy
124. **(j)** Electroconvulsive therapy
125. **(e)** Henoch schönlein purpura
126. **(h)** Sickle cell crisis
127. **(i)** Acute gastroenteritis
128. **(m)** Diabetes mellitus
129. **(h)** Sickle cell crisis
130. **(d)** Appendicitis
131. **(d)** Naproxen
132. **(d)** Naproxen
133. **(b)** Colchicine
134. **(k)** Probenecid
135. **(f)** Paracetamol
136. **(d)** Naproxen
137. **(h)** Hyperthyroidism
138. **(f)** Hyperprolactinaemia
139. **(f)** Hyperprolactinaemia
140. **(b)** Endometriosis
141. **(j)** Inflammatory bowel disease
142. **(i)** Diverticulitis
143. **(a)** Acute appendicitis
144. **(h)** Psoas haematoma
145. **(c)** Ectopic pregnancy
146. **(b)** Hypoglycaemia
147. **(h)** Subacute combined degeneration
148. **(i)** Wernicke's encephalopathy
149. **(k)** Herpes simplex encephalitis
150. **(e)** Hypercapneic encephalopathy
151. **(g)** Metastatic carcinoma
152. **(e)** Ankylosing spondylitis
153. **(a)** Prolapsed intervertebral disc

154.	**(d)**	Spinal stenosis	177.	**(a)**	Migraine
155.	**(j)**	Paget's disease	178.	**(c)**	Senile macular degeneration
156.	**(m)**	Narcotic overdose	179.	**(b)**	CRVO
157.	**(j)**	Meningococcal meningitis	180.	**(e)**	RD
158.	**(d)**	Renal failure	181.	**(h)**	Cardiac neurosis
159.	**(g)**	Typhoid	182.	**(b)**	MI
160.	**(c)**	Phaeochromocytoma	183.	**(g)**	Aortic aneurysm
161.	**(i)**	Acute pericarditis	184.	**(d)**	Pneumothorax
162.	**(g)**	Mitral regurgitiation	185.	**(e)**	Oesophageal reflux
163.	**(c)**	Valvular aortic stenosis	186.	**(f)**	Urinary catheter
164.	**(j)**	Tricuspid regurgitation	187.	**(h)**	IV pamidronate
165.	**(g)**	Mitral regurgitiation	188.	**(d)**	Adequate IV fluids
166.	**(f)**	Epidermolysis bullosa	189.	**(e)**	IV glucose and insulin
167.	**(d)**	Chicken pox	190.	**(b)**	IV methylprednisolone
168.	**(b)**	Bullous pemphigoid	191.	**(g)**	Sarcoidosis
169.	**(k)**	Pemphigus	192.	**(h)**	Multiple myeloma
170.	**(e)**	Dermatitis herpetiformis	193.	**(j)**	Phosphate depletion
171.	**(c)**	Donepezil	194.	**(e)**	Tertiary hyperparathyroidism
172.	**(g)**	Levodopa	195.	**(c)**	Primary hyperparathyroidism
173.	**(i)**	Riluzole	196.	**(f)**	Prednisolone
174.	**(a)**	Baclofen	197.	**(a)**	Enalapril
175.	**(h)**	Propranolol	198.	**(d)**	Phenytoin
176.	**(d)**	Optic neuritis	199.	**(i)**	Simvastatin
			200.	**(c)**	Clonidine

General Medical Council PLAB Test Part 1

Full Name

Test Centre/Date

- Use pencil only • Make heavy marks that fill the lozenge completely
- Write your candidate number in the top row of the box to the right **and** fill in the appropriate lozenge below each number
- Given **one** answer only for each question

Do not Write in this space

Section C

Section C

SOME COMMON ANTIBODIES

1. Anti TSH (Anti microsomal) antibodies—Hashimoto's thyroiditis, **Grave's disease**, Juvenile lymphocytic thyroiditis.
2. Anti thyroglobulin antibodies—**Hashimoto's thyroiditis**, Myxoedema.
3. cANCA–Wegeners granulomatosis.
4. pANCA–Crescentic glomerulonephritis, Systemic vasculitides, Ulcerative Colitis.
5. c/p ANCA–Churg Strauss syndrome.
6. Anti ds DNA–SLE.
7. Anti parietal cell antibody–Pernicious anaemia, Atrophic gastritis.
8. Anti acetylcholine receptor antibody–Myasthenia gravis.
9. Anti reticulin antibody–Coeliac disease, Crohn's disease.
10. Anti smooth muscle antibody–Chronic active hepatitis, Idiopathic cirrhosis, Viral infections.
11. Anti streptolysin antibody–Rheumatic fever, Poststreptococcal glomerulonephritis.
12. Anti mitochondrial antibody–Primary biliary cirrhosis.
13. Rheumatoid factor–Rheumatoid arthritis, Sjögren's syndrome, Felty's syndrome.
14. Anti Ribonuclear Protein (RNP)–Mixed connective tissue disorder.
15. Anti centromere antibody–CREST syndrome, systemic sclerosis.
16. Anti basement membrane antibody–Goodpasture's syndrome.
17. Anti haemoglobin antibody–Diguglielmo's disease (Erythromyelosis)
18. Donath Landsteiner antibody–Mumps, Measles, Chicken pox, Syphilis.
19. ASCA (Anti Saccharomyces Cerevisiae antibody)–Crohn's disease.
20. Anti LKM (Liver–kidney–microsomal) antibody–Autoimmune hepatitis type II.
21. ANCA–Primary sclerosing cholangitis.
22. Anti nuclear antibody–SLE, Juvenile rheumatoid arthritis.
23. Anti cardiolipin antibody–Antiphospholipid syndrome, SLE with thrombosis.
24. Anti Ro–SLE, Sjögren's.
25. Anti La–SLE, Sjögren's.
26. Anti Scl 70–Diffuse cutaneous scleroderma.
27. Anti Jo-1–Polymyositis, lung involvement.
28. Anti histone antibody-SLE.
29. Anti endomyseal and α-gliadin antibody–Coeliac disease.

SOME IMPORTANT INCUBATION PERIODS

1.	Staphylococcus aureus	1-6 hrs
2.	Cholera	3 hrs-5 days
3.	Clostridium botulinum	12-36 hrs
4.	E coli	12 hrs to 3 days
5.	Influenza	1-4 days
6.	Rotavirus	1-7 days
7.	Plague	1-7 days
8.	Shigella	1-7 days
9.	Gonorrhoea	2-10 days
10.	Relapsing fever	2-10 days
11.	Yellow fever	2-14 days
12.	Typhus	2-21 days
13.	Typhoid	3-21 days
14.	Poliomyelitis	~ 7 days
15.	Measles	7-21 days
16.	E. histolytica	7-28 days
17.	G. lamblia	7-28 days
18.	Rabies	9-90 days
19.	Syphilis	9-90 days
20.	Chicken pox	11-21 days
21.	Falciparum malaria	12 days
22.	Mumps	14-21 days
23.	Rubella	14-21 days
24.	Hepatitis A	2-6 weeks
25.	Infectious mononucleosis	4-5 weeks
26.	Hepatitis B	1-6 months
27.	Scabies	6 weeks
28.	Creutzfeldt Jacob disease	10-20 years

not virus ? is it ?

SOME ADVERSE EFFECTS OF DRUGS

1. *Metformin*–Lactic acidosis, Metallic taste, Pain abdomen.
2. *Amiodarone*–Pulmonary fibrosis, Thyrotoxicosis, Peripheral neuropathy
3. *Amphotericin B*–Type I Renal Tubular Acidosis (Distal RTA).
4. *Acetazolamide*–Type II Renal Tubular Acidosis (Proximal RTA).
5. *Carbamazepine*–Agranulocytosis, Rash, Neurotoxicity, Hyponatraemia.
6. *Clozapine*–Agranulocytosis.
7. *Carbimazole*–Agranulocytosis.
8. *Cimetidine*–Impotence.
9. *Cyclophosphamide*–Haemorrhagic cystitis, Alopecia.
10. *Diamorphine*–Constipation.
11. *OCPs*–DVT.
12. *Amoxicillin*–Stevens Johnson syndrome, Pseudomembranous colitis.
13. *Insulin*–Lipodystrophy.
14. *Porcine Insulin*–Development of anti insulin antibodies.
15. *Troglitazone*–Fulminant hepatic failure.
16. *Acarbose*–Flatulence.
17. *Chlorpromazine*–Impotence, Extrapyramidal effects, Increased Prolactin levels.
18. *Lithium*–Thirst, Polyuria, Tremors, Rashes, Hyperthyroidism (if toxicity), Hypothyroidism (long term use).
19. *Haloperidol*–Neurolept malignant syndrome.
20. *Quinine*–Cinconism-Urinary retention, Ringing of ears, Heart block.
21. *Amitriptyline*–Anticholinergic side effects, Dry mouth, Tremors, Blurring of vision.
22. *Phenytoin*–Ataxia, Nystagmus, Tremors, Dystonia, Gum hypertrophy, Hirsutism.
23. *Sodium valproate*–Weight gain.
24. *Captopril*–Renal failure, Dry cough.
25. *Frusemide*–Hypokalaemia.
26. *Gentamycin*–Ototoxicity and Nephrotoxicity.
27. *Methylsergide*–Retroperitoneal fibrosis.
28. *Bromocriptine*–Retroperitoneal fibrosis, Postural hypotension, Raynaud's phenomenon.
29. *Rifampicin*–Hepatitis.
30. *Isoniazid*–Hepatitis, Peripheral neuritis.
31. *Pyrazinamide*–Hepatitis, Increased uric acid levels.
32. *Ethambutol*–Optic neuritis, Increased uric acid levels.
33. *Streptomycin*–Ototoxicity, Hepatotoxicity.
34. *Simvastatin*–Hepatitis, Rhabdomyolysis.
35. *Aspirin*–Tinnitus, Vertigo, Dehydration, Hyperventilation, Reye's syndrome.
36. *Digoxin*–Yellow green visual haloes, Arrhythmia, Decreased cognition.
37. *Danazol*–Weight gain, Facial hair, Decreased breast size, Dyspareunia, Atrophic vaginitis.
38. *Progestogens*–Breakthrough bleeding, Weight gain, Prolonged amenorrhoea.
39. *Paracetamol*–Jaundice, Encephalopathy (due to liver failure).
40. *Clomiphene citrate*–Abdominal pain, Hot flushes, Visual disturbances, Breast tenderness.
41. *Sildenafil*–Blue tinted vision.
42. *Methanol*–Blindness, Metabolic acidosis, Pulmonary oedema.

PRESCRIBING IN PREGNANCY

	1st trimester	2nd trimester	3rd trimester	Comments
1. ACE inhibitors	C/I	C/I	C/I	
2. Cephalosporins	safe	safe	safe	
3. Chloramphenicol	C/I	C/I	C/I	Grey baby
4. Chloroquine	safe as prophylaxis	safe as prophylaxis	safe prophylaxis	syndrome
5. Erythromycin	safe	safe	safe	
6. Glibenclamide	safe	safe	C/I	
7. Griseofulvin	C/I	C/I	C/I	
8. Heparin	safe	safe	safe	
9. Inhaled beta agonists	safe	safe	safe	
10. Metformin	C/I	C/I	C/I	
11. Metoclopramide	safe	safe	safe	
12. Nitrofurantoin	C/I	C/I	C/I	
13. Paracetamol	safe	safe	safe	
14. Penicillin derivatives	safe	safe	safe	
15. Streptomycin	C/I	C/I	C/I	Ototoxic effect
16. Tetracycline	C/I	C/I	C/I	Affects bone and teeth
17. Theophyllines	safe	safe	Increased risk of neonatal jaundice	
18. Trimethoprim-Sulphamethoxazole	—	—	C/I	
19. Warfarin	C/I	safe	C/I	
20. Zidovudine	safe	safe	safe	Treatment with drug decreases risk of congenital infection

C/I*-Contraindicated

SOME COMMON ANTIDOTES

1. *Phenothiazine*–Procyclidine/Orphenandrine.
2. *Benzodiazepines*–Flumazenil.
3. *Beta blockers*–Atropine → Glucagon if atropine fails.
4. *Organophosphates*–Atropine, Pralidoxime.
5. *Botulism toxin*–Botulinum Antitoxin.
6. *Digoxin*–Digoxin Specific Fab antibody fragments.
7. *Iron*–Desferrioxamine.
8. *Cyanide*–Dicobalt edetate, O_2, Amyl nitrite, Sodium nitrite.
9. *Carbon monoxide*–Hyperbaric Oxygen, Mannitol if raised ICT.
10. *Warfarin*–Phytomenadione.
11. *Opiates*–Naloxone.
12. *Carbon tetrachloride*–Acetylcysteine.
13. *Paracetamol*–N-Acetylcysteine, Methionine.
14. *Salicylate*–Activated charcoal → Alkaline diuresis.
15. *Ecstacy*–Activated charcoal.
16. *Paraquat*–Activated charcoal.
17. *Cocaine*–Amyl nitrate by inhalation.
18. *Ethylene glycol*–Haemodialysis, Ethanol.
19. *Inhalation of organic solvents*–Methylene blue.
20. *Lead*–DMSA, Sodium calcium edetate.
21. *Arsenic*–Dimercaprol, DMSA.
22. *Methanol*–Ethanol.
23. *Mercury*–DMPS.
24. *Phenothiazine or Butyrophenone dystonia*–Benztropine, Procyclidine.

TUMOUR MARKERS

1. Alfa-fetoprotein–Hepatocellular carcinoma, Teratoma, Open neural tube defects.
2. CA 19-9–Colorectal carcinoma, Pancreatic carcinoma.
3. CD 25–Hairy cell leukaemia, Adult T cell leukaemia.
4. CD 30–Hodgkin's, anaplastic large cell lymphoma.
5. CA 125–Ovarian carcinoma.
6. CA 153–Breast carcinoma, benign Breast disease.
7. Chorio Embryonic Antigen–Colorectal carcinoma, Mucinous cystadenoma ovary.
8. HCG–H. mole, Choriocarcinoma.
9. Neurone Specific Enolase–Small cell carcinoma lung, Neuroblastoma.
10. Placental Alkaline Phosphatase–Seminoma.
11. Prostate Specific Antigen–Prostatic carcinoma, Benign prostatic hypertrophy.
12. Calcitonin–Medullary carcinoma thyroid.
13. S-100–Malignant melanoma.
14. Urinary 5 HIAA–Carcinoid tumour.
15. Urinary HVA, HMMA–Phaeochromocytoma.
16. LDH–Lymphoma, Ewings sarcoma.
17. Acid Phosphatase–Prostatic carcinoma.

SOME IMPORTANT DRUG INTERACTIONS

1. Increased effect of drug — Due to the drug

Increased effect of drug	Due to the drug
i. Aminoglycosides	Loop diuretics, Cefalosporins.
ii. Antidiabetics	Alcohol, β-blockers, MAO inhibitors.
iii. Azathioprine	Allopurinol.
iv. β-blockers	Verapamil
v. Carbamazepine	Erythromycin, Isoniazid, Verapamil.
vi. Cyclosporin	Erythromycin.
vii. Digoxin	Amiodarone, Diuretics, Quinine, Verapamil.
viii. Lithium	Thiazide diuretics.
ix. Phenytoin	Chloramphenicol, Isoniazid, Sulfonamides.
x. Theophyllines	Ciprofloxacin, Erythromycin, Contraceptive steroids, Propranolol.
xi. Warfarin	Alcohol, Amiodarone, Aspirin, Chloramphenicol, Ciprofloxacin, Co-trimoxazole, Erythromycin, Metronidazole, NSAIDs, Phenytoin, Tetracyclines, Thyroxine.

2. Decreased effect of drug — Due to the drug

Decreased effect of drug	Due to the drug
i. Sulfonylureas	Rifampicin.
ii. ACE inhibitors	NSAIDs.
iii. β-blockers	NSAIDs.
iv. Contraceptive steroids	Antibiotics, Barbiturates, Carbamazepine, Phenytoin, Rifampicin.
v. Cyclosporin	Phenytoin.
vi. Diuretics	NSAIDs (especially indomethacin).
vii. Phenytoin	Carbamazepine.
viii. Theophyllines	Barbiturates, Carbamazepine, Phenytoin, Rifampicin.
ix. Warfarin	Barbiturates, Carbamazepine, Phenytoin, Rifampicin.

3. Cimetidine potentiates the actions of Theophylline, Warfarin, Lignocaine, Amitriptyline, Propranolol, Phenytoin, Metronidazole.

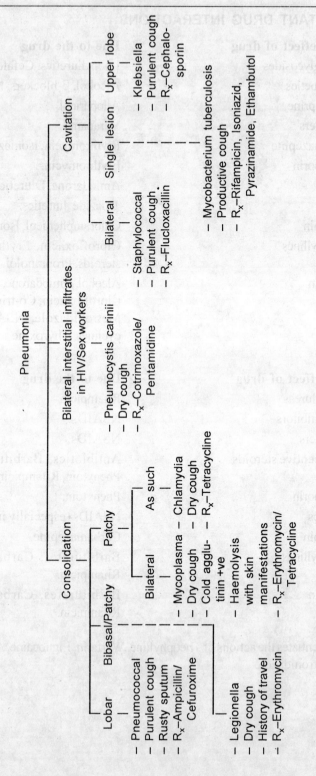

Pneumonia

Cavitation

Single lesion
- Upper lobe
  - Klebsiella
  - Purulent cough
  - R_x–Cephalo-
    sporin

Bilateral
- Staphylococcal
- Purulent cough.
- R_x–Flucloxacillin

- Mycobacterium tuberculosis
- Productive cough
- R_x–Rifampicin, Isoniazid,
  Pyrazinamide, Ethambutol

Bilateral interstitial infiltrates
in HIV/Sex workers
- Pneumocystis carinii
- Dry cough
- R_x–Cotrimoxazole/
  Pentamidine

Consolidation

Patchy

As such
- Chlamydia
- Dry cough
- R_x–Tetracycline

Bilateral
- Mycoplasma
- Dry cough
- Cold agglu-
  tinin +ve
- Haemolysis
  with skin
  manifestations
- R_x–Erythromycin/
  Tetracycline

Bibasal/Patchy

Lobar
- Pneumococcal
- Purulent cough
- Rusty sputum
- R_x–Ampicillin/
  Cefuroxime

- Legionella
- Dry cough
- History of travel
- R_x–Erythromycin

ECG

Normal

a. PR interval	0.12-0.20 sec
b. QRS complex	< 0.12 sec duration
c. QT interval	0.38-0.42 sec
d. Normal axis is between	$-30°$ and $+90°$
e. Q wave	< 0.04 sec wide and < 2 mm deep

i. Prolonged PR interval–1st degree heart block, Hypokalaemia.
ii. Shortened PR interval–Wolff—Parkinson—White syndrome.
iii. Large QRS complex–Ventricular hypertrophy.
iv. Low voltage QRS complex–Hypothyroidism, COPD, Pulmonary embolism, Bundle branch block, Myocarditis, Heart muscle diseases, Pericardial effusion, Pericarditis.
v. Prolonged QT interval–Acute MI, Myocarditis, Bradycardia, Head injury, Hypothermia, Hypokalaemia, Hypocalcaemia, Hypomagnesaemia, Drugs (Macrolides, Amiodarone, Antihistamines, Tricyclics, Quinidine, Sotalol).
vi. Shortened QT interval–Hypercalcaemia.
vii. ST elevation–Acute MI, Prinzmetal's angina, Acute pericarditis (saddle-shaped), Left ventricular aneurysm.
viii. ST depression–Digoxin, Myocardial ischaemia.
ix. T inversion
   a. In V_1-V_3—RBBB, Pulmonary embolism, RVH.
   b. In V_2-V_5—Subendocardial MI, HOCM, SAH, Lithium.
   c. In V_4-V_6—Ischaemia, LVH, LBBB.
x. Absent P wave–Atrial fibrillation, sinoatrial block, junctional (AV nodal) rhythm.

ECG changes in various settings

i. RBBB–QRS > 0.12 sec, 'RSR' and dominant R in V_1, inverted T wave in V_1-V_3, deep wide S wave in V_6.
ii. LBBB–QRS > 0.12 sec, 'M' pattern in V_5, inverted T wave in I, aVL, V_5-V_6.
iii. Right Ventricular Hypertrophy–dominant R in V_1, inverted T wave in V_1-V_3, deep S wave in V_6.
iv. Left Ventricular Hypertrophy–R wave in V_6 > 25 mm, S wave in V_1 + R wave in V_6 > 35 mm.
v. Right Atrial Hypertrophy–Peaked P waves.
vi. Left Atrial Hypertrophy–Bifid P waves.
vii. Hyperkalaemia–Tall, tented T waves, widened QRS complex, absent P waves, 'Sine wave' appearance.
viii. Hypokalaemia–Small T waves, prominent U waves, prolonged PR interval, depressed ST segment, pseudo-P-Pulmonale.
ix. Hypercalcaemia–Short QT interval.
x. Hypocalcaemia–Long QT interval, small T waves.

xi. Hypothermia–J waves.

xii. Digoxin effect–ST depression, inverted T wave in V_5-V_6.

xiii. Left Axis Deviation–Left anterior hemiblock, inferior wall MI.

xiv. Right Axis Deviation–Pulmonary embolism, Anterolateral MI, Left posterior hemiblock, Dextrocardia.

xv. Atrial Fibrillation–Absent P waves, irregularly irregular QRS complexes.

xvi. Atrial Flutter–'Sawtooth' baseline, regular QRS complexes.

JVP

i. Large a wave
  i. Pulmonary hypertension
  ii. Pulmonary stenosis
  iii. LVH.
ii. Cannon a wave:
  i. Complete heart block
  ii. Atrial flutter
  iii. Nodal rhythm
  iv. Ventricular arrhythmias or ectopics.
iii. Absent a wave
  i. Atrial fibrilliation.
iv. Large v wave–Tricuspid regurgitation.
v. Slow y descent:
  i. Tricuspid stenosis
  ii. Right atrial myxoma.
vi. Rapid deep y descent:
  i. Severe tricuspid regurgitation
  ii. Constrictive pericarditis.
vii. Accentuated x descent–Constrictive pericarditis (with high plateau of JVP).
viii. Raised JVP with no pulsation–SVC obstruction.
ix. Raised JVP with normal waves' pattern:
  i. Fluid overload
  ii. Right heart failure.

MODE OF INHERITANCE

Autosomal Dominant	*Autosomal Recessive*
1. Gilbert's syndrome	1. Tay Sachs disease
2. Familial hypercholesterolemia	2. Cystic fibrosis
3. Hereditary haemorrhagic telangiectasia	3. Wilson's disease
4. Achondroplasia	4. Sickle cell anaemia
5. Hereditary angioneurotic oedema	5. Infantile polycystic kidney disease
6. Hereditary spherocytosis	6. *β Thalassaemia
7. Huntington's chorea	7. Hurler's syndrome
8. Von Willebrand's disease	8. Glycogen storage disease
9. Osteogenesis imperfecta	9. Gaucher's disease
10. Criggler Najjar Type II syndrome	10. Criggler Najjar Type I syndrome
11. Adult polycystic kidney disease	11. Fanconi syndrome
12. Marfan's syndrome	12. Generalized albinism
13. Acute intermittent porphyria	13. Congenital cretinism
14. Noonan syndrome	14. Ataxia telangiectasia
15. Tuberous sclerosis	15. Homocystinuria
16. Neurofibromatosis	16. Phenylketonuria
17. Otosclerosis	17. α_1 antitrypsin deficiency
18. Retinoblastoma	

X linked Dominant	*X linked Recessive*
1. Fabry's disease	1. Colour blindness
2. Alport's syndrome	2. Christmas disease
3. Vitamin D resistant rickets	3. Haemophilia A
	4. Duchenne's muscular dystrophy
	5. Glucose 6 phosphate dehydrogenase deficiency

SOME IMPORTANT NAMED SIGNS

1. **Babinski sign** : Plantars upwards (positive)—seen in **UMN** lesions (lesions in cerebral cortex, internal capsule or corticospinal tracts).

2. **Chvostek's sign** : Neuromuscular excitability. Tapping over parotid gland causes facial muscles to twitch—seen in **HYPOCALCAEMIA.**

3. **Trousseau's sign** : Carpopedal spasm (wrist flexion with fingers drawn inwards) if brachial artery occluded with BP cuff—seen in **HYPOCALCAEMIA.**

4. **Corrigan's sign** : Carotid Pulsation—seen in **AORTIC REGURGITATION.**

5. **de Musset's sign** : Head nodding—seen in **AORTIC REGURGITATION.**

6. **Quincke's sign** : Capillary pulsation in nail bed—seen in **AORTIC REGURGITATION.**

7. **Duroziez's sign** : Femoral diastolic murmur—seen in **AORTIC REGURGITATION.**

8. **Traube's sign** : Pistol shot sound over femoral arteries—seen in **AORTIC REGURGITATION.**

9. **Cullen's sign** : Periumbilical discolouration—seen in **ACUTE PANCREATITIS.**

10. **Grey Turner's sign** : Flanks' discolouration—seen in **ACUTE PANCREATITIS.**

11. **Homan's sign** : Increased resistance to forced foot dorsiflexion—seen in **DVT.**

12. **Kernig's sign** : Pain and resistance on passive knee extension and hip flexion—seen in **MENINGITIS.**

13. **Brudzinski's sign** : Hips flex on bending the head—seen in **MENINGITIS.**

14. **Kussmaul's sign** : JVP increases with inspiration—seen in **CONSTRICTIVE PERICARDITIS, CARDIAC TAMPONADE.**

15. **Ewart's sign** : Large **PERICARDIAL EFFUSION** compressing left lower lobe of the lung.

16. **Lasegue's sign** : Painful straight leg raising on supine and is less than 45°–seen in **LUMBAR DISC PROLAPSE** causing nerve root irritation.

17. **Levine sign** : Clenched fist placed over sternum—seen in **CARDIAC PAIN.**

18. **Lhermitte's sign** : Paraesthesiae in limbs on flexing the neck—seen in **MULTIPLE SCLEROSIS.**

19. **Uhthoff's sign** : Visual defects on exercising/increase in temperature—seen in **MULTIPLE SCLEROSIS.**

20. **Murphy's sign** : Pain and arrest of inspiration when fingers placed on **Right Upper Quadrant**—seen in **ACUTE CHOLECYSTITIS.**

21. **Rovsing's sign**   : Pain more in **RIF** when **LIF** is pressed—seen in **ACUTE APPENDICITIS.**

22. **Troissier's sign**   : Enlarged left supraclavicular lymph node (Virchow's node)— seen in **CARCINOMA STOMACH.**

23. **Winterbottom sign**   : Enlargement of pasterior cervical lymph node—seen in **TRYPANOSOMIASIS** (Sleeping sickness).

24. **Setting sun sign**   : Seen in—**KERNICTERUS.**

25. **Positive Draw(er) sign** : Seen in—**ANTERIOR CRUCIATE LIGAMENT RUPTURE.**

26. **Positive Setback sign** : Seen in—**POSTERIOR CRUCIATE LIGAMENT RUPTURE.**

27. **Bell's sign**   : Weakness or paralysis of the facial muscles on one side with failure of eye closure and upward deviation of the eye as this is attempted—seen in **FACIAL NERVE PALSY.**

28. **Austpitz sign**   : Pinpoint bleeding on removal of scales—seen in **PSORIASIS.**

29. **Hutchison's sign**   : Nose tip involvement implies involvement of nasociliary branch of the trigeminal nerve—seen in **OPHTHALMIC SHINGLES.**

30. **Battle's sign**   : Bruising over the mastoid—seen in **FRACTURE BASE OF SKULL.**

31. **Russel's sign**   : Calluses on the back of the hand due to its repeated abrasion against incisors during inducement of vomiting—seen in **BULIMIA.**

32. **Froment's paper sign**   : On holding a piece of paper between thumb and finger there is flexion of the thumb's distal phalanx on trying to pull apart— seen in **ULNAR NERVE INJURY.**

33. **Schwartz's sign**   : A pink tinge to the tympanic membrane—seen in **10%** of cases of **OTOSCLEROSIS.**

DERMATOLOGICAL CONDITIONS

1. Acanthosis nigricans — Adenocarcinoma stomach, Prostatic carcinoma
2. Alopecia areata — Autoimmune disease (e.g.vitiligo), Addison's disease, Pernicious anaemia
3. Bullous Pyoderma gangrenosum — Leukaemia, Myeloma
4. Bazin's disease — Skin TB
5. Cafe-au-lait spots — Neurofibromatosis
6. Dermatitis herpetiformis — Coeliac disease
7. Dermatomyositis — Bronchial carcinoma, Breast carcinoma, Genitourinary carcinoma in females
8. Eczema craquele — Myxoedema
9. Eruptive xanthomata — Hereditary dyslipidaemic disease
10. Erythema chronicum migrans — Lyme disease
11. Erythema marginatum — Rheumatic fever
12. Erythema multiforme — Herpes simplex, Mycoplasma, Sulphonamides, Penicillins, Anticonvulsants
13. Erythema nodosum — Ulcerative colitis, Crohn's disease, Sarcoidosis, TB, OCPs, Dapsone, Sulphonamides, Leprosy
14. Facial butterfly rash — SLE
15. Granuloma annulare — Diabetes mellitus
16. Lupus vulgaris — Skin TB
17. Livedo reticularis — SLE, PAN
18. Malassezia furfur — Pityriasis versicolor
19. Migratory thrombophlebitis — Carcinoma tail of Pancreas
20. Mycosis fungoides — Cutaneous T cell lymphoma
21. Necrobiosis lipoidica — Diabetes mellitus
22. Pretibial myxoedema — Hyperthyroidism
23. Pyoderma gangrenosum — Ulcerative colitis, Crohn's disease, Autoimmune hepatitis, Wegener's granulomatosis, Myeloma, Rheumatoid arthritis
24. Slapped cheek — Rubella, Erythema infectiosum
25. Toxic epidermal necrolysis — Anticonvulsants, Sulphonamides, Penicillins, Allopurinols, NSAIDs.

FITNESS TO DRIVE IN UK

1. Avoid driving for 1 week
   - i. Post-operative angioplasty
   - ii. Pacemaker implant
   - iii. Treated syncope

2. Avoid driving for 4 week
   - i. Uncomplicated MI
   - ii. Q wave MI

3. Avoid driving for 1 month
   - i. Controlled arrhythmia
   - ii. After starting insulin

4. Avoid driving for 6 month
   - i. Untreated, undiagnosed syncope
   - ii. When on antiepileptic withdrawal

5. Avoid driving for 1 year
   - i. TIA/Stroke
   - ii. Seizure when awake
   - iii. Seizure when asleep (unless the seizure was >3 years ago)

6. Inform DVLA
   - i. All diabetics
   - ii. All epilepsies
   - iii. Unexplained blackouts
   - iv. Multiple sclerosis
   - v. Parkinson's
   - vi. MND
   - vii. Recurrent TIAs/Stroke
   - viii. Mild Dementia or Psychosis

7. Driving to be stopped
   - i. Binocular vision < 120°
   - ii. Incomplete monocular vision
   - iii. Angina occuring at wheels/rest
   - iv. Disabling giddiness, vertigo or ataxia
   - v. Severe dementia or psychosis
   - vi. Severe mental or behavioural disorder
   - vii. Alcohol/Drug/Chemical dependency
   - viii. Frequent hypoglycaemic attacks

8. Can drive
   - i. Mild dementia
   - ii. Vision 6/9 in better eye and 6/12 in the other eye (even with glasses)
   - iii. Vision 3/60 in each eye without glasses

SOME IMPORTANT TESTS

1. Short ACTH stimulation test (Synacthen test) : Addison's disease
2. Overnight dexamethasone suppression test : Cushing's syndrome
3. Direct Coomb's test : Immune mediated haemolysis
4. Osmotic fragility test : Membrane abnormality causing haemolysis e.g. Hereditary spherocytosis
5. Ham's test : Paroxysmal nocturnal haemoglobinuria
6. Kveim test : Sarcoidosis
7. Monospot test (Paul—Bunnell test) : Infectious mononucleosis
8. Ochner's test : Median nerve neuropathy
9. Rinne's test : Deafness
10. Weber's test : Deafness
11. Schilling test : Vitamin B_{12} deficiency
12. Schirmer's test : Keratoconjunctivitis sicca
13. Romberg's test : Gait disturbance due to abnormal joint position sense
14. Schuffner agglutination test : Weil's disease
15. Phalen's test : Carpal tunnel syndrome
16. Tinel's test : Carpal tunnel syndrome
17. Enterotest : Giardiasis
18. Treadmill exercise test : Suspected IHD
19. Trendelenburg test : a. Incompetence of sapheno-femoral junction in varicose vein
      b. Instability of hip
20. 2-glass urine test : Urethritis
21. Weil-Felix test : Typhus
22. Clinitest : Urine test for reducing agents e.g. galactosaemia
23. Tensilon test : Myasthenia gravis
24. Schick test : Diphtheria
25. Widal test : Typhoid
26. Leishmanin test : Leishmaniasis
27. Pathergy test : Behcet's disease
28. Secretin test : Zollinger—Ellison syndrome
29. Glucose tolerance test : Acromegaly
30. Insulin tolerance test : Hypopituitarism (to assess effect on cortisol and GH)
31. Single breath test : Early lung damage due to smoking/occupational lung disease

32.	Urea breath test	: *H pylori*
33.	CLO test	: *H pylori*
34.	Whiff test	: Bacterial vaginosis
35.	Cover test	: Squint e.g. manifest/latent
36.	Guthrie test	: Phenylketonuria
37.	Kleihauer test	: Antepartum haemourrhage
38.	Mc Murray's test	: Pedunculated meniscal tears at the knee
39.	Lachman's test	: Cruciate ligament injury at the knee
40.	Pivot shift test	: Cruciate ligament injury at the knee
41.	Marcus Gunn test	: Afferent defect in optic pathway
42.	Casoni intradermal test	: Hydatid disease
43.	Ortolani test	: Congenital dislocation of hip
44.	Hallpike test	: Benign positional vertigo
45.	Talbot's test	: Anterior uveitis
46.	Thomas test	: Fixed flexion deformity e.g. lower limbs
47.	Sweat test	: Cystic fibrosis
48.	Clonidine suppression test	: Phaeochromocytoma
49.	Water deprivation test	: Diabetes insipidus
50.	Mantoux test	: Tuberculosis
51.	Heaf test	: Tuberculosis
52.	Tine test	: Tuberculosis
53.	Tilt test	: Orthostatic hypotension in diabetic autonomic neuropathy
54.	Deoxyuridine suppression test	: Vitamin B_{12} or folate deficiency
55.	TPHA test	: Syphilis
56.	FTA-ABS test	: Syphilis
57.	Lepromin test	: Leprosy
58.	Lewis-Prusik test	: Raynaud's phenomenon

MEDIAL ETHICS IN UK

- A person's advance refusal of treatment should be respected if he can take in and retain treatment information believe the information, weigh the information balancing risks and needs.
- Valid consent is **Voluntary, Informed** and **made by a competent individual**.
- When a patient lacks capacity to give consent, a treatment can be discontinued (e.g. Passive Euthanasia) where its use is no longer considered to be in best interest of the patient.
- Active Euthanasia is not allowed even if the patient wants it and is competitive enough to decide.
- It is **Legal** to give or withhold consent on behalf of an **incapable** patient by a kin. Patient is incapable if incapable of acting, making decisions, communicating, understanding or remembering decisions.
- In casualty treatment can be immediately started to an incapable adult also, to save his life or safeguard his health.
- **In Netherlands**– Euthanasia (Active) is allowed if patient has made a voluntary and well considered request and that suffering is unbearable and without prospect of improvement or relief. The act should be both **Autonomous** and **Beneficent**. Dont simply kill the patient if they say they are tired of living.
- Competent patients aged 18 years or above the have right to refuse treatment.
- Parents/Guardians of incompetent patients < 18 years can consent for treatment on patients' behalf.
- In case of patients who are incompetent and > 18 years, treatment is done in their best interest in case parents or guardians are not available.
- Best interest is determined by consultation with relatives and those involved in care of the patient.
- A patient aged 16 or > can give consent to medical treatment.
- A patient < 16 years can give consent if they can demonstrate that they are competent to do so.
- If patient < 16 years refuses consent, doctor should consult with their parents or guardians and the courts if necessary. Treatment may go ahead if it is in the best interest of the patient.
- 'Common Law' covers emergency situations. Doctors can treat patients immediately in situations where it is assumed that consent would be given and if delay to obtain consent would cause serious harm to the patient.
- **Negligence**– could be due to
  i. Failure to diagnose
  ii. Failure to treat
  iii. Failure to warn of risks involved in the treatment.
- To initiate claim procedure, the patient must prove that :
  i. Doctor owed them a duty of care.
  ii. Doctors' standard of care was less than that should be expected by a reasonable doctor in that post.
  iii. Negligence caused them harm/injury which they would not otherwise have sustained.
- Doctors have a duty to protect patients, if they suspect that they themselves or a colleague poses a risk to the welfare of the patients e.g. is incompetent due to drug abuse, or carries a serious communicable disease.

- Doctors **must inform** their **employers** and the GMC if they have ever committed certain offences, or been investigated for fitness to practice issues ("except Parking Tickets!!")
- Patients should receive treatment for their condition regardless of how much they contributed to their ill health.

Death certificate/summary

- If you are unsure about the cause of death, speak to a senior before completing the death certificate.
- Do not complete a cremation form until death certificate has been issued.
- If the death is notified to the Coroner/Procurator Fiscal, the next of kin should be informed that a postmortem may be necessary– relatives **cannot** prevent if from taking place.
- If a postmortem is desired for other reasons (e.g. research), relatives must first give their consent and be told accurate information about what exactly will happen to all parts of the body including organs and tissues.

Organ donation

People can indicate that they would like to donate their organs after their death by joining the donor register and carrying out a donor card. This is **not** a legally binding agreement and **Relatives should be consulted before organs are taken out**.

- Valid informed consent should be taken from patients before commencing any examination, investigation or treatment.
- **Always obtain** consent from a patient before performing an examination. Failure to do so may be considered assault/crime.
- For simple blood tests implied consent is taken but for HIV testing explicit consent must be obtained.
- Consent from a patient must be taken before discussing their case with a third party.
- Confidentiality should be breached only in exceptional circumstances (e.g. if husband is HIV positive: wife should be told either by husband himself and if he does not tell her, the doctor should.)
- If the doctor feels that parents/guardians are wrong to refuse consent for their child, they can apply to the courts for permission to treat.
- Administering treatment without consent could be regarded as a crime.
- A patient with a mental disorder can be involuntarily detained for assessment and treatment (without their consent).
- So long as the intervention is directly or indirectly a form of 'treatment' for the mental disease, it can be allowed under the Mental Health Act.
- Patient with clear cut suicidal tendency should not be prescribed TCAs as he may be collecting the drugs for overdosage. He should be referred to a psychiatrist.
- Detention of psychiatric patients (i) By doctor or police officer is allowed for 72 hrs; (ii) By mental nurse is allowed for 6 hrs.
- Doctors who pose a risk to patients due to their own psychiatric condition should be advised to stop practising until they are well enough to return to work and if they do not stop against advice then action should be taken.

- Abortion in UK is illegal unless covered by one of the conditions under the abortion act.
- Fathers have no legal right to decide whether their unborn child should be aborted or not.
- Obtaining informed consent is an in-depth procedure, which involves giving information about what you are going to do, and of any risks involved.
- Admission of psychiatric patients without their consent or wishes:

	Applicant	Doctors	Duration
1. For Assessment	Relative/social worker	Two (i) Psychiatrist (ii) GP	28 days. No renewal. Seperate application for extension.
2. Emergency Assessment	Relative/social worker	One GP	72 hrs. Patient may appeal to a Mental Health Review tribunal to overturn the section order.
3. For treatment	Nearest relative/ social worker	Two	6 months. 6 months renewal can be done.

- In UK, children who are considered to be 'Gillick competent' can give consent to treatment but they cannot refuse it.
- Those children who are not 'Gillick competent' require parental consent to treatment. In these cases it is still considered good practice to involve the child as far as possible in any decision making progress.
- The HFEA regulates the use of stored ova and embryos.
- GMC guidance advises that you must not use your position as a doctor to establish emotional relationships with your patients.

REFERENCE–INTERVALS

Measuremet				Reference Interval

Arterial Blood Gases

1. pH		7.35	–	7.45
2. PaO_2			>	10.6 kPa
3. $PaCO_2$		4.7	–	6 kPa
4. Base excess			±	2 mmol/L
5. Hydrogen ion		36	–	44 mmol/L

Note: 7.6 mm Hg = 1 kPa (atmospheric pressure *≈ 100 kPa)

CSF Analysis

1. Cells			≤	5 cells/mm^3
2. Chloride		120	–	170 mmol/L
3. Glucose		2.5	–	4.0 mmol/L
4. Total protein		100	–	400 mg/L

Haematology

1. Haemoglobin	M	13.5	–	18.0 g/dL
	F	11.5	–	16.0 g/dL
2. Red cell count	M	4.5	–	6.5×10^{12}/L
	F	3.9	–	5.6×10^{12}/L
3. Packed red cell volume (PCV)	M	0.40	–	0.54 l/L
or haematocrit	F	0.37	–	0-47 l/L
4. Mean cell volume (MCV)		76	–	96 fL
5. Mean cell haemoglobin (MCH)		27	–	32 pg
6. Mean cell haemoglobin concentration (MCHC)		30	–	36 g/dL
7. White cell count (WCC)		4.0	–	11.0×10^9/L
8. Neutrophils		2.0	–	7.5×10^9/L;
				(40-75% WCC)
9. Lymphocytes		1.3	–	3.5×10^9/L;
				(20-45% WCC)
10. Eosinophils		0.04	–	0.44×10^9/L;
				(1-6% WCC)
11. Basophils		0.0	–	0.10×10^9/L
				(0-1% WCC)
12. Monocytes		0.2	–	0.8×10^9/L
				(2-10% WCC)
13. Platelet count		150	–	400×10^9/L
14. Reticulocyte count		0.8	–	2.0% ($25-100 \times 10^9$/L)
15. Prothrombin time				
(Factors I, II, VII and X)		10	–	14 seconds
16. Activated partial thromboplastin time		35	–	45 seconds
(Factors VIII, IX, XI and XII)				
17. Thrombin time		10	–	15 seconds
18. Bleeding time			<	8 min
19. INR		0.9	–	1.2
20. CRP			<	10 mg/L

21.	Erythrocyte sedimentation rate	M	0	–	5 mm/hr
		F	0	–	7 mm/hr
22.	Fibrinogen		1.5	–	4.0 g/L
23.	Vitamin B12		250	–	900 ng/L

Bio Chemistry

1.	Adrenocorticotrophic hormone (ACTH)			<	80 mg/L
2.	Alanine aminotransferase (ALT)		5	–	35 iu/L
3.	Albumin		35	–	50 g/L
4.	Aldosterone		100	–	500 pmol/L
5.	Alkaline phosphatase		30	–	300 iu/L (adults)
6.	α–Amylase		0	–	180 somogyiu/dL
7.	α–fetoprotein			<	10 ku/L
8.	Aspartate transaminase		5	–	35 iu/L
9.	Bicarbonate		24	–	30 mmol/L
10.	Bilirubin		3	–	17 mmol/L (0.25-1.5 mg/100/ml)
11.	Calcium (ionized)		1.0	–	1.25 mmol/L
12.	Calcium (total)		2.12	–	2.65 mmol/L
13.	Chloride		95	–	105 mmol/L
14.	Cholesterol		3.9	–	< 6 mmol/L
15.	HDL		0.9	–	1.93 mmol/L
16.	LDL		1.55	–	4.44 mmol/L
17.	VLDL		0.128	–	0.645 mmol/L
18.	Cortisol (A.M.)		450	–	700 mmol/L
19.	Creatine kinase (CK)	M	25	–	195 iu/L
		F	25	–	170 iu/L
20.	Creatinine (related to lean body mass)		70	–	≤ 150 µmol/L
21.	Ferritin		12	–	200 µg/L
22.	Follicle-stimulating hormone (FSH)		2	–	8 u/Lin (luteal); ovulatory peak 8-15 follicular phase and males 0.5-5.0 ; Post menopausal > 30
23.	γ–glutamyl transpeptidase	M	11	–	51 iu/L
		F	7	–	33 iu/L
24.	Glucose (fasting)		3.5	–	5.5 mmol/L
25.	Glycated (glycosylated) haemoglobin		5	–	8%
26.	Growth Hormone			<	20 mu/L
27.	Iron	M	14	–	31 µmol/L
		F	11	–	30 µmol/L
28.	Lactate dehydrogenase (LDH)		70	–	250 iu/L
29.	Luteinizing hormone Premenopausal: (LH)		3	–	13 U/L; Follicular 3-12; Ovulatory peak 20-80; Luteal 3-16; Postmenopausal > 30

30.	Lead		<	1.8 mmol/L
31.	Magnesium	0.75	–	1.05 mmol/L
32.	Osmolality	278	–	305 mosmol/kg
33.	Phosphate (inorganic)	0.8	–	1.45 mmol/L
34.	Potassium	3.5	–	5.0 mmol/L
35.	Prolactin	M	<	450 u/L
		F	<	600 u/L
36.	Prostate specific antigen (PSA)	0	–	4 nanograms/mL
37.	Protein (total)	60	–	80 g/L
38.	Sodium	135	–	145 mmol/L
39.	Thyroid-stimulating hormone	0.5	–	5.7 mu/L
40.	Thyroxine (T_4)	70	–	140 nmol/L
41.	Thyroxine (free)	9	–	22 pmol/L
42.	Total iron-binding capacity	54	–	75 µmol/L
43.	Triiodothyronine	1.2	–	3.0 nmol/L
44.	Triglyceride	0.55	–	1.90 mmol/L
45.	Urate	M	210	–	480 µmol/L
		F	150	–	390 µmol/L
46.	Urea	2.5	–	6.7 mmol/L

Urine Analysis

1.	Cortisol (free)		<	280 nmol/24 hrs
2.	Osmolality	350	–	1000 mosmol Kg
3.	Phosphate (inorganic)	15	–	50 mmol/24 hrs.
4.	Potassium	14	–	120 mmol/24 hrs.
5.	Protein		<	150 mg/24 hrs.
6.	Sodium	100	–	250 mmol/24 hrs.
7.	Hydroxy indole acetic acid	16	–	73 µmol/24 hrs.
8.	Hydroxy methyl mandelic acid	16	–	48 µmol/24 hrs.
9.	17-oxogenic steroids	M	28	–	30 µmol/24 hrs.
		F	21	–	66 µmol/24 hrs.

WHO SAID THIS IS THE END?

Medicine is an unexhaustive subject. This book has made a sincere attempt to provide you with sufficient material that would make you confortable with the PLAB exam pattern. We regret any errors and request you to come up with suggestions to improve upon this book. You can mail your contributions to the following address: peepee160@rediffmail.com

If you think your require more mock test papers for practising, wait, for we are soon-coming up with a book of mock papers with solutions and detailed explanations.

There are certain things you ought to remember while walking through the road to success:

i. An aim in life is the only fortune worth finding. Any man who knows just what it is that he wants, has already gone a long way towards attaining it.

ii. Believe in yourself.

> *"Start by doing what is necessary, then what is possible,*
> *and suddenly you are doing the impossible."*
> — St. Francis of Assisi
>
> *Don't be a man of words, become a man of action.*
> *Don't just "tell" the world that you can do it – "show" it!*
> *And just cut out that word 'Impossible' from your vocabulary.*

Remember: The winner is always a part of the answer and the loser is always a part of the problem. A winner would make it happen, where as a loser will let it happen. Which one are you?

iii. *Perseverance:* Anyone can make an attempt to start, but only those who persist, will FINISH. Unless you are willing to make personal sacrifices, you can never achieve great success. The test of a man is the fight he makes, the way he faces fate's blows and keeps moving on.

> *"The kite of success rises against the wind of adversity– not with it!"*

Some men are successful as long as someone else stands at their back encourage them, and some men are successful inspite of Hell!

Make your choice.

iv. *Cooperation and Team-work:* Always study in a group. Two minds at work are better than one. And in a positive environment of competition, even a marginal performer's output goes up. No man can rise to fame without carrying others along with him. It just can't be done, And when you find yourself at the top of the ladder of success, you are never alone because no one can climb to genuine success without taking others along.

And just keep in mind that nothing is so contagious as enthusiasm, that can even move stones.

v. Nothing is as detrimental as over-confidence. I would congratulate you if you have been successful, but not if you are not able to forget how successful you have been, because then I would pity you.

> *Just keep the hard work on.*
> *Hoping to see all our readers as SHO'S in the hospitals in UK.*

Dinesh Khanna